LEADING EVIDENCE-BASED PRACTICE AND QUALITY IMPROVEMENT INITIATIVES IN ADVANCED NURSING PRACTICE

LEADING EVIDENCE-BASED PRACTICE AND QUALITY IMPROVEMENT INITIATIVES IN ADVANCED NURSING PRACTICE

A COMPETENCY-BASED APPROACH

Jayne Jennings Dunlap
Texas Woman's University
&
Julee Briscoe Waldrop, Editors
Duke University

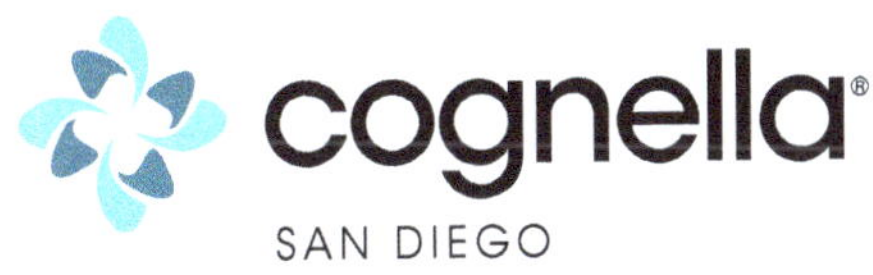

Bassim Hamadeh, CEO and Publisher
Amanda Martin, Executive Publisher
Amy Smith, Associate Editorial Manager
Casey Hands, Senior Production Editor
Emely Villavicencio, Senior Graphic Designer
Kylie Bartolome, Licensing Specialist
Natalie Piccotti, Director of Marketing
Kassie Graves, Senior Vice President, Editorial
Alia Bales, Director, Project Editorial and Production

ISBN: 9798823344623

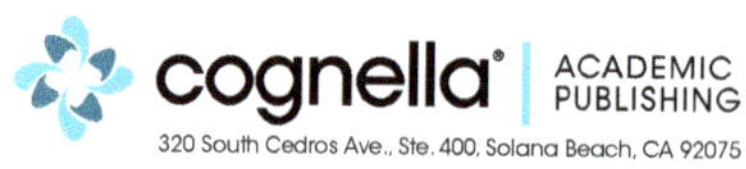

To my soulmate, Brian, who shepherds our family so well. To our parents, John and Jolie and Eddie and Karen, all leaders in their own right who have modeled 90 years of marriage, meaningful work, and faithful parenting. To our sisters: Joanna (Asa Sr.), Amy (Todd), and Mandy (Andrew). You are gifted leaders who make the world better through your service to others. And our next generation: Addie, Weston, Violet, Asa Jr., Emmett, Rory, Jack, Travis, Madisyn, Gavin, and Gracelynn Jayne. You are precious to me.

To my mentor, Julee, who speaks the truth and diligently guides me and others as a nurse practitioner, educator, editor, and admirable friend.

To nurse leaders: You are the architects of the future. Lead your teams well and step up to the important work that may only get done if you rise to the challenge. Have courage and lead by example with a pioneering spirit.

—Jayne Jennings Dunlap

To Jayne, whose visionary ideas and belief in me allowed me to believe in myself. To believe that I could use my voice even beyond the ways I was currently doing so (as an educator and editor in chief of *The Journal for Nurse Practitioners*) and avid Letter to the Editor writer. She challenges me to think so big, always asking why not us? Why not indeed. Why not has brought me on extraordinary journeys and in the end, it is the journey that matters most.

To all the nurses, nursing students, nurses in advanced roles, and my many mentors and supportive colleagues too numerous to mention.

My family, my parents, Vic and Betsy Briscoe, who also believe in me and continue to worry that I do too much. My children, Cabe and Dallas, and their wonderful spouses and my two amazing grandchildren, Penny and Oliver, who keep me young in spirit and dreaming of new adventures.

—Julee Briscoe Waldrop

BRIEF CONTENTS

DETAILED CONTENTS

CHAPTER 4 The Leadership Role of the Advanced Nurse in Searching for Evidence 65

Heather Carter-Templeton, Niki Cobb, Erin Whitaker, Tracy Brewer, and Julee Briscoe Waldrop

CHAPTER 5 Leading Critical Appraisal of Quantitative Evidence 85

Julee Briscoe Waldrop, Garry J. Brydges, Ninotchka Brydges, Jayne Jennings Dunlap, Tracy Brewer, and Melissa Hessock

CHAPTER 7 Leading the Appraisal of Other Types of Evidence to Inform Best Practices 143

Julee Briscoe Waldrop, Jayne Jennings Dunlap, Jennifer Woo, Melissa Hassock, and Tracy Brewer

CHAPTER 8 Incorporating the Patient Perspective in Quality Care 171

Elizabeth Walters and Julee Briscoe Waldrop

CHAPTER 11 Leading Evaluation of EBPQI Initiatives 241

Julee Briscoe Waldrop and Elizabeth Walters

CHAPTER 12 Dissemination Transcending the Discipline 261

Rosalie Mainous and Jayne Jennings Dunlap

Foreword

It was such a pleasure to read this first edition of *Leading Evidence-Based Practice and Quality Improvement Initiatives in Advanced Nursing Practice: A Competency Based Approach*, coedited by Jayne Jennings Dunlap and Julee Briscoe Waldrop. This book is written *for* students and a welcome addition to the currently available books on evidence-based practice (EBP) or quality improvement (QI). The authors have focused on providing students with a comprehensive and cogent roadmap that will help them throughout their career as a nurse in advanced practice.

The authors skillfully use several heuristics to make it easier for students to apply what they are reading about. One is the use of tables to compare and contrast (e.g., how to rate and report the quality of the evidence from the literature). Another is the use of mini case studies for the concept being discussed. Discussion questions at the end of each chapter require the student to think about what they have learned and how they will use that knowledge. The authors also use two examples throughout the book to provide exemplars for students to apply the various concepts in the chapters. One example is administrative (i.e., turnover and attrition in staff) and one is clinically focused (i.e., vaccination rates in children after COVID-19) focused.

This book does an admirable job of helping students differentiate research, EBP, and QI. This differentiation is important as students get into practice and are expected to lead teams who are engaging in initiatives to improve care. Another unique chapter in the book gives the students some understanding of how to appraise evidence outside of the peer-reviewed literature such as expert opinion, whitepapers, economic evaluations, and so on. These are all also placed in a table and compared to enhance understanding. I learned a lot reading this chapter. Another excellent chapter deals with the concepts of patient preferences—an often talked about concept integral to EBP but rarely broken down and expanded upon. The impact of how cultural differences on standard EBP can affect outcomes is well delineated. The authors also take the opportunity to help the student reflect on their own understanding of culture and cultural humility by providing specific steps the reader can take to deepen their understanding and skills working with patients from other cultures.

Another chapter focuses on dissemination—and doesn't limit the discussion to peer-reviewed papers. The authors also include posters, podcasts, and blogs. The discussion about authorship is highly relevant and will be so useful as students and faculty think through disseminating the final scholarly project report.

The focus on leadership throughout this book is unmistakable. Several of the chapters address the graduate-prepared nurse and the expectations of others for their leadership.

The final chapter is excellent and again reinforces the role of graduate-prepared nurses as leaders in the profession. The authors discuss mentorship, team building, self-awareness (a crucial skill for any leader), as well as conflict management. A very interesting discussion on legacy (an often-neglected topic) is also included. The discussion questions in this and all the chapters will help students to reflect and apply what they have learned.

In summary, this book is unique in how it focuses on students' learning and their understanding of complex topics. I would also posit that most faculty will themselves learn a great deal, as I did, while using this book in class. Faculty can use the examples, case studies, and discussion questions to guide discussion boards and/or student presentations. This book fills a gap in this literature and does so in a contemporary way. I know students will find it useful not just when they are in their courses but throughout their career.

Marion E. Broome, PhD, RN, FAAN
Dean Emerita and Ruby Wilson Professor of Nursing Emerita,
Duke University

Editors' Note to Readers

Message from Jayne

As Julee and I completed coediting for our first textbook, *Introduction to Evidence-Based Practice and Quality Improvement for Professional Nursing Practice: A Competency-Based Approach* for nurses entering the profession (level I) in 2023, we were humbled by the positive reviews and wide-reaching support for the text as a needed guide for new and seasoned nurses participating on evidence-based practice and quality improvement (EBPQI) teams. I had recently taken over interim oversight of Texas Woman's University's Doctor of Nursing Practice (DNP) program just as Julee stepped out of her DNP oversight role at Duke University. Julee and I talked about how much we wished there was an EBPQI textbook with a leadership focus for advanced (level II) students. We agreed this vital work was needed, deciding we might take it on together someday.

Despite this plan, I kept being reminded of the need for an advanced book throughout my interactions with nursing graduate faculty, students, and community partners. I finally began to think about whether it would be possible to create a leveled text for nurses entering or already positioned in advanced roles and specialties to complete a first-of-its-kind leveled textbook set, capturing the breadth of what our profession strives to achieve today. I considered how much I would have loved the opportunity to get my hands on that type of guidebook during my own master's or DNP coursework and how I wish current students across advanced nursing-focused programs had that type of needed resource now. One day, Julee vocalized a similar thought during our weekly meeting, stating that a derivative work, building on the foundational work we had already created and leveling the content up for nurse leaders, could meet this critical need. At that moment, I decided that we shouldn't wait, feeling strongly compelled that we could choose to start on the text you now have to explore. The truth was, even though it would be hard work on the heels of our first textbook, I knew the need was urgently upon us professionally, and I wanted to keep going with Julee as my editor partner. As soon as I clicked out of the Zoom meeting with Julee that day, I began working on the textbook proposal and the table of contents. One week later, I sent the proposal to Julee and asked her if she was up for it. We could see that this work was positioned to truly help reach a worthy readership of nurse leaders (you!) who will have an enormous impact that will transcend the nursing profession toward sustainable health care improvements.

Advanced nurses have historically been limited in roles and specialties by various barriers. In the spirit of tomorrow, we present this text to you, hoping that by engaging with the content you will be better equipped to lead interprofessional and even interdisciplinary teams to positive practice change. Julee and I wrote and edited this as two advanced practice nurses striving to keep patients at the forefront of all evidence-based decisions. We have at least one contributing author ambassador from each advanced practice role and advanced nursing specialty to ensure that this content will be relevant to you regardless of your future advanced focus. Throughout this text, we use the term "advanced nursing practice" (ANP) to capture all of you collectively as one group of nurse leaders.

Writing and editing this book has solidified an essential personal and professional lesson for me. Don't wait for the perfect time when something important needs to be done and it doesn't look like anyone else will step up to do it. Find and secure the necessary support matrix and resources, start on the good work, and stay focused on progress. As we did with the first textbook, Julee and I continued to prioritize our loved ones in our unique life stages and maintained self-care throughout this writing project to the best of our ability. We encourage you to engage in a wellness focus as leaders as well. Leadership-focused wellness boxes are located at the end of each chapter, and you can also explore your personalized evidence-based improvement plan in Appendix B.

We invite you to refresh your knowledge of the critically appraising research and other evidence and prepare to dive deeply into EBPQI leadership through an advanced competency-based approach (see Appendix A). EBPQI will be the core method you use to lead teams in practice change initiatives throughout your career in ANP. We hope you will find Appendix C's completed critical appraisal tools helpful in your practical leadership EBPQI journey as you guide your team in adherence to evidence-informed practice improvements. Adventure awaits.

****

Message from Julee

This textbook is personal. I have taught nurses in graduate nursing programs for 30 years and struggled to understand the issues nurses were having in practice, as leaders, and advanced practice registered nurses (APRNs) to find their unique contribution to the health care system. In the last 10 years, I began to figure it out. With the help of great colleagues (including Jayne and many of the authors of chapters in this book) I now have a vision for nurses in advanced nursing roles. My vision is that every nurse who earns a graduate degree will be able to demonstrate competency in understanding and appraising research reports and lead an EBPQI initiative or robust program evaluation or actively address a policy issue. Once consistency of these outcomes occurs, nurses in advanced roles will be able to cement our rightful place in health care. Our practice partners will know what we are capable of doing beyond direct patient care, that we can have a positive impact on populations and systems, and that by doing so improve value for patients, practitioners, and health care systems. Come be part of my vision! This textbook will show you the way.

****

Note: We recognize that gender is not binary and that all genders identities are represented in the field of nursing. In this textbook we use cisgender terms for ease of reading.

Acknowledgments

We sincerely thank our nurse leader chapter contributors and book reviewers for their high level of commitment and great contributions to this work. Their meaningful additions and recommendations undoubtedly strengthened this project for our readership, who will shape the contour and direction of the nursing profession for years to come.

We are uniquely grateful to DonnaLee Frega, PhD, RN, for her continued excitement and expert editing of this book project.

Reviewers

Celeste M. Baldwin, PhD, MS, APRN-CNS, GAHN
Regis College

Beatriz G. Bautista, DNP, APRN, FNP-BC, CDCES
University of Texas Rio Grande Valley

Cynthia D. Beckett, PhD, RNC-OB, LCCE, LSS-BB, CHRC, EBP-C
The Ohio State University, College of Nursing

Bonnie H. Bowie, PhD, RN, MBA, FAAN
Seattle University College of Nursing

L. Amy Giles, DNP, CNM, LSMC, FACNM
Louise Herrington School of Nursing, Baylor University

CHAPTER 1

Preparing to Lead Evidence-Based Practice and Quality Improvement

Jayne Jennings Dunlap and Julee Briscoe Waldrop

KEY CONCEPTS

Advanced nursing practice
Leadership
Spirit of inquiry
Research
Evidence-based practice
Quality improvement
Competencies

LEARNING OBJECTIVES

1. Explore the evolution of nursing research, evidence based practice, and quality improvement related to advanced nursing practice.
2. Differentiate between and integrate research, evidence based practice, and quality improvement.
3. Identify the advanced nursing practice role as an EBPQI team leader.
4. Introduce EBP models and a new EBPQI model.
5. Discuss future directions for EBPQI within and beyond advanced nursing practice.

> To be "in charge" is certainly not only to carry out the proper measures yourself but to see that everyone else does so too; to see that no one either willfully or ignorantly thwarts or prevents such measures. It is neither to do everything yourself nor to appoint a number of people to each duty, but to ensure that each does that duty to which he is appointed.
>
> —Florence Nightingale, *Notes on Nursing: What It Is, and What It Is Not*

Introduction

"What made you decide to pursue an advanced degree?" is a question we often ask the graduate students who enroll in our advanced nursing practice programs. In response, many report that they became frustrated with the limitations of their current professional nursing role and wish to do more to help patients. For example, a student who had worked as a bedside nurse in a busy intensive care unit described a night when three patients coded (experienced cardiac arrest) simultaneously. Her patient was the third for whom a code was called and thus had to wait to receive crucial care from the two advanced practice registered nurses (APRNs) on duty. This student recalled that while attempting to help her patient within the scope of her practice as an RN, she contemplated returning to school to enhance her education and abilities. Such stories present poignant reminders of the purpose behind our vocational goals as nurses and serve as a call to continue learning.

As a practicing nurse, you surely have many stories of your own on positive and negative care experiences. We encourage you, as you begin this journey, to pause and reflect on your choice to pursue further education. Allow your memories and reasons to drive your progress toward the commendable goal of entering advanced nursing practice. You may want to write your purpose statement for pursuing an advanced degree in nursing and place it somewhere visible as a reminder of your personal motivations.

We are delighted that you have decided to enhance your professional role! The contents of this textbook will equip you, in your future role as an advanced nursing practice leader, to achieve health care system improvements through **evidence-based practice** (EBP) and **quality improvement** (QI). Although EBP and QI are different processes, we will often refer to them together (EBPQI) because their synergism is needed to make sustainable practice changes for continuous improvement in health and health care.

In addition to a review of research fundamentals, you will be introduced to advanced EBPQI-focused nursing practice competencies (i.e., what you can do or demonstrate). These competencies will serve as a foundation on which to build system-level changes in your advanced nursing practice specialty (e.g., administration/practice leadership, informatics, population/public health, or health policy) or through your advanced practice nursing role (certified clinical nurse specialist, certified nurse practitioner, certified nurse midwife, certified registered nurse anesthetist). We will use the term "advanced nursing practice" (ANP) consistently to make clear that the material you learn is designed for use across all ANP specialties and roles.

You are entering ANP at an important time when nursing programs are transitioning to competency-based education (American Association of Colleges of Nursing, 2021); this means that earning your degree will depend on your successful demonstration of required competencies rather than solely on your completion of courses and clinical rotations. Stakeholders now know exactly what to expect from an ANP graduate, so let's get started!

Why Do We Need EBP and QI?

Harm often occurs during health care. Almost 25% of all hospitalized patients experience an adverse event (Bates et al., 2023). Many errors are caused by the use of outdated, inaccurate, or nonevidence-based practices that fall below care standards. To reduce the risk of harm, we must use EBP and consistently pursue QI. The need for EBPQI leaders (like you!) will continue to increase as the complexity of the health care system grows.

As a nurse, you are already a valuable EBPQI team member because you likely can identify the current problems in your workplace and support EBPQI practice change in various ways. As you prepare to assume an ANP position, you will move into a leadership role to ensure that EBPQI is instituted across your health care setting, often at a systems level with notable scalability. We need nurse leaders who are strongly committed to EBPQI to lead teams to improve the quality and safety of health care.

Although most research-based ANP programs focus on skills for conducting original research, this textbook teaches you how to explore and appraise current evidence that supports EBPQI initiatives. First, we review the differences between and interrelatedness of research and EBPQI. Much historical and discipline-wide confusion exists around these key processes, and we want you to enter your leadership position with a clear understanding of the evidence continuum. Next, we review the evolution and fundamental concepts of research and EBPQI using a modern framework that will help you throughout our journey.

Evolution of Nursing Research, EBP, and QI

You probably were given an introduction to nursing research as part of your prelicensure nursing program. Perhaps you were taught that Florence Nightingale was the first nurse researcher and used evidence to improve practice (quite true; Mackey & Bassendowski, 2017), but you may not have learned that in the mid-20th century, nursing fought to be recognized as a separate scientific discipline by arguing that a discipline is formed by scientists, scholars, and practitioners who share a common perspective on an empirical world. Nurses decide which issues are relevant to nursing and what questions are asked (researched), which is the domain of a discipline (Visintainer, 1986). Concurrently with this debate, in the 1950s and 60s, academic nursing developed more doctoral programs as well as pre- and postdoctoral fellowships to train nurse researchers. It was not until 1985, however, that the federal government established the National Institute of Nursing Research (NINR) (www.ninr.nih.gov/) within the National Institutes of Health. The NINR has been the major funder of nursing research since its inception. In alignment with the Future of Nursing Report (National Academies of Science, 2020), the NINR's research priorities are to support research that improves health equity.

Today, nursing research (the scientific study of new phenomena) includes clinical research, health systems research, outcomes research, and nursing education research. The new knowledge generated by nurses on these topics is evidence that nurses at the advanced level can and must use to lead initiatives to enhance the quality of care provided to patients, improve health care systems, and advocate for policies that impact populations.

Review of Research Basics

Nurse researchers seek to answer questions about solutions that are not yet known. To find answers to their questions, nurse researchers develop and test hypotheses. **Hypotheses** are simply statements about what the researcher expects their study's outcome will be. Hypothesis testing includes statistical analysis. The goal of **statistical analysis** is to determine that the results are not due to chance.

Research methodologies can be divided broadly into two categories, quantitative and qualitative, based on the type of results they produce. **Quantitative research** generally produces numerical results, and qualitative research produces narrative (word-based) results. All research includes variables. **Variables** are characteristics that can be measured, such as age or income (or even a complex construct such as the quality of life). In a specific research study, researchers label the variables as dependent or independent according to their hypothesis (what they expect will happen in answer to their research question). A variable is labeled **independent** if the researcher expects it to influence another variable. The variable that is expected to be influenced is labeled the **dependent** variable. Here is a trick to help you remember: A baby's weight is "dependent" on (influenced by) its milk intake. How much milk a mother can produce is "independent" of the infant's weight.

Quantitative research designs are further categorized as experimental or observational. **Experimental research** involves the researcher's manipulation of independent variables with the objective of finding out what effect they have on the dependent variable. Because there are often additional variables that could impact the dependent variable (which may or may not be considered in the study), experimental studies include a **control group**. In the control group, the researcher does not manipulate the independent variable. At the end of the experiment, the dependent variable is measured in both groups, and results from both groups are compared using statistical analysis to determine whether there is any statistically significant difference in outcomes.

When a research study uses human subjects, the researcher must choose **criteria** to determine which types of subjects will be included or excluded from the study. A thoughtful choice of criteria allows the researcher to determine whether the study's results can be **generalized** (considered applicable) to a broader population of people beyond those in the study. If the sample of participants in the study is random (meaning that everyone who participates in the study has a random chance of being placed in either the experimental group or the control group), the experiment is classified as a **randomized controlled trial** (RCT). A common theme in research evaluation is that a RCT always produces the highest quality of evidence. Results from RCTs are thought to have the least bias and, therefore, to reveal the answer to the research question closest to the truth. Accordingly, the results are accepted as generalizable and can be applied to everyone. However, this consideration is problematic because a biased choice of inclusion criteria can compromise generalizability to the wider population. For example, many current drug-based therapies are based on past RCTs and subsequent systematic reviews that were comprised almost entirely of subjects who were White men. Although these RCTs included few women and even fewer subjects who were Black, Indigenous, or people of color (BIPOC), their results were unwisely considered applicable across diverse populations.

Furthermore, due to advances in genetics and genomics, we now know that individualized care may be better than care that works for most people, as previously thought. It is important to note that Indigenous healers and ancient therapeutic systems such as ayurveda and traditional Chinese medicine have understood the importance of individualized care for thousands of years. Researchers must always be aware of the ways our personal values and social context might influence research perspectives and choices.

Common **observational research** study designs include cross-sectional, cohort, and case-control studies (see Figure 1.1). **Cross-sectional studies** examine a phenomenon of interest at one point in time. Surveys or questionnaires are frequently used in cross-sectional studies to collect information on a specific topic. **Cohort studies** follow a group of people over time and collect data from them at various points over time. A cohort study can be **retrospective** (look at a person's history) or **prospective** (follow people in the cohort into the future). Often, participants in a cohort study have something in common, such as where they live or a certain diagnosis. **Case-control studies** compare people with a specific exposure or condition (case) to a control group of people who are without the exposure or condition but similar in as many other aspects as possible.

BOX 1.1: QUANTITATIVE RESEARCH EXAMPLE

During the COVID-19 pandemic, some policies created to protect people from infection, such as stay-at-home orders, may have resulted in consequences beyond their intent, especially for multimorbid elderly patients. This cohort study followed a group of 82 complex multimorbid elderly patients living in a community in Spain for a year, assessing them every 3 months. The researchers aimed to describe changes in many aspects (variables) of the participants' health and health care, including nursing care and nursing diagnoses. Functional outcomes reported in the study included statistically significant increases in nursing diagnoses related to impairment of physical mobility and ambulation, constipation, and the ability to dress oneself. Despite living with family members and having caregivers, which allowed them to stay in their community, patients' health and use of health care services declined (Ruzafa-Martinez et al., 2023).

Qualitative research differs from quantitative research in that it seeks to describe and understand a phenomenon in depth, adding to what is already known. Qualitative research aims to present a fuller understanding of what a specific phenomenon means to the people it affects (e.g., how it feels to live with a chronic condition such as diabetes or to lose a loved one to cancer).

Qualitative studies are often the precursor to quantitative studies. When little is known about a phenomenon, a full description of it can provide the knowledge needed to develop more specific quantitative studies to fill in the knowledge gaps. There are many variations and methods in nursing research besides these basics. You will learn more about evaluating their quality and the strength of their results in Chapters 6 and 7.

BOX 1.2: QUALITATIVE RESEARCH EXAMPLE

Improvement initiatives in health care do not always succeed. In one study (Nilsen et al., 2020), researchers aimed to investigate the characteristics of changes that health professionals deemed successful. The research team conducted semi-structured interviews with 30 health care professionals (physicians, RNs, and assistant nurses) in a Swedish health care system. Interview questions were developed based on the existing literature. The interviewer invited participants to describe their experiences and perceptions of any health care changes, large or small, that had impacted their work. The recorded and transcribed narratives were analyzed, and three primary categories were revealed: (a) having an opportunity to influence the change, (b) being prepared for the change, and (c) valuing the change. The study concluded that when these three criteria are considered in addition to whether a change will benefit patients, the change has a greater chance of success.

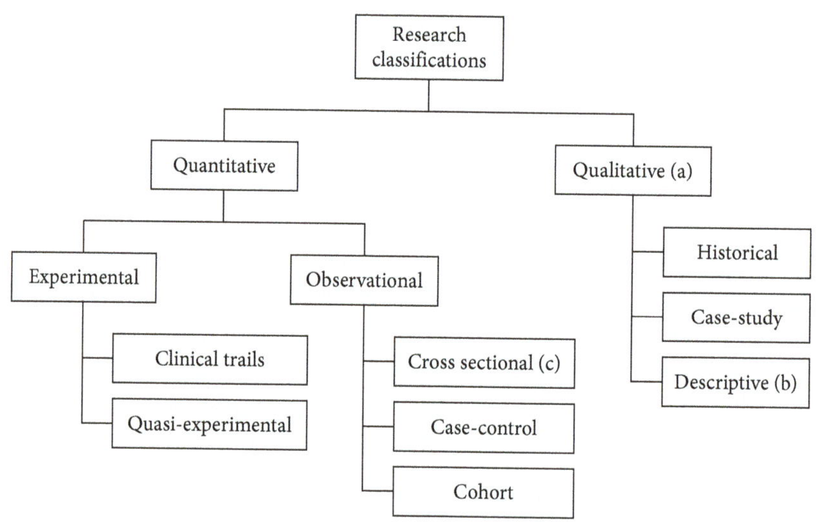

(a) There are many types of qualitative studies, but these are the most common in nursing research.
(b) Descriptive studies can also be quantitative research.
(c) Cross-sectional designs are also used in qualitative research.

FIGURE 1.1 Classification of research.

Evidence-Based Practice

At this level of your education and experience, you likely are familiar with certain important aspects of EBP: use of the best available research, clinical expertise, and consideration of patient/family preferences and/or values (Table 1.1). In nursing, EBP is described as a problem-solving approach best accomplished within the context of care (Fineout-Overholt et al., 2005). The basic-level EBP competencies (adequate knowledge and skills) for practicing registered nurses were developed in 2014 (Melnyk et al., 2014) and are used today. A subsequent study (Melnyk et al., 2018) on nurses' achievement of the 13 EBP competencies revealed that much progress remains to be made. Results revealed that no competency averages reached the *competent* to *very competent* range, with most falling in the *needs improvement* category. The goal for all nurses is to achieve these competencies. As a nurse leader, you will need to consider how you might facilitate improvement in these competencies in those who report to you. Additional competencies have been developed for advanced nursing practice (Melnyk et al., 2014). This textbook will be your reference and guide as you become competent in EBP or EBPQI at the advanced level (see Table 1.2).

TABLE 1.1 EBPQI Process Steps, Descriptions, and Chapter Location

Step in the EBPQI Process	Description	More Information
0	Cultivate a spirit of inquiry	Chapters 1 and 2
1	Identify the problem Ask the question	Chapters 2 and 3
2	Search for the best evidence-based research and other evidence	Chapters 4
3	Critically appraise the evidence	Chapters 5, 6, and 7
4	Integrate the evidence with your clinical expertise and patient preferences. Implement a model (EBP, QI, or EBPQI)	Chapters 8
5	Implement the practice change and evaluate the outcomes	Chapter 10 Chapter 11
6	Disseminate the outcome(s)	Chapter 12

Fineout-Overholt et al. (2005)

TABLE 1.2 Steps in EBP Process for Advanced Nursing Practice

1.	Questions clinical practice
2.	Describes clinical problems using internal evidence
3.	Participates in forming questions
4.	Participates in searches of external evidence
5.	Participates in critically appraising pre-appraised evidence
6.	Participates in critically appraising research studies for practice
7.	Participates in the synthesis of evidence
8.	Collects practice data
9.	Integrates evidence into EBP changes
10.	Implements practice change based on three components of EBP
11.	Evaluates practice changes
12.	Disseminates best practices
13.	Participates in strategies to sustain EBP culture
	Additional Advanced Competencies (notice the verb changes)
14.	Systematically conducts an exhaustive search for external evidence to answer clinical questions
15.	Critically appraises relevant pre-appraised evidence
16.	Integrates a body of external evidence from nursing and related fields with internal evidence in making decisions about patient care
17.	Leads transdisciplinary teams in applying synthesized evidence to initiate clinical decisions and practice changes to improve the health of individuals, groups, and populations
18.	Generates internal evidence through outcomes management and EBP implementation projects for the purpose of integrating best practices
19.	Measures processes and outcomes of evidence-based clinical decisions
20.	Formulates evidence-based policies and procedures
21.	Participates in the generation of external evidence with other health care professionals
22.	Mentors others in evidence-based decision-making and the EBP process
23.	Implements strategies to sustain an EBP culture
24.	Communicates best evidence to individuals, groups, colleagues, and policy makers

Source: Melnyk et al. (2013).

Nurses are not the only health care professionals who must be competent in EBP practices. Because health care is complex and requires a team of professionals to provide the best care, all must be competent in EBP. A systematic review (Saunders et al., 2019) of systematic reviews (n = 11) reported that practicing health care professionals' self-reported knowledge and beliefs about EBP were at a moderate to high level; however, as we know, gaining knowledge about something does not always result in changing one's actions or behaviors accordingly. Much EBP implementation, evaluation, and sustainable practice is still lacking.

Evidence-Based Practice Models and Frameworks

Models that support the process of putting evidence into practice have been developed and are being used routinely in many health care settings. All models generally include the steps of the EBP process (see Table 1.1). If you look closely, you will find the nursing process in most models!

A systematic review of evidence-based practice models and frameworks (Dusin et al., 2023) identified 19 that were appropriate for health care settings; all begin with the identification of a problem, the development of a clinical question, and a search for evidence. Interestingly, only four of these 19 models and frameworks include the critical component of patient preferences and values, which constitutes a third of the definition of EBP! Application of evidence is an area in which the models differ in detail and guidance. The ability to evaluate evidence critically was noted as a crucial skill for EBP expertise. This textbook will be a great resource for developing your EBP skills so that you can mentor others in the health care team. The following are brief overviews of examples of EBP models.

Rosswurm and Larrabee (1999) developed one of the first models for EBP. Their linear model assumes that change occurs in the following orderly, stepwise fashion:

Step 1 identifies the problem and assesses the current status.

Step 2 focuses on identifying potential interventions and selecting outcome indicators.

Step 3 includes searching the evidence (research), critique and synthesis, and determination of feasibility.

Step 4 is planning for implementing the proposed change.

Step 5 includes piloting, implementing, evaluating, and determining whether to adapt, adopt, or reject the practice change.

The ACE star model, developed in 2004, is similar in simplicity, leaving much room for interpretation. The first point on the star represents *discovery research*, and the other points (in clockwise order) stand for *evidence summary*, *translation guidelines*, *practice integration*, and *process-outcomes evaluation*. The ACE model was revolutionary in helping to distinguish research from EBP and properly position these two paradigms on the evidence continuum. Although this model was created almost 2 decades ago, little has been published on its use, and a sustainability component is lacking, which highlights the need for EBP model evolution (Stevens, 2015).

The IOWA model for evidence-based practice was published in 2001 (Titler et al., 2001) and most recently revised and validated in 2017 (Iowa Model Collaborative et al., 2017). This model is popular in many organizations, and we will use it in Chapter 10 of this textbook in an example of practice change implementation. Because this model contains decision points, you might think of it as a decision tree. The IOWA model begins, as most models do, with identifying the **triggering issue** (i.e., the problem to be addressed) and guides users to develop a **purpose statement** based on this issue. Next, you must determine whether addressing the issue you have chosen is an institutional priority. If your proposed practice change will not be an institutional priority, you need to reconsider and find another opportunity for change on which you can focus (there is no shortage of issues needing improvement in health care). When you have identified a problem for which finding and implementing a solution is an institutional priority, it is time to form a team. As an advanced nurse, you will be able to lead such a team!

First, you will search the evidence (the existing research) for potential solutions to the triggering issue you have chosen. Next, you will collect, critically appraise, and synthesize the available evidence. Once you have all this information assembled, you must ask (and answer) an important question: Is there enough evidence to support a change in practice? It is irresponsible to change practice without enough evidence to support a change. Let's suppose the answer is *no*, or *not yet*. In this case, your team can consider doing further research to develop the evidence needed. If there is sufficient evidence to support change, you can move forward to design and pilot the proposed practice change. This stage in the process will involve many activities! You will need to engage stakeholders (persons with a stake in the current [and future] way of doing things) as well as prepare materials and collect data. Once the data has been collected and the outcomes evaluated, you must make one final decision: Is the practice change appropriate for permanent adoption? If it is not, consider alternatives. If it is, you can integrate it into the system and continue to monitor the effects. Last, disseminate the results so that others can benefit from your findings.

The Center for Evidence-Based Practice at Johns Hopkins' (n.d.) model focuses on problem solving in interprofessional teams. This model involves making an inquiry using a practice question, identifying evidence (research) to translate your findings into best practice, reflecting and learning as practice improvements are made, and returning to the inquiry. Many tools to guide your practice are available free of charge from the website, including a decision tree (for determining whether there is a need for the project), a work plan, a Population, Intervention, Comparison, Outcome (PICO) question guide, a stakeholder analysis and communications tool, a hierarchy-of-evidence guide, critical appraisal tools, evidence summary and synthesis table templates, translation, and an action planning tool.

Unlike the previously described process-focused models for EBP, the ARCC model is a system-wide framework meant to advance and sustain EBP across the entire health care system (Melnyk et al., 2017). This model is, therefore, more complex and begins with an organizational assessment of the current EBP culture. To advance EBP within health systems, a group of EBP mentors must be in place. Without this leadership level to educate, guide, and support others as they implement change into practice, the outcomes of improved care, reduced costs, and increased clinician satisfaction are much less likely to occur.

TABLE 1.3 EBP Models

Model	Links and Resources
IOWA model	Iowa Model Collaborative. (2017). Iowa model of evidence-based practice: Revisions and validation. *Worldviews on Evidence-Based Nursing, 14*(3), 175–182. https://doi.org/10.1111/wvn.12223
Model of EBP change	Rosswurm, M. A., & Larrabee, J. H. (1999). A model for change to evidence-based practice. *Image—The Journal of Nursing Scholarship, 31*(4), 317–322. https://doi.org/10.1111/j.1547-5069.1999.tb00510.x
Johns Hopkins evidence-based practice model	Dang, D. & Dearholt, S. (2022). *Johns Hopkins nursing evidence-based practice model and guidelines* (4thed.). Sigma Theta Tau International. https://www.hopkinsmedicine.org/evidence-based-practice/model-tools
Advancing research and clinical practice through close collaboration	Melnyk, B. M., Fineout-Overholt, E., Giggleman, M., & Choy, K. (2017). A test of the ARCC© model improves implementation of evidence-based practice, health care culture, and patient outcomes. *Worldviews on Evidence-Based Nursing, 14*(1), 5–9. https://doi.org/10.1111/wvn.12188
ACE star model of EBP	Stevens, K. R. (2004). ACE star model of EBP: Knowledge transformation. Academic Center for Evidence-based Practice, University of Texas Health Science Center at San Antonio. https://uthscsa.edu/nursing/research/resources-scholarly-support/star-model

Quality Improvement

You might think that quality improvement (QI) is a recent innovation, but it is not. As with research and evidence-based practice, Florence Nightingale (1859) is credited with being the first nurse to practice quality improvement; however, Ignaz Semmelweis was another early pioneer of QI. During the 1800s, in a teaching hospital in Vienna, Semmelweis observed that there were far fewer infections and deaths among patients of midwives than of physicians. Initially, he resisted the notion that the routine hand washing performed by midwives contributed to preventing infection or the transfer of infection from patient to patient; he performed studies to determine whether anything else could account for his observations. Finally, after performing what might be considered the first controlled trial, he was forced to admit that the results demonstrated that handwashing was an effective intervention in limiting the spread of infection. Unfortunately, his ideas were extremely unpopular, and his work was largely ignored. Over 20 years later, researchers whose names you may find more familiar (Pasteur, Koch, Lister) were credited for exploring and promoting antiseptic techniques (Best & Neuhauser, 2004).

QI did get a big boost when, in 1999, the Institute of Medicine (now the National Academies of Science) published a report entitled *To Err Is Human: Building a Safer Health System* (Institute of Medicine's Committee on Quality of Health Care in America, 2000), which highlighted the significant problem of safety in the health care system and the harm to patients and care workers caused by errors. In a follow-up report, *Crossing the Quality Chasm: A New Health System for the 21st Century* (Institute of Medicine, 2001), goals were formulated to improve the quality of care provided by the U.S. health care system along with specific principles to guide improvement, including a recommendation for the "Six Aims for Improvement": care that is safe, timely, effective, efficient, equitable, and patient-centered (STEEEP). You will learn more about quality standards in Chapter 2.

A model for improvement introduced and developed by Edwards Deming, a celebrated engineer and manufacturing statistician of the 20th century, included plan-do-study-act (PDSA) cycles (see Figure 1.2) as an integral part of problem solving (Langley et al., 2009). Process improvement methodologies such as LEAN and Six Sigma use similar principles. All improvement methods are based on the following fundamental questions:

- What are we trying to accomplish?
- How will we know whether a change is an improvement?
- What change can we make that will result in an improvement?

You will learn more about quality and safety, the model for improvement, why you need data to know whether a change has occurred, and statistical process control (how to measure something to know whether there is an improvement) in Chapters 2 and 9.

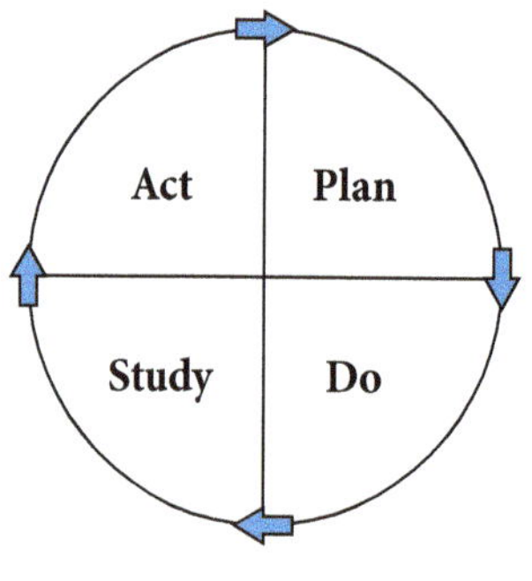

FIGURE 1.2 PDSA cycle.

Differentiating Research, EBP, and QI

There is a lethal gap between what is known about achieving improvement and the actual use of knowledge for this purpose. Despite a wealth of research evidence that indicates the need for its implementation into practice, far too often important work ends up on a shelf or within digital databases untouched rather than being broadly and consistently applied to health care practice—a sobering lost opportunity. However, more than 2 decades of implementation research, EBP, and QI have led to decreased care gaps in some areas. For example, cancer care evidence-to-practice gaps have narrowed from 17 to 15 years (Khan et al., 2021). Unfortunately, at this slow rate, it will take well over the next 100 years to close these costly health care gaps.

As a future leader in ANP, you must understand how research, EBP, and QI are defined to learn how these paradigms differ and are interconnected (see Table 1.4). Although some definition variability exists, consistent use of research, EBP, and QI language and terminology across academic and clinical settings is essential (Dunlap et al., 2024). Research is a systematic scientific process to establish facts and generate new knowledge or theory. EBP is a process used to review, critically appraise, and translate the latest external evidence (data generated from scientific research studies) into practice recommendations. EBP teams use (a) the best available research (external evidence), (b) clinical experience, and (c) patient preferences/values to inform clinical decision-making. QI uses rapid cycles of change in practice to improve processes or outcomes. QI relies on internal evidence (data generated from your own clinical setting or organization) and typically does not involve a systematic search and critical appraisal of evidence. For more information on internal and external evidence, see Chapter 4.

TABLE 1.4 Comparative Representation of Research, EBP, and QI Paradigms for Competency-Based Education

	Research	EBP	QI
Function	Generates new knowledge; replicates evidence; tests or generates theory; improves methods or instrumentation	Translates evidence to recommend best practice	Identifies a problem and incorporates local evidence to improve process and/or outcomes
Methods	Qualitative/quantitative designs, mixed methods	Evidence search	Identify measurements, enact changes, and analyze results to improve systems
Questions	May be directional or nondirectional; can be research questions and/ or hypotheses	PICO (population, intervention, comparison, outcome); PPCO (problem, population, change, outcome)	SMART aims (specific, measurable, actionable, relevant, timely)

(Continued)

TABLE 1.4 *(Continued)*

	Research	EBP	QI
Focus	New knowledge; replication of former findings; revelations in big data; generation or testing of theory; lived experience	Critical appraisal of current evidence with synthesis	Continuous process improvement, element of time
Process	Uses a variety of research methods and designs to dictate procedure	Produces outcomes through implementation of a practice change in a narrow population through integration of best external evidence, patient/family values, and clinician expertise	Produces internal evidence to evaluate the performance of systems and processes and improve outcomes in the (local) setting
Reliability	May yield highly reliable measures with consistent approach; related concept is validity (the accuracy of the measure)	Reliable if considered trustworthy, credible, and applicable to the problem	Attempts to increase reliability (greater reliability means less error)
Generalizability/ Transferability	May be generalizable in quantitative methodologies; seeks transferability if using qualitative methods	Not generalizable but may have transferability	Not generalizable but may have transferability
Significance	Focus is on statistical significance or a better understanding of phenomena	Clinical/practical significance	Clinical/practical significance, displayed visually in run or statistical control charts over time

Source: Dunlap et al. (2024).

Research aspires to produce generalizable results (findings that can be generalized to a population beyond the participants in the study). Less understood but equally important is the **transferability** of research results. When research results determine that an intervention is effective, these results should be implemented into general practice. This is often where the gap between knowledge and the application of knowledge occurs. Research findings can take 15 years or more to be adapted into general practice (Morris et al., 2011). Granted, research conducted in a controlled setting with participants chosen because they meet specific criteria is not quite an accurate reflection of everyday nursing

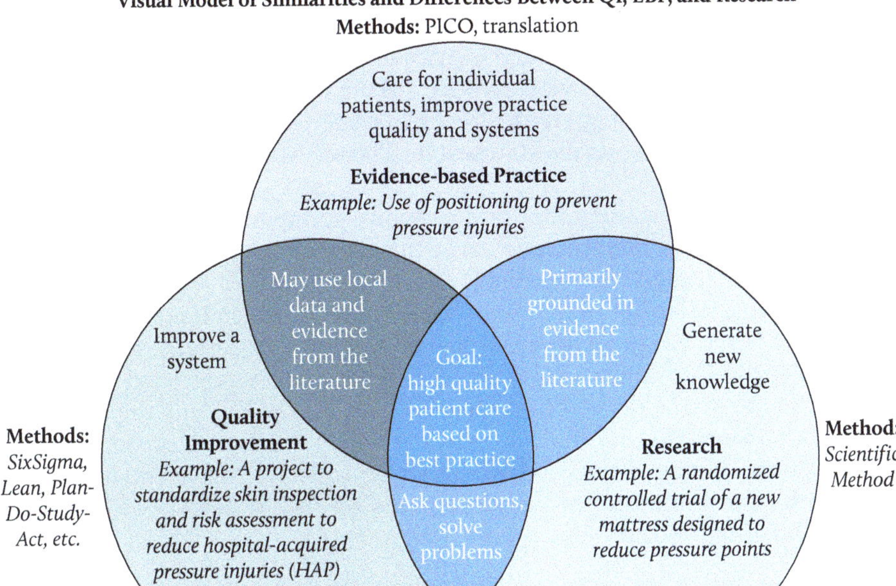

FIGURE 1.3 Visual model of similarities and differences between research, EBP, and QI.

practice. Nonetheless, as nurses in leadership roles, you will be challenged to shorten this timeline, and putting evidence into practice in your workplace is one way to do it!

Be prepared for some resistance. As nurses put research results into practice in their settings, the results of their QI efforts may be criticized for not being generalizable because the participants (all the patients affected by the practice change) are not representative of the broader population. This criticism is unjust. An evidence-based QI initiative that has worked in one organization can be transferred and adapted to another so long as the core of the intervention remains the same. For example, following best-practice recommendations, a newborn infant should receive their first hepatitis B vaccine (core intervention) before discharge from the hospital (American Academy of Pediatrics, Committee on Infectious Diseases & Committee on Fetus and Newborn, 2017); however, various aspects of the intervention can differ, such as the use of standing orders, who obtains informed consent, or the specific schedule of vaccine administration after birth (Damschroder et al., 2009). Although not always generalizable, EBP and QI work is highly transferable, with clinical and practical significance. This will be discussed further in Chapter 12.

Implementation science and translational science are areas of research focus that are commonly referred to interchangeably with EBP and/or QI and often need clarification. **Implementation science** is research that focuses on studying the methods and strategies that facilitate the uptake of research into practice, and **translational science** is research focused on understanding the scientific and operational principles underlying each step of the translational process (Nilsen, 2015). Additionally, it's important for you to remember that the term "study" should be used synonymously with research. The terms "project" and "initiative" describe EBP and QI endeavors. "Project" may be used to describe research, but "study" should not describe other project types. You may see these terms used interchangeably in the literature; however, the distinction is important to understand in an ANP leadership position.

There is an overlap between research, EBP, and QI, which is represented well in Figure 1.3 (Grys, 2022); all have the goal of high-quality patient care. Integration of EBP and QI frameworks is evolving due to the urgent need to sustain EBP improvements. Evidence-based QI (EBP-I) blends the EBP and improvement processes by integrating internal and external evidence into the decision-making about practice change (Hempel et al., 2022; Levin et al., 2010). The mountain model is the first framework to fully integrate EBP and QI as EBPQI (Figure 1.4; Waldrop & Dunlap, 2024).

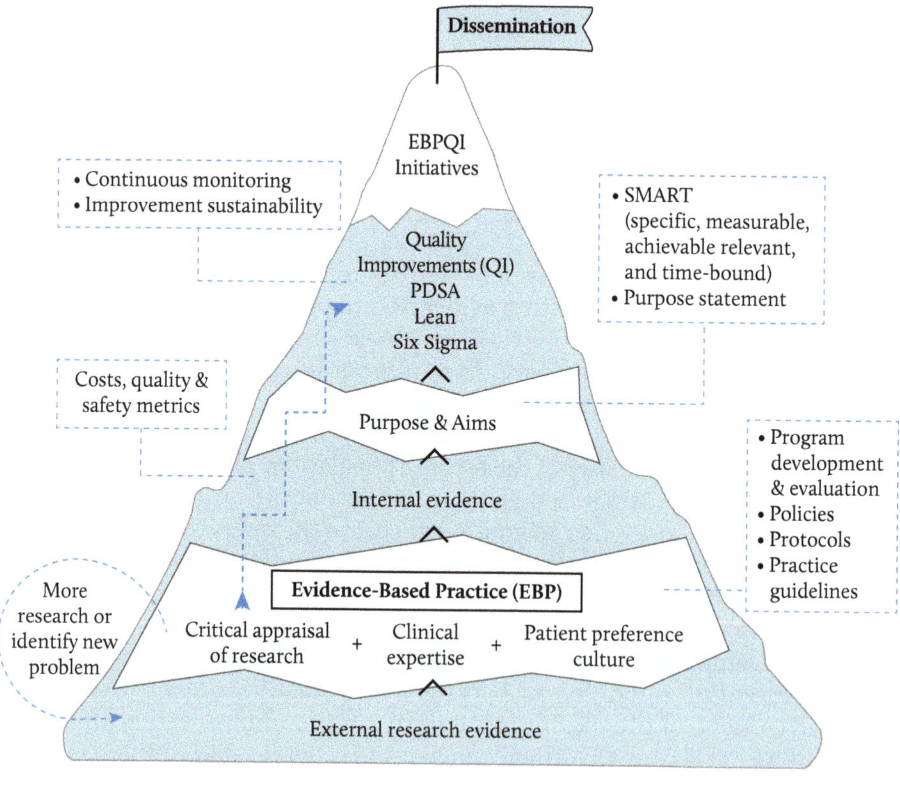

FIGURE 1.4 The mountain model for EBPQI initiatives.

The Mountain Model for EBPQI

Having described the fundamental differences among research, EBP, and QI, we are ready to introduce you to the mountain model for EBPQI. This model comprehensively integrates the EBP and QI processes to inform timely EBPQI initiatives (see Figure 1.4), and we will use it throughout this textbook.

In the mountain model, research is the foundation upon which all improvements in health and health care must be built. Using this research foundation, the first level above the base of the mountain is EBP (i.e., applying research, clinical expertise, and patient preference in your practice). At this level of the mountain, you can use any of the many EBP processes and protocols mentioned (Table 1.3) or others. Stopping at this level, with just recommendations for practice, limits the usefulness of research. At the next level, QI, you will use external and internal evidence as well as patient preference to (a) make successful and sustainable practice change and (b) identify outcomes or measures (SMART aims) that demonstrate that the practice change has made a difference (e.g., in costs, quality, or safety metrics). Working upward through these levels will produce an EBPQI initiative culminating in the dissemination (sharing) of your efforts with others. This integral part of EBPQI, illustrated by the mountain summit flag, is paramount. It ensures that we don't keep reinventing the same things and can learn from and build on best practices for making a positive difference in health and health care (Waldrop & Dunlap, 2024).

The fundamental knowledge and skills that you are learning at this moment in your graduate nursing program will enable you to face current health care challenges with evidence-based support. As you gain leadership experience and advance in your pursuit of excellence in practice, you will likely transition from serving as an EBPQI team member to the team leader. After earning your graduate degree in your chosen role or specialty in ANP, you will be qualified to lead initiatives that improve population health, health system processes, and care delivery. Large and complex research projects are often conducted by a nurse who has earned a Doctor of Philosophy (PhD) degree or by a person with an advanced science degree with additional education and training in research methodology. These backgrounds prepare individuals to lead diverse teams and work with professionals from various disciplines to complete studies that will provide nurses with new scientific information to translate into clinical practice. Although all nurses should have a clear EBP understanding and engagement, often the largest or most complex projects are conducted by a nurse who has earned a DNP degree, which prepares one to be an expert in EBPQI.

Research, EBP, and QI projects are often carried out by a team of professionals (see Figure 1.5). Nurses at all levels can participate as team members. Nurses who are experts in a specific area (e.g., Masters of Science in Nursing (MSN)-prepared pediatric nurse practitioners in acute care, certified nurse educators) frequently contribute their expertise. The best teams are generally those which incorporate diversity in background and experience. The most pressing problems in health care need to be addressed by teams assembled to ensure different paradigm expertise and a multidisciplinary approach.

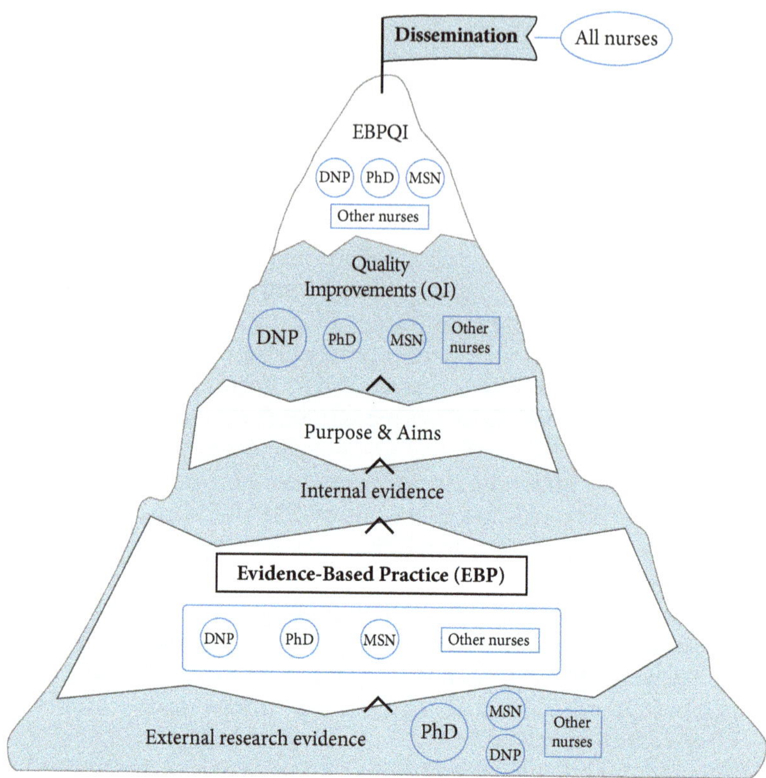

FIGURE 1.5 Nurses' roles in EBPQI.

BOX 1.3: A PERSONAL CASE STUDY BY JAYNE

"They're going to intubate my mom!"

I was very concerned when I received this text message from a friend whose middle-aged mother, in relative physical health, had been hospitalized with pneumonia 2 weeks prior.

"It's just a precaution. She's getting tired, and this will allow her to rest and recover," she tried to assure me; however, this rationale did not bring me much reassurance. The facility where the patient was receiving care held numerous excellence designations, yet I was keenly aware that medical errors are common in hospitals. I knew that my friend needed a support person as she attempted to advocate for her mom.

My friend was waiting outside the hospital when I arrived an hour later. Her mother had already been intubated. Fortunately, at my suggestion, she had visited with her mother before the intubation, in what would be their last verbal exchange. In the patient's room, we were greeted with a beeping alarm.

"What does that sound mean?" my friend asked.

I checked the patient and the machine to which she was tethered. The alarm indicated low blood pressure. My heart sank as I pressed the call light. A nurse arrived and titrated medication to increase the patient's blood pressure. He explained that low blood pressure was to be expected but was unable to explain why. He suggested that we ask the physicians when they rounded the next morning. At that point, I requested to speak with a provider.

Soon after, a nurse practitioner (NP) appeared who had cared for the patient in collaboration with the hospitalist team and physician for several days. The patient's daughter was able to ask all of her questions, and afterward the NP offered to show her the patient's chest X-rays. We gathered around the computer to review the complete series of X-rays from her mother's multiweek hospital stay. To my horror, the most recent image, taken just hours earlier to confirm airway placement following intubation, revealed the whiteout presence of several infiltrations. The dinging alarm signaling low blood pressure had suggested to me that the patient might have sepsis (an overwhelming systemic infection). Now, looking at the images, I knew that she was in trouble and hoped there would be a path forward through a partnership with the health care team.

"Have the cultures come back yet?" I asked. A long pause followed before the NP answered, "We didn't get any cultures."

We stood in silence as the patient's daughter stared at us. Obtaining cultures before starting antibiotics for worsening pneumonia in hospitalized patients with declining status is a standard of care (CDC, 2023). Blood and sputum cultures isolate the infective pathogen and ensure that the treatment used will be effective. If a particular infective agent is antibiotic resistant, for instance, this will be indicated in the findings of the cultures, allowing timely medication adjustments or changes to be made. Because culture results typically take 2–3 days to grow, broad-spectrum antibiotics are initiated immediately after obtaining culture specimen samples to increase the likelihood of proper treatment and eventual recovery from infection. Broad-spectrum antibiotics had been started days prior for this patient, but the critical step of obtaining cultures had been missed, and the patient was now deteriorating.

The NP and I realized that the health care team had been caring for their patient without complete information, and time was no longer on her side. Hoping that her guess would prove correct, the NP placed an order for Flagyl (an antibiotic to stop the growth of certain bacteria and parasites) and an urgent order to have cultures drawn. My friend still believed that her mother's intubation was simply a precautionary measure, so I explained that the patient was in some trouble and encouraged her to visit her mother with her husband and children. Nonplussed, she notified her entire family and some close friends, many of whom came to visit. During this time, she was able to communicate with her mom using a notepad. Her mother wrote that she believed she would recover and be discharged home, but her status soon became unstable. The out-of-state family arrived but could only watch helplessly as their loved one was placed on extracorporeal membrane oxygenation (ECHMO) and taken to surgery. Afterward, she experienced cardiac arrest repeatedly. The surgical team vocalized no understanding of how or why cardiac arrest occurred; they only told the family to wait for improvement and give the patient time. I can still picture her body lying face down and retroverted while the health care team continued extraordinary measures to revive her. The health care team continued to treat the patient with full life support, even after there were no longer signs of brain function. "She's too young. This is just pneumonia. I don't understand," family members lamented, but finally, at the recommendation of the still-shocked health care team, they decided to withdraw care, and the patient died immediately. The next day, my friend received a call from the hospital with her mother's culture results. *Candida*—a fungus that cannot be cured with traditional broad-spectrum antibiotics. The patient's family and her health care team were left to wonder how different her outcome might have been with adherence to EBP.

Think about when the practice and process breakdown(s) occurred in the situation described in this personal case study and how these could have been avoided or prevented through EBPQI. At what points could the NP have intervened? We challenge you, as a future EBPQI leader, to critically consider how ANP leaders are empowered to uncover care plans that do not align with standards of care.

Future Responsibilities for Advanced Nursing Practice

The most effective drivers of change are nurses—nurses who care; are problem solvers; can reach people where they live, work, or play; and are culturally aware and always learning. Nurse leaders who know how to use evidence in a systematic way to improve problems can do so in many different spaces. For example, nurses are impacting populations as they gain traction in the areas of policy and politics. As of 2023, there are 72 nurses serving as state legislators across 36 U.S. states. This represents a decrease from previous years—down from 97 nurses serving in 39 states in 2013. These nurse legislators include both state representatives and senators, with many serving on health-related and finance committees. Nurse representation in state legislatures remains critical for advocating healthcare reform, nursing workforce issues, and patient care policies, yet there is still room for growth in their political presence (Brusie, 2024). As of 2024, there are currently three nurses serving in the U.S. House of Representatives. These include notable figures such as Lauren Underwood, who represents Illinois' 14th district, and Jennifer Kiggans, who represents Virginia's 2nd district. These nurse representatives bring valuable healthcare experience to legislative decision-making, particularly in areas like healthcare policy, access, and maternal health. No nurses have yet served in the U.S. Senate, which highlights the ongoing need for more representation of healthcare professionals in Congress (Summers, 2022). Congresswoman Lauren Underwood of Illinois has been a vocal champion for improving health disparities related to maternal mortality. The Black Maternal Health Caucus's (n.d.) Momnibus Act includes 13 individual bills that seek investments that address the drivers of health disparities in the

United States. There are many examples of nurses in official governing roles and unofficial volunteer roles in towns and cities nationwide. Two advanced practice nurses founded *Healing Politics*, a campaign school for nurses. Healing Politics' mission, according to the website's home page, is to "inspire, motivate, recruit, and train nurses and midwives to run for elected office up and down the ballot while building a future of civic engagement within the profession." They held their first campaign school in 2023.

WELLNESS IN ACTION: READING

Reading serves as a knowledge gateway, and the science and evolution of reading continues to be widely researched (Petscher et al., 2020). We challenge you, as an adult learner, to continue (or re-engage with) reading regularly. EBPQI requires substantial reading to understand, appraise, and apply the state of the science. We hope that you will be interested not only in scientific literature but in reading for pleasure, that you will solidify your reading habit, and that you will be a reading role model for others. Consider the recommended reading practices, which have enriched our personal and professional lives:

- Plan to buy or borrow books or periodicals that are interesting to you.
- Visit your local library or e-library to explore and access a variety of titles.
- Subscribe to reading sources that pique your interest and curiosity.
- Set a reading goal (e.g., two books per month). This could apply to audiobooks, paperbound books, or a mixture of both.
- Listen to an audiobook while engaging in a physical activity or ride a stationary bike while reading to stimulate physical and mental well-being.
- Host a book or journal club and discuss what you are reading.
- Track the number of books you read for the purpose of accountability and encouragement.

WRAPPING UP

We owe it to the public to ensure proper population care provision. Research, EBP, and QI are all required to support optimal patient and population care. Upon entering your ANP role or specialty, you will likely be called upon to lead EBPQI. The knowledge and skills you are learning now will prepare you for this important challenge. Our patients, communities, and the nursing profession are counting on you to prepare for this vital task. It is critical that you learn the fundamentals of the different paradigms (research, EBP, and QI) so that you will be equipped to actively lead teams in practice improvement throughout health care settings. It is also important to remember that although this textbook employs a competency-based approach, the underlying caring practice of nursing, which has been a part of our rich discipline history, should be emphasized throughout holistic health care leadership. Competency and caring by ANP leaders are needed to ensure optimal health care outcomes.

REFLECTION QUESTIONS

1. As a future EBPQI leader, how can you ensure that patients are kept at the center of care?
2. After you complete your advanced graduate nursing program, how will you continue to grow and learn more about EBPQI?
3. How does a fundamental understanding of research and EBPQI influence your vocational pursuit?

REFERENCES

American Academy of Pediatrics Committee on Infectious Diseases, & Committee on Fetus and Newborn (2017). Elimination of Perinatal Hepatitis B: Providing the First Vaccine Dose Within 24 Hours of Birth. *Pediatrics, 140*(3), e20171870. https://doi.org/10.1542/peds.2017-1870

American Association of Colleges of Nursing. (2021). *The essentials: Core competencies for professional nursing education.* https://www.aacnnursing.org/AACN-Essentials

Bates, D. W., Levine, D.M., Salmasian, H., Syrowatka, A., Shahian, D. M., Lipsitz, S.,Zebrowski, J. P., Myers, L. C., Logan, M. S., Roy, C. G., lannaccone, C., Frits M. L., Volk, L. A., Dulgarian, S., Amato, M. G., Edrees, H. H., Sato, L., Folcarelli, P., Einbinder, J. S., Reynolds, M. E., &ort, E. (2023). The safety of inpatient health care. *New England Journal of Medicine, 388*, 142–153. https://doi.org/10.1056/NEJMsa2206117

Best, M., & Neuhauser, D. (2004). Ignaz Semmelweis and the birth of infection control. *Quality & Safety in Health Care, 13*(3), 233–234. https://doi.org/10.1136/qshc.2004.010918

Brusie, C. (2024). Nurses in politics: Leaders who started at the bedside. https://nurse.org/news/nurses-in-politics

Centers for Disease Control and Prevention. Hospital Sepsis Program Core Elements. Atlanta, GA: US Department of Health and Human Services. https://www.cdc.gov/sepsis/hcp/core-elements/

Damschroder, L. J., Aron, D. C., Keith, R. E., Kirsh, S. R., Alexander, J. A., & Lowery, J. C. (2009). Fostering implementation of health services research findings into practice: A consolidated framework for advancing implementation science. *Implementation Science, 4*, 50. https://doi.org/10.1186/1748-5908-4-50

Dunlap, J., Waldrop, J. B., & Mainous, R. O. (2024). Differentiation and integration of research, evidence-based practice, and quality improvement. *Journal of Nursing Education.* https://doi.org/10.3928/01484834-20240514-01

Dusin, J., Melanson, A., & Mische-Lawson, L. (2023). Evidence-based practice models and frameworks in the health care setting: A scoping review. *BMJ Open, 13*(5), e071188. https://doi.org/10.1136/bmjopen-2022-071188

Fineout-Overholt, E., Melnyk, B. M., & Schultz, A. (2005). Transforming health care from the inside out: Advancing evidence-based practice in the 21st century. *Journal of Professional Nursing: Official Journal of the American Association of Colleges of Nursing, 21*(6), 335–344. https://doi.org/10.1016/j.profnurs.2005.10.005

Grys, C. A. (2022). Evidence-based practice, quality improvement, and research: A visual model. *Nursing, 52*(11), 47–49. https://doi.org/10.1097/01.NURSE.0000889812.89287.45

Hempel, S., Bolshakova, M., Turner, B. J., Dinalo, J., Rose, D., Motala, A., Fu, N., Clemesha, C. G., Rubenstein, L., & Stockdale, S. (2022). Evidence-based quality improvement: A scoping review of the literature. *Journal of General Internal Medicine, 37*(16), 4257–4267. https://doi.org/10.1007/s11606-022-07602-5

Institute of Medicine & Committee on Quality of Health Care in America. (2021). *Crossing the quality chasm: A new health system for the 21st century.* National Academies Press. https://doi.org/10.17226/10027

Institute of Medicine's Committee on Quality of Health Care in America. (2000). *To err is human: Building a safer health system* (L. T. Kohn, J. M. Corrigan, & M. S. Donaldson, Eds.). National Academies Press. http://www.ncbi.nlm.nih.gov/books/NBK225182/

Iowa Model Collaborative, Buckwalter, K. C., Cullen, L., Hanrahan, K., Kleiber, C., McCarthy, A. M., Rakel, B., Steelman, V., Tripp-Reimer, T., & Tucker, S. (2017). Iowa model of evidence-based practice: Revisions and validation: Iowa model-revised. *Worldviews on Evidence-Based Nursing, 14*(3), 175–182. https://doi.org/10.1111/wvn.12223

Johns Hopkins Medicine, Center for Evidenced-Based Practice. (n.d.). *A problem-solving approach to clinical decision making.* https://www.hopkinsmedicine.org/evidence-based-practice

Khan, S., Chambers, D., & Neta, G. (2021). Revisiting time to translation: Implementation of evidence-based practices (EBPs) in cancer control. *Cancer Causes & Control, 32*(3), 221–230. https://doi.org/10.1007/s10552-020-01376-z

Langley, G. J., Moen, R. D., Nolan, K. M., Nolan, T. W., Norman, C. L., & Provost, L. P. (2009). *The improvement guide: A practical approach to enhancing organizational performance* (2nd ed.). Jossey-Bass.

Levin, R. F., Keefer, J. M., Marren, J., Vetter, M., Lauder, B., & Sobolewski, S. (2010). Evidence-Based Practice Improvement: Merging 2 Paradigms. *Journal of Nursing Care Quality, 25*(2), 117–126. https://doi.org/10.1097/NCQ.0b013e3181b5f19f

Mackey, A., & Bassendowski, S. (2017). The history of evidence-based practice in nursing education and practice. *Journal of Professional Nursing, 33*(1), 51–55. https://doi.org/10.1016/j.profnurs.2016.05.009

Melnyk, B. M., Fineout-Overholt, E., Giggleman, M., & Choy, K. (2017). A test of the ARCC© model improves implementation of evidence-based practice, health care culture, and patient outcomes. *Worldviews on Evidence-Based Nursing, 14*(1), 5–9. https://doi.org/10.1111/wvn.12188

Melnyk, B. M., Gallagher-Ford, L., Long, L. E., & Fineout-Overholt, E. (2014). The establishment of evidence-based practice competencies for practicing registered nurses and advanced practice nurses in real-world clinical settings: Proficiencies to improve health care quality, reliability, patient outcomes, and costs. *Worldviews on Evidence-Based Nursing, 11*(1), 5–15. https://doi.org/10.1111/wvn.12021

Melnyk, B. M., Gallagher-Ford, L., Zellefrow, C., Tucker, S., Thomas, B., Sinnott, L. T., & Tan, A. (2018). The first U.S. study on nurses' evidence-based practice competencies indicates major deficits that threaten health care quality, safety, and patient outcomes. *Worldviews on Evidence-Based Nursing, 15*(1), 16–25. https://doi.org/10.1111/wvn.12269

Morris, Z. S., Wooding, S., & Grant, J. (2011). The answer is 17 years, what is the question: Understanding time lags in translational research. *Journal of the Royal Society of Medicine, 104*(12), 510–520. https://doi.org/10.1258/jrsm.2011.110180

National Academies of Sciences, Engineering, and Medicine. (2021). *The future of nursing 2020–2030: Charting a path to achieve health equity.* National Academies Press. https://doi.org/10.17226/25982

Nightingale, F. (1859). *Notes on nursing: What it is, and what it is not.* Harrison, 59, Pall Mall, bookseller to the Queen.

Nilsen, P. (2015). Making sense of implementation theories, models and frameworks. *Implementation Science, 10*(1), 53. https://doi.org/10.1186/s13012-015-0242-0

Nilsen, P., Seing, I., Ericsson, C., Birken, S. A., & Schildmeijer, K. (2020). Characteristics of successful changes in health care organizations: An interview study with physicians,

registered nurses and assistant nurses. *BMC Health Services Research, 20*(1), 147. https://doi.org/10.1186/s12913-020-4999-8
Petscher, Y., Cabell, S. Q., Catts, H. W., Compton, D. L., Foorman, B. R., Hart, S. A., Lonigan, C. J., Phillips, B. M., Schatschneider, C., Steacy, L. M., Terry, N. P., & Wagner, R. K. (2020). How the science of reading informs 21st-century education. *Reading Research Quarterly, 55*(1), S267–S282. https://doi.org/10.1002/rrq.352
Rosswurm, M. A., & Larrabee, J. H. (1999). A model for change to evidence-based practice. *Image--the journal of nursing scholarship, 31*(4), 317–322. https://doi.org/10.1111/j.1547-5069.1999.tb00510.x
Ruzafa-Martinez, M., García-González, J., Morales-Asencio, J. M., Leal-Costa, C., Hernández-Méndez, S., Hernández-López, M. J., Albarracín-Olmedo, J., & Ramos-Morcillo, A. J. (2023). Consequences of the Covid-19 pandemic on complex multimorbid elderly: Follow-up of a community-based cohort. SAMAC3 study. *Journal of Nursing Scholarship, 55*(4), 792–804. https://doi.org/10.1111/jnu.12860
Saunders, H., Gallagher-Ford, L., Kvist, T., & Vehviläinen-Julkunen, K. (2019). Practicing health care professionals' evidence-based practice competencies: An overview of systematic reviews. *Worldviews on Evidence-Based Nursing, 16*(3), 176–185. https://doi.org/10.1111/wvn.12363
Stevens, K. (2015). *Stevens star model of knowledge transformation.* https://www.uthscsa.edu/sites/default/files/2018/aaa_star_model_single_ppt_1.pdf
Summers, L. (2022). Is there a nurse in the house? Or the senate? *American Nurse,* https://www.myamericannurse.com/is-there-a-nurse-in-the-house-or-the-senate
Titler, M. G., Kleiber, C., Steelman, V. J., Rakel, B. A., Budreau, G., Everett, L. Q., Buckwalter, K. C., Tripp-Reimer, T., & Goode, C. J. (2001). The Iowa model of evidence-based practice to promote quality care. *Critical Care Nursing Clinics of North America, 13*(4), 497–509.
U.S. House of Representatives, Black Maternal Health Caucus. (n.d.). *The Momnibus Act.* https://blackmaternalhealthcaucus-underwood.house.gov/Momnibus
Visintainer, M. A. (1986). The nature of knowledge and theory in nursing. *Image: The Journal of Nursing Scholarship, 18*(2), 32–38. https://doi.org/10.1111/j.1547-5069.1986.tb00539.x
Waldrop, J. & Jennings Dunlap, J. (2024). The mountain model for evidence-based practice quality improvement initiatives. *The American Journal of Nursing, 124*(5), 31–37.

IMAGE CREDITS

Fig. 1.1: Jayne Jennings Dunlap and Julee Briscoe Waldrop, *Introduction to Evidence-Based Practice and Quality Improvement for Professional Nursing Practice: A Competency Based Approach*, p. 6. Copyright © 2024 by Cognella, Inc. Reprinted with permission.
Fig. 1.2: Source: https://implementation.fpg.unc.edu/wp-content/uploads/Active-Implementation-Overview.pdf.
Fig. 1.3: Crystal A. Grys, "Evidence-Based Practice, Quality Improvement, and Research: A Visual Model," *Nursing*, vol. 52, no. 11. Copyright © 2022 by Wolters Kluwer Health.
Fig. 1.4: Julee Waldrop and Jayne Jennings Dunlap, "Setting the Stage for Clear Understanding of Research, Evidence-Based Practice, and Quality Improvement," *Introduction to Evidence-Based Practice and Quality Improvement for Professional Nursing Practice: A Competency Based Approach,* p. 12. Copyright © 2024 by Cognella, Inc. Reprinted with permission.
Fig. 1.5: Julee Waldrop and Jayne Jennings Dunlap, "Setting the Stage for Clear Understanding of Research, Evidence-Based Practice, and Quality Improvement," *Introduction to Evidence-Based Practice and Quality Improvement for Professional Nursing Practice: A Competency Based Approach,* p. 15. Copyright © 2024 by Cognella, Inc. Reprinted with permission.

CHAPTER 2

Advancing Quality and Safety

Bradi B. Granger, Staci S. Reynolds, and Julee Briscoe Waldrop

KEY CONCEPTS

Institute of Medicine (IOM) landmark publications

Quintuple aim

National safety goals

Quality improvement

Root cause analysis

Key dimensions of health care quality (STEEEP)

System levels of quality context (micro, meso, macro)

Just culture

Identifying health care problems

LEARNING OBJECTIVES

1. Explore the background of health care quality and safety.
2. Identify the nurse leader's role in ensuring quality and safety in advanced practice.
3. Discuss the impacts of just culture and event reporting in health care.

"Quality is not an act [or an episode], it is a habit."

—Aristotle

Introduction

What is quality in health care, and how do we recognize it? The purpose of this chapter is to introduce you to the background and underlying principles of health care quality, particularly in regard to safety. The success and sustainability of quality improvement in health care depend on the quality and safety evidenced at three levels: (a) the *micro* level, which includes the immediate clinical team; (b) the *meso* level, which includes the organization (e.g., the entire hospital); and (c) the *macro* level, which includes the broader sociopolitical context within which care is delivered. As a nurse with an advanced degree, you can impact quality at all three levels! It is important that you understand how your practice as well as various contextual factors impact the quality and safety of patient care at each level. For example, as a nursing leader on a clinical unit (i.e., at the micro level), your influence on the unit's culture and readiness to implement EBPs can play a major role in bringing about improvements. Similarly, as a leader at the meso level, your influence on hospital-based policies, the growth of the organization, and the range of provided services can impact the ability to improve care. Finally, at the macro level, which may include many hospitals, communities, or payment systems across locations, your work and involvement with such factors as environmental pressures, demography of the populations served, or the accessibility of locations of affiliated hospitals and clinics (e.g., in urban versus rural areas) can significantly impact the quality of health care (Fulop & Robert, 2015). Health care quality can be improved not only in hospital settings but in outpatient settings such as clinics, community health centers, and public health departments. Let's consider an example of using advanced nursing practice to improve the quality and safety of care in a busy neuroscience intensive care unit (ICU; see Box 2.1).

BOX 2.1: PROGRESSIVE MOBILITY

Nurse practitioner (NP) Jarvis knows that immobility in the ICU can lead to preventable patient harm such as pressure injuries, atelectasis, pneumonia, and decline in physical function, as well as longer hospital stays. She has noticed that although an increasing number of patients are becoming debilitated due to immobility, the multidisciplinary team does not discuss patient mobility status during bedside rounds. NP Jarvis considers this issue with her colleagues, including another advanced practice nurse who is a clinical nurse specialist (CNS), and together they develop and initiate (a) an early mobility screening tool and (b) a protocol that shows the roles and responsibilities of multidisciplinary team members related to providing early mobility care. Consequently, a "mobility" section is added to the provider note template in the electronic health record, which allows providers to document patient-specific barriers to mobility along with a daily mobility plan of care. An online educational module is developed to educate all staff members on the new process. NP Jarvis, the CNS, and the nursing unit manager collaborate to develop a unit-based gaming competition in which staff who consistently perform early mobility practices are entered in a raffle to win prizes and acknowledged during the unit's daily huddle. This comprehensive and collaborative approach enables NP Jarvis to lead an EBPQI initiative that increases mobility and fosters a culture of safety and collaboration within the ICU (Jarvis et al., 2023).

As a nurse in an advanced leadership role, you are well positioned to understand the measurement and foundational evidence that supports contemporary quality measures in the United States and abroad. Not surprisingly, the goals for health care quality are universal and have been established or adopted by the National Academy of Medicine (formerly the Institute of Medicine [IOM]) and the World Health Organization (WHO). If you are knowledgeable about standards of care quality and how they are measured, you will be able to identify substandard practices in need of improvement. Chapter 9 explores measurement methodologies and step-by-step strategies, and Chapter 11 discusses how to create an evaluation plan to determine the impact of EBPQI initiatives in clinical practice. In this chapter, we address several foundational questions about quality, including the following:

- What is health care quality?
- How is health care quality measured?
- What resources are available to help clinicians provide quality health care?
- What are the barriers to providing evidence-based quality health care?
- How do we identify quality deficits?

Note that Chapter 9 discusses how to prioritize and improve quality deficits identified in health care.

What Is Health Care Quality?

Background of Health Care Quality

In recent decades, there have been many contributions to health care quality improvement and safety in the United States. These efforts have resulted in (a) the establishment of numerous organizations, government agencies, and private foundations devoted to driving the national quality agenda and (b) the production and implementation of a plethora of new terms, guidelines, and quality metrics (which may seem confusing and unclear). A bit of background should help to clarify when and why these initiatives came about.

The roots of health care quality and safety can be traced back to the 1800s (Figure 2.1), when Florence Nightingale (1863) collected and reported data that identified an association between poor hospital conditions and high rates of mortality among soldiers in the Crimean War. Nightingale's findings helped her improve the quality-of-care provision through (what we now know as) EBPs such as frequent handwashing, exposure to natural light, clean drinking water, and other basic sanitation measures (Nightingale, 1985).

In the early 1900s, Ernest Codman, a surgeon at Massachusetts General Hospital, tracked surgical patients and documented their outcomes to determine the cause of complications, including deficits in surgeon proficiency or the hospital's efficiency (Altan et al., 2022). Codman's advocacy for tracing poor surgical outcomes to their source was not always popular with his fellow practitioners or hospital administrators, but his work to improve health care quality assurance and control across levels is now credited for the standardization of surgical practices and the eventual development of The Joint Commission in 1951 (Chun & Bafford, 2014).

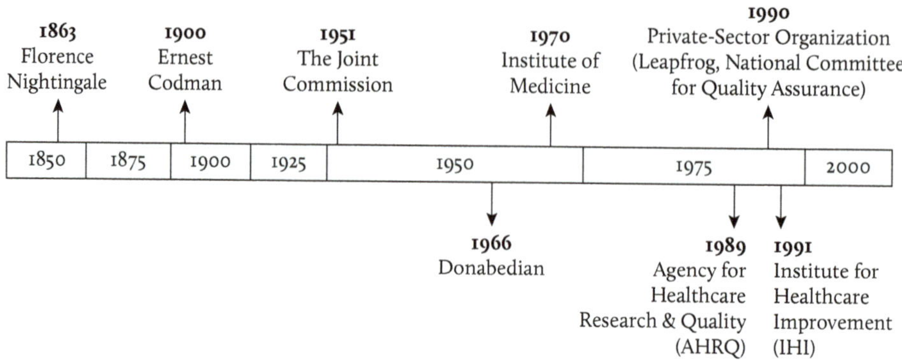

FIGURE 2.1 Timeline of seminal events in the history of health care quality.

In 1966, Avedis Donabedian published "Evaluating the Quality of Medical Care," which added elements of structure, process, and outcomes to the evaluation of quality of care (Glickman et al., 2007). Shortly thereafter, the IOM launched seminal work focused on quality and safety. In 1989, the Agency for Healthcare Research and Quality (AHRQ) was created in response to reports of misuse and overuse of treatments, as well as variations in practice. In 1991, Dr. Donald Berwick (1991a) founded the Institute for Healthcare Improvement (IHI), a repository of resources that provide guidance to clinicians who conduct QI initiatives (Berwick, 1991b). A nonprofit organization called The Leapfrog Group was founded in 1998 by a group of independent business leaders in response to the increasing cost and poor quality of health care; this organization aims to give consumers a stronger voice to support positive change within the U.S. health care system, champion transparency in health care, and collect evidence to promote informed consumer choices.

Two landmark reports highlighted serious issues in U.S. health care and provided a profound continued impetus for change. The IOM's Committee on Quality of Health Care in America published the transformative report *To Err Is Human: Building a Safer Health System* in 2000, followed by *Crossing the Quality Chasm: A New Health System for the 21st Century* in 2001; these reports noted that medical errors were causing up to 98,000 deaths annually. As the need for improved health care quality gained a spotlight, health care institutions, organizations, and the government joined efforts to improve the quality of patient care, including through reimbursement and payment models based on high-quality care delivery (Porter, 2009).

Definition of Health Care Quality

Many organizations in the United States focus on health care quality, yet each has a slightly different definition of quality. For instance, AHRQ describes the foundation of quality health care as doing the right thing at the right time, in the right way for the right person, with the best possible results. Quality health care often involves striking a balance between the avoidance of health care overuse (e.g., providing unnecessary tests, the indiscriminate use of antibiotics), underuse (e.g., failure to provide needed screenings or procedures), or misuse (e.g., prescribing multiple drugs despite dangerous interactions). The WHO defines quality of care as the degree to which health services for individuals and populations increase the likelihood of desired health outcomes. In a concept analysis of health care quality, including a review of 42 articles, Allen-Duck et al. (2017) defined health care quality as "the provision of effective and safe care, reflected in a culture of excellence, resulting in the attainment of optimal or desired outcomes" (p. 381).

The Health Care Quality Framework

The six domains of health care quality, a framework first published by the IOM in 2001, continues to drive the national quality agenda across all public and private sectors (IOM's Committee on Quality of Health Care in America, 2001). The six domains (safety, timeliness, effectiveness, efficiency, equity, and patient centeredness) comprise the acronym STEEEP. There is no established hierarchy among the domains, nor is their importance linear; in fact, the volume of evidence, metrics, measures, and indicators for each domain is highly variable. In 2022, the model was revised to depict person centeredness as a ring encompassing all health care quality (see Figure 2.2). Also in 2022, the impact of the *environment* on health was added to the model, creating a seventh domain and a fourth "E" in the acronym to ensure an eco-friendly focus on care (Nunday et al., 2022)

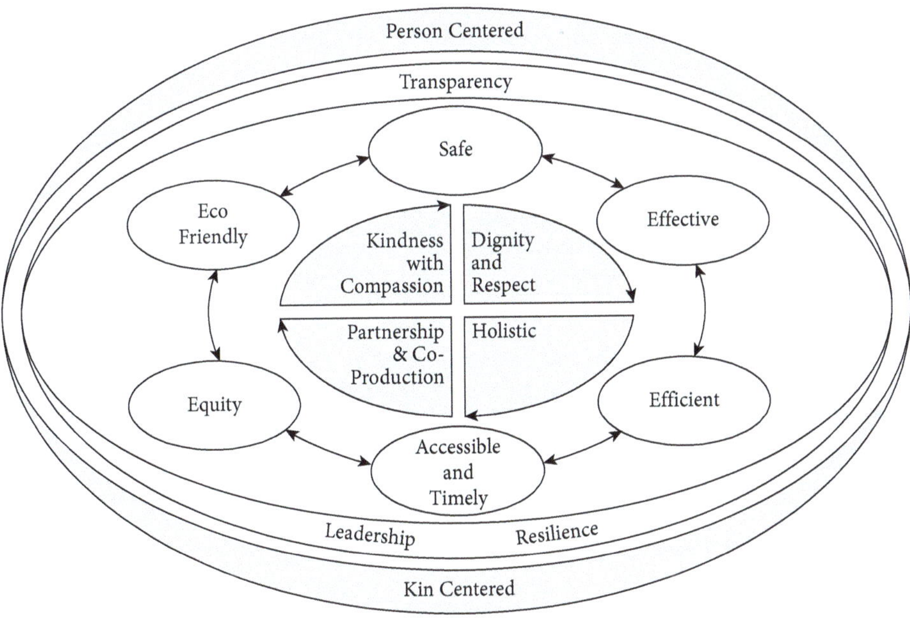

FIGURE 2.2 Seven domains of health care quality.

TABLE 2.1 STEEEEP Definitions and Examples

Domain	Definition	Example of Domain in ANP
Safe	Avoiding harm to patients from the care that is intended to help them	A nurse midwife provides instruction in complementary pain management practices during labor to decrease the use of medications that might impact the infant at birth
Timely	Reducing wait times, and possibly harmful delays, for persons who are receiving or providing care	A clinic manager with an advanced degree develops a process to improve patient flow between clinic, lab, and the bronchoscopy suite
Effective	Providing appropriate services based on scientific knowledge only to patients who may benefit from them (avoiding underuse and misuse, respectively)	A nurse practitioner safely prescribes opioids to a patient who was in a motorcycle accident by adhering to state and national guidelines
Efficient	Avoiding waste, including waste of equipment, supplies, ideas, and energy	A certified registered nurse anesthetist reduces waste in the operating room by using smaller vials of propofol for surgical cases
Equitable	Providing care that does not vary in quality because of personal characteristics such as gender, ethnicity, geographic location, or socioeconomic status	An informaticist develops clinical decision support tools within the electronic health record to guide clinicians in ordering evidence-based tests for all patients
Eco-friendly	Maintaining a hospital environment that minimizes risks to patients and local communities (e.g., addressing energy use and waste disposal management)	A clinical nurse specialist leads a program to reduce the amount of nonbiohazard waste put into the red trash can, which is only meant for biohazard waste
Patient-centered	Providing care that is respectful of and responsive to individual patient preferences, needs, and values and ensuring that patient values guide all clinical decisions	A nurse educator with an advanced degree provides tailored, individualized education to patients diagnosed with hematologic malignancies prior to treatment

(see Table 2.1). Most recently, the national agenda has shifted toward identifying and addressing inequities in health care delivery and accessibility; this shift will likely impact priorities and funding, and (one hopes) will result in scientific development and clinical practice to ensure the equity of quality care.

The Quintuple Aim

Berwick et al. (2008) defined a framework for high-quality care known as the triple aim: (a) improving the *individual experience* of health care, (b) improving the *health of the populations*, and (c) reducing the *per capita costs* of health care. A fourth aim, achieving *meaning in work*, was eventually included, so the framework became known as the quadruple aim (Bodenheimer & Sinsky, 2014). In 2021, achieving *health equity* was added as a fifth aim (Nunday et al., 2022). The quintuple aim requires all health care team members to be highly effective and engaged, provide equitable care, and have a sense of meaning and accomplishment in their contributions. The editors have added wellness boxes at the end of each chapter because they strongly believe in clinician well-being!

Health Equity

In 2021, the National Academies of Science (NAS, 2021) published its third report in a series to guide nursing as a profession for the next 10 years. *The Future of Nursing 2020–2030: Charting a Path to Achieve Health Equity* challenges nurses to accept responsibility for addressing the huge inequities in our health care system, particularly those related to social determinants of health (SDoH). Social determinants of health are "conditions in the environments in which people are born, live, learn, work, play, worship, and age [which] affect a wide range of health, functioning, and quality-of-life outcomes and risks." Only 20% of health is determined by the provision of health care in a hospital setting or through interactions with health care personnel in a clinic or community. A broader 80% of health is determined by conditions in and features of the social environment, including economic stability, the physical environment, education, nutrition, support systems, and accessibility of health services (see Figure 2.3).

Health disparities are associated with SDoH and can be important indicators of equity. Health equity and health disparities are closely related but not causal. Health disparities are differences in health or key determinants of health (e.g., education, safe housing, and freedom from discrimination) that adversely

Economic Stability	Neighborhood and Physical Environment	Education	Food	Community and Social Context	Health Care System
Employment Income Expenses Debt Medical bills Support	Housing Transportation Safety Parks Playgrounds Walkability Zip code/ geography	Literacy Language Early childhood education Vocational training Higher education	Hunger Access to healthy options	Social integration Support systems Community engagement Discrimination Stress	Health coverage Provider availability Provider linguistic and cultural competency Quality of care

Health Outcomes
Mortality, Morbidity, Life expectancy, Health care expenditures, Health status, Functional limitations

FIGURE 2.3 SDoH and related health outcomes.

affect marginalized or excluded groups. According to the National Center for Chronic Disease Prevention and Health Promotion, health equity is achieved when every person has the opportunity to attain his or her full potential, and no one is disadvantaged from achieving this potential because of social position or other socially determined circumstances (CDC, n.d,).

It is important to reflect on how SDoH impact health equity for the patients or populations to whom you provide care; when a presenting health problem is strongly associated with SDoH, simply treating its symptoms will not address (and may perpetuate) the root causes of the problem. You can lead work that addresses complex social problems on a broader scale as a nurse with an advanced degree than as a direct care nurse. Remember that your attitudes, beliefs, and behaviors impact everyone to whom and with whom you provide care. With this in mind, let's consider evidence-based strategies for a sample case (Box 2.2).

BOX 2.2: CASE STUDY

Michael is a 65-year-old Black male with end-stage renal disease. He is currently on hemodialysis and is treated at the dialysis clinic 3 days weekly. Due to his disability and frequent dialysis visits, Michael is unable to work. He lives in an apartment by himself and is sometimes late with his rent. Given the rising cost of food, Michael is unable to purchase the healthy food he needs and typically eats cheeseburgers from a local fast-food restaurant. The neighbor who has been driving him to his dialysis visits recently mentioned that they will soon be moving to another state in order to be closer to their grandchildren. Michael worries about how he will get to his dialysis appointments without his neighbor's assistance.

We are confident that you identified several SDoH issues in this case, but let's discuss an obvious one: limited access to health care. After Michael's neighbor moves, he may lack transportation and financial resources to get to the dialysis clinic. An inability to receive hemodialysis can lead to multiple adverse events such as hyperkalemia, arrhythmia, myocardial infarction, or death.

Limited access to health care is a sweeping problem, but you can commit to addressing it by seeking related evidence and potential solutions for your patient(s). Chapter 3 will show you how to begin. As a leader in advanced nursing practice, perhaps you could implement a tool such as the Core 5 Determinants of Health Screening Tool within your clinic to screen patients for various SDoH and provide those in need with community resources (e.g., bus passes), thereby improving the equity and quality of their care. Remember, equitable care is one of the STEEEEP domains of health care quality!

Environment

SDoH intersect with the environment. The negative effects of climate change often have the greatest impact on populations who have contributed the least to the problem. For example, you have probably heard news reports about older people dying in heat waves. Over the past 20 years, temperature change has led to a 53.7% increase in health-related deaths in people over 65 years of age (Watts et al., 2021). What can be done about this problem? How can systems be changed to help prevent such deaths?

As you might guess, nurses were early advocates of improving the environment to improve health. Florence Nightingale published work on the topic of ventilation and light in 1859, and in 1986, the International Council of Nurses (2013) released its first position statement urging nurses to actively address environmental issues. The mission of the Alliance of Nurses for Health Environments is to promote an "understanding that optimal health requires good nutrition, adequate mobility, a healthy environment, and social support. Nurse members are committed to taking evidence-based action to improve the health of themselves and others while also healing the planet" (Nurses Drawdown, n.d., para. 2). By engaging in responsible personal practice (see Wellness Box), you can inspire others. Working together, nurses can improve the problems of climate change, but it will take all of us to make a difference.

Affordable Care Act

In 2010, President Barack Obama signed the Affordable Care Act (ACA) with the intent of modernizing the U.S. health care system. In 2011, the Centers for Medicare and Medicaid Services (CMS) released the final rules for accountable care organizations (ACOs), which were established to guide health care providers and hospitals toward more coordinated, higher quality, patient-centered care. Health care quality and safety issues continue to be researched and addressed as the need for improvement in various areas, or domains, of care are recognized.

How Is Health Care Quality Measured?

Quality is measured through measurable key quality indicators. Many key quality indicators are defined and measured by external organizations, and some are defined and measured internally within a health care system. Examples of quality indicators that are defined and measured by external organizations include those that impact (a) quality and patient safety, such as length of stay, health care–associated infections (HAIs), falls, pressure injuries, or readmission rates; (b) patients' experiences of or satisfaction with their health care; and (3) the people and environments within health care organizations, such as staff turnover or the percentage of employees with specialty certification or a specific degree (e.g., initiatives for direct care nurses to obtain a bachelor of science in nursing (BSN), percentage of advanced practice nurses who enter practice with a Doctor of Nursing Practice (DNP). Many measurements by external organizations have financial implications. For example, theoretically, a patient should not develop an HAI while hospitalized if EBPs are followed; therefore, if this circumstance occurs, the hospital may not receive reimbursement from CMS for care related to the infection. Quality indicators that have financial implications are generally given high priority by health care systems. Other quality indicators may be defined and measured internally, such as a finance and growth domain, including the percentage of agency or travel nurses used; the volume of surgical procedures; or the volume of admissions and discharges.

Contemporary oversight of quality in health care is organized by the federal executive branch of government under the Department of Health and Human Services (DHHS; Figure 2.4). The DHHS includes divisions that are responsible for various aspects of health care quality, education, regulation, and funding (see Table 2.2). The overarching goal of the DHHS and its operating divisions

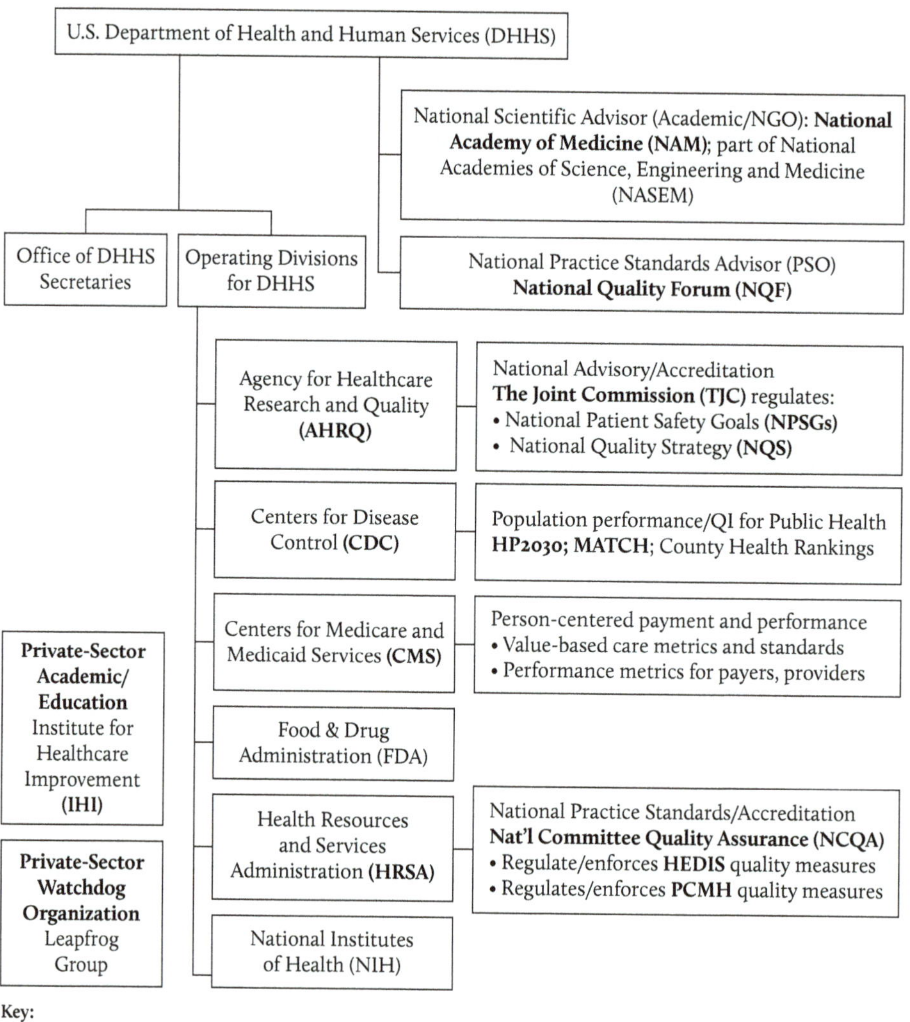

FIGURE 2.4 Organizational hierarchy for creation, regulation, and enforcement of quality. NPSG: national patient safety goals; HEDIS: Health care Effectiveness Data and Information Set; PCMH: patient-centered medical home.

is to provide the highest quality of care to patients and their families across all settings. Information about individual agencies can be found on their websites. Let's review several of the external organizations in the United States that define and measure the quality indicators used in health systems.

TABLE 2.2 DHHS Quality Oversight Agencies and Organizations

Agency or Organization	Acronym	Purpose and Website
Department of Health and Human Services	DHHS	Oversees the functions, roles, responsibilities, and reporting relationships of 12 federal operating divisions, six of which are directly responsible for various aspects of health care quality, education, regulation, and funding https://www.hhs.gov/
National Academy of Medicine	NAM	Nonprofit, nongovernmental organization that generates evidence-based recommendations, reports on key issues impacting health, and develops *The Future of Nursing Reports*, which provide direction for the nursing workforce https://nam.edu/
National Quality Forum	NQF	Not-for-profit organization that works to catalyze improvements in health care through NQF-selected measures and standards that enhance value, safety, and patient outcomes https://www.qualityforum.org/
Agency for Healthcare Research and Quality	AHRQ	Federal agency charged with improving the safety and quality of health care for all Americans; resources include the Comprehensive Unit-Based Safety Program (CUSP) method (https://www.ahrq.gov/hai/cusp/index.html) and TeamSTEPPS® (a curriculum that helps optimize patient outcomes by improving communication and teamwork among all health care members) https://www.ahrq.gov/
The Joint Commission	TJC	Not-for-profit organization that establishes quality standards, evaluates performance of individual health care organizations, and provides education to organizations to support continuous quality improvement; TJC accreditation is a DHHS requirement for financial reimbursement of CMS funding. TJC-implemented national patient safety goals (NPSG) include the following: ▪ Identify patients correctly. ▪ Prevent infection. ▪ Improve staff communication. ▪ Identify patient safety risks. ▪ Prevent mistakes in surgery. ▪ Use medicines safely. ▪ Use alarms safely. https://www.jointcommission.org

(*Continued*)

TABLE 2.2 *(Continued)*

Agency or Organization	Acronym	Purpose and Website
Centers for Disease Control and Prevention	CDC	The nation's leading science-based organization dedicated to protecting the public's health; nurses have access to useful resources through the CDC's website https://www.cdc.gov/
Centers for Medicare and Medicaid Services	CMS	Federal agency that provides health coverage to more than 160 million people through Medicare, Medicaid, the Children's Health Insurance Program, and the Health Insurance Marketplace; CMS works in partnership with the entire health care community to improve quality, equity, and outcomes in the health care system https://www.cms.gov/
Health Resources and Services Administration	HRSA	Oversees quality and accreditation for programs that serve the underserved (e.g., by providing discounts on prescription drugs to safety net providers or facilitating organ, bone marrow, and cord blood transplantation for those unable to access these types of specialty care) https://www.hrsa.gov/
National Committee Quality Assurance	NCQA	Develops and enforces quality standards such as the Healthcare Effectiveness Data and Information Set (HEDIS), which is a comprehensive set of performance measures designed to provide purchasers and consumers with information needed for reliable comparison of health plan performance https://www.ncqa.org/
Institute for Health Care Improvement	IHI	Nonprofit organization that improves health care worldwide by providing tools and resources through training sessions, conferences, and advisory services https://www.ihi.org/
Leapfrog Group	Leapfrog	Organization that supports informed health care decisions and promotes high-value care through transparency of health care data; the Leapfrog Hospital Safety Grade is a composite score made up of 22 evidence-based measures of patient safety https://www.leapfroggroup.org/

The Joint Commission

TJC defines many of the quality indicators used in U.S. hospitals. Every few years, TJC visits hospitals to ensure that standards and quality protocols are being followed. It has identified several NPSGs that hospitals must follow, including identifying patients correctly (e.g., ensuring that the correct patient receives a surgical procedure or treatment), using alarms and medications safely, and preventing mistakes in surgery (other NPSGs can be found in Table 2.2). Additionally, health care systems and hospitals can seek specialty designations through TJC. For example, a neuroscience division can become designated as a comprehensive stroke center, showing that they follow best practices related to the care of patients recovering from stroke. Nurses with advanced degrees are key players in TJC site visits because they can discuss and demonstrate how evidence-based standards are being followed, as well as role-model best practices and mentor staff who may feel intimidated by TJC site visits.

National Healthcare Safety Network

The National Healthcare Safety Network (NHSN), part of the CDC, is the nation's most widely used tracking system for HAIs. There are several infections that hospitals track per NHSN's definitions, including central line-associated bloodstream infections (CLABSI), catheter-associated urinary tract infections (CAUTI), surgical site infections (SSI), ventilator-associated events (VAE), and *Clostridioides difficile* (*C. diff*). These infections cause harm to patients and can have financial implications; as such, they are a high priority for health care systems.

National Database for Nursing Quality Indicators

The National Database for Nursing Quality Indicators, or NDNQI, is an external organization focused on indicators that are impacted by the quality of nursing care (also known as "nurse-sensitive outcomes"). This database provides quarterly and annual benchmark reporting on indicators such as falls, pain assessment, pressure injuries, restraint prevalence, and infections. The data are benchmarked to similar hospitals and units; for example, a surgical stepdown unit would be provided comparison data from other surgical stepdown units, or a large academic medical center would be provided comparison data from other large academic medical centers (Montalvo, 2007).

Patient and Employee Satisfaction

Most of the organizations we have described focus on quality and patient safety indicators. HCAHPS, or the Hospital Consumer Assessment of Healthcare Providers and Systems, is a survey developed by the CMS and AHRQ to measure patients' satisfaction and perspectives on the quality of health care; an organization's reimbursement by the CMS is tied to how well its survey scores reflect high patient satisfaction. There are survey tools for inpatient (hospital) and outpatient experiences. Here are some examples of questions on the inpatient HCAHPS survey:

- How often did you get help as soon as you wanted it after hitting the call button?
- How often did you get help going to the bathroom?
- How often did nurses explain things in a way you could understand?

Questions on the HCAHPS are designed to provide measurements in several domains: care received from nurses and physicians, experiences in the hospital, the hospital environment (e.g., cleanliness, level of noise), and care when discharged from the hospital. Another patient satisfaction survey, referred to as the "Press Ganey" after the company that developed it (www.pressganey.com/), is used by many hospitals and health care organizations to identify areas for improvement.

Another metric that can indirectly impact patient quality and safety is health care staff satisfaction. Evidence has demonstrated that satisfied employees are more likely to stay at their current place of employment (Pressley & Garside, 2023). Successful employee retention can save an organization the expense of hiring and training new staff. To determine how employees feel about their employment, organizations often request that they complete "climate surveys" that include questions about issues such as safety, diversity, equity, inclusion, and belonging. The results from these surveys can be used to identify areas for improvement.

Our overview of how quality is measured by common external organizations is by no means an exhaustive list. As an advanced nursing practice leader, you will be responsible for understanding these metrics, how they are measured, and how your unit/clinic/area is performing in terms of quality indicators. Further on in this chapter, we discuss how to identify potential opportunities for improvement related to these indicators.

What Resources Do Clinicians Have to Provide Quality Care?

There are many resources available that outline EBPs to reduce variation in practice and improve the quality and safety of care; these include clinical practice guidelines, resources from national organizations such as the CDC, EBP bundles, and local hospital policies and procedures. As a leader in ANP, you must ensure that these EBPs in clinical care are always followed precisely. For example, the nurse practitioner leading a heart failure clinic would need to ensure that heart failure guidelines published by the American Heart Association are easily retrievable and followed by all staff in the clinic. Similarly, the CNS serving an inpatient oncology unit might need to educate staff nurses on how to access and search the hospital's online policy database for evidence-based policies and procedures. Many of the external organizations mentioned previously (e.g., IHI, CDC, AHRQ) have online education and resources that are widely available to help clinicians provide quality care.

Professional nursing organizations are engaged in improving the quality and safety of health care. In 2014, the American Academy of Nursing was the first nursing organization to partner with other medical and health care organizations, such as the American Board of Internal Medicine, to encourage conversations about which EBPs in health care should be considered of current value. See Table 2.3 for examples of nursing organizations and nurse-led endeavors focused on improving quality.

TABLE 2.3 Nursing Organizations and Initiatives Focused on Improving Quality in Health Care

Organization	Initiative	Description	For more information
Institute of Pediatric Nursing	Choosing Wisely campaign	Encourages patients and nurses to question health care practices and identify the evidence behind them	https://ipedsnursing.org/choosing-wisely
American Nurses Association	National Alliance for Quality Care (NAQC) Quality and Safety Education for Nurses (QSEN)	NAQC works in tandem with QSEN to advance high-quality, patient-centered health care	https://www.nursingworld.org/practice-policy/naqc/
Registered Nurses Association of Ontario	Best practice guidelines (BPG)	Systematically developed evidence-based recommendations for nursing practice	https://rnao.ca/bpg/guidelines
American Organization of Nursing Leadership (AONL) / American Association of Critical Care Nurses (AACN)	Healthy Work Environment	Has developed nine elements of a healthy work environment that contribute to high-quality and safe patient care (e.g., adequate numbers of qualified nurses present, shared decision making at all levels)	https://www.aonl.org/elements-healthy-practice-environment

What Are Barriers to Providing Evidence-Based Quality Health Care?

Although there are many resources to guide clinicians in providing evidence-based quality care, there are also many barriers. In 1991, researchers developed the BARRIERS to Research Utilization Scale, a 29-item tool that uses a 4-point Likert scale (1 = *barrier to no extent*, 4 = *barrier to a great extent*) to identify common barriers to EBP within four domains (i.e., the adopter, organization, innovation, or communication). Characteristics of the adopter include the nurse's research values, skills, and awareness; this domain measures barriers such as whether the nurse does not perceive the value of research findings, feels incapable of evaluating or using research, or is unwilling to change. Characteristics of the organization include barriers and limitations within the setting itself; this domain measures barriers related to leadership and colleague support, as well as inadequacies within the facility. Characteristics of the innovation (or the EBP change) measures barriers related to the quality of the research that supports the change in practice. Lastly, characteristics of the communication domain pertain to how the EBP change is presented; barriers in this domain include implications that findings lack clarity or relevance to the nurse's practice. The BARRIERS to Research Utilization Scale is over 30 years old, but it continues to be relevant in practice and has been used numerous times to identify major barriers within local nursing contexts (see Box 2.3).

BOX 2.3: EXAMPLE OF BARRIERS TO RESEARCH UTILIZATION SCALE

D'Sa and Varghese (2020) conducted a cross-sectional study with 175 surgical nurses at a tertiary care hospital in Saudi Arabia to identify nurses' self-reported perceptions of barriers to research utilization. They found that the characteristics of the *organization* (mean = 2.65; SD = 0.55) were rated as the highest barrier among staff; the question with the highest individual mean (mean = 2.96, SD = 0.97) was "There is insufficient time on the job to implement new ideas." Findings were interpreted as a lack of institutional support for research utilization; therefore, the institution may need to consider implementing initiatives to reduce this barrier.

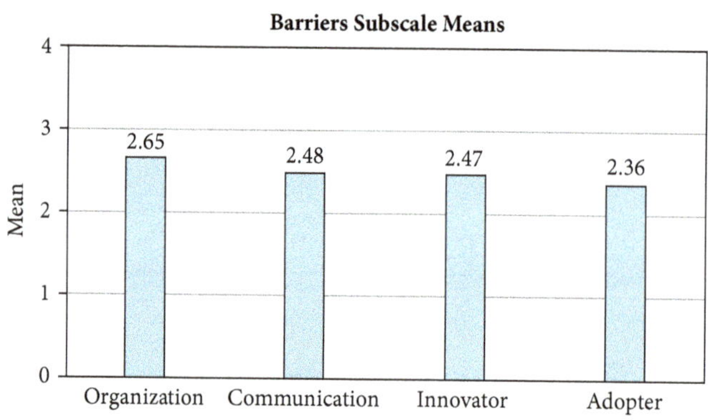

FIGURE 2.5 BARRIERS subscale means.

Missed Nursing Care

The concept of "missed nursing care" reflects challenges associated with providing evidence-based, quality care. Missed nursing care refers to care that is delayed, partially completed, or not completed at all. A care omission, or care left undone, is harder to measure than an error (e.g., a medication error) but can be equally harmful. Most studies on care omissions are cross-sectional surveys that ask nurses to self-report how often they do not complete specific aspects of care. In one study, only 15% of nurses surveyed said that they always reported care left undone (Ulrich & Kear, 2014). Similarly, a retrospective review of 100 patient charts found that between 8%–84% of 32 identified care tasks had been partly or fully omitted during each patient's stay (Saar et al., 2021). Care omissions are harder to track and not likely to be reported by staff; however, collecting and trending this data can identify systematic errors that can be corrected to improve the quality of care.

Care that is missed is often basic, foundational nursing care such as ambulation, turning, education, and hygiene (e.g., brushing teeth, bathing). Nurses have stated that reasons for missed care include inadequate staffing, lack of adequate time (e.g., to ambulate a patient around the unit), or becoming habitually negligent about performing a task (e.g., brushing patients' teeth; Kalisch, 2006). In 2009, Kalisch developed a missed nursing care model based on the Donabedian framework of structure-process-outcome. Structures that may influence missed nursing care include characteristics at the macro, meso, and micro levels; for example, hospital characteristics (e.g., bed size and location) along with unit characteristics (e.g., unit culture and amount of nurse staffing) can lead to missed nursing care that impacts both patient and staff outcomes. Missed nursing care can contribute to poor quality indicators such as falls, infections, and pressure injuries and can impact job satisfaction and turnover rates. Missed care, combined with barriers, can contribute to suboptimal quality of care provided to patients. As leaders in ANP, you will be able to impact many of these barriers. For example, as a nursing manager, you can help set the tone of the culture on the unit to decrease barriers and missed nursing care.

How Do We Identify Specific Clinical Problems (Quality Deficits)?

You now have a sense of the big picture of quality metrics, but as a nursing leader, how can you identify health care problems? There are practice-focused ways to identify health care problems:

- Your observations or personal experiences—what you see and hear in your daily practice—will often provide your first insight into a problem that should be addressed.
- A coworker may come to you with a concern.
- A patient may alert you to an issue that is worrisome from their perspective.
- You may realize that you or others lack the knowledge to attend to a specific patient care need. Perhaps the standard of care has recently been changed, and your unit has not made corresponding updates in practice to meet the new standard. Perhaps you have attended a conference or professional organization meeting and heard about a new practice that has improved care elsewhere.

The problem you identify may be broad and chronic or small and specific to your organization or unit. When you think you have found a problem, ask yourself, "What evidence do I have to support that this is a problem?"

Your workplace will provide a variety of locations in which to search for evidence. Many problems in health care organizations, especially hospitals, are tracked by the national/international safety and quality organizations described previously in this chapter. Data on how well an organization meets their standards is often available to the public. Such benchmarking allows potential patients and other interested groups to compare certain aspects of quality (e.g., between hospitals, or between health care organizations) to make an informed choice about where they wish to receive (and pay) for their care (see Box 2.4). This type of benchmarking data also provides hospitals and health care systems with guidance on how best to focus their quality improvement efforts. Additional information about benchmarking is discussed in Chapter 9.

BOX 2.4: EXAMPLE QUALITY CARE INDICATORS DASHBOARD

HAIs	United Acres Hospital	State Average	National Average	Areas for Improvement
CLASBI	1.22	2.0	1.0	X
CAUTI	0.5	1.5	1.0	
Surgical site infection (SSI)	1.8	2.0	1.0	X
Ventilator-associated event	2.0	1.5	1.0	X
C. diff	0.4	1.0	1.0	

CAUTI = catheter-associated urinary tract infection; CLABSI = central line - associated bloodstream infection

Adverse Events

Despite advances and improvements in quality over the past few decades, the prevalence of adverse events and patient harm continues to present hospitals with opportunities for improvement. A study by Bates et al. (2023) found evidence of patient harm in nearly one in four hospital admissions, and 25% of this harm was preventable; such findings highlight the need for an ongoing focus on quality and safety in health care. Decades ago, the main takeaway from the IOM report *To Err Is Human* was that errors responsible for harm were primarily due to systems problems rather than human errors. Human errors occur when the conduct of an individual or group unintentionally causes (or could have caused) an undesirable outcome (IOM, 2000). Human errors are inevitable, even among the most conscientious nurses who consistently practice the highest care standards, and typically result from a system(s) failure or process breakdown (Marx, 2001). Although humans do commit errors, a focus on making health care systems safer continues to be of paramount importance.

TJC conducts evaluations of health care organizations with the purpose of inspiring them to uphold the highest standards of quality and safety and pursue continuous quality improvement. To identify opportunities for improvement, hospitals accredited by TJC keep track of adverse events, especially sentinel events. A sentinel event (also known as a "never" event) is a patient safety event that results in death, permanent harm, or severe temporary harm. These events are often high on an organization's list of problems needing a solution. As you will see in future chapters, nurses in leadership play a critical role in preventing events that pose harm.

Health care organizations try to prevent sentinel events by collecting data on adverse events and near misses. Reports that generate this information are commonly referred to as "incident reports" and can be submitted by any team member; many hospitals have online incident reporting systems so that staff can easily submit events in real time. An adverse event is any event that resulted in an undesirable outcome not caused by the underlying disease process. Of particular importance, but often overlooked and underreported, are near misses and close calls. A near miss or close call is an event that could have resulted in a patient injury but did not due to mere chance (Agency for Healthcare Research and Quality, n.d.). TJC describes a near miss as a patient safety event that didn't make it to the patient (Marks et al., 2013). As a nurse in an advanced role, you have likely experienced or witnessed multiple near misses in your career. It is important to pay attention to these close calls and encourage others to do so as well. You should view them as symptoms of areas that require attention rather than as proof that health care system safeguards are effective. Intention to report near misses is associated with patient safety culture. Ignoring a near miss only increases the chance that a patient will be harmed next time (Yang et al., 2023).

Incident reports should trigger a nonpunitive (not aimed at punishment) investigation of the situation with a focus on improving the system to prevent recurrence (rather than on finding someone to blame). Health care workers are often reluctant to report incidents or near misses because they fear retaliation. One way systems can address such reluctance is to establish a "just culture."

Just Culture

The concept of "just culture" was an underlying principle of the *To Err Is Human* report. Just culture is an industry-related concept based on systems thinking, which assumes that mistakes are not solely the fault of individuals but rather are a product of the organizational culture; therefore, organizational mistakes affecting workplace safety are investigated through a lens of justice and problem solving versus blame and punishment (Boysen, 2013).

A "just culture" supports the reporting of all types of errors (adverse events, near misses, omissions in care) because the organization understands and emphasizes that mistakes are generally the result of a faulty culture or systems failure rather than individual misconduct. Reports are encouraged because they help the organization to improve processes and systems to prevent or decrease the occurrence of errors. Health care leaders have a duty to (a) recognize the inevitability of errors, (b) design systems that decrease the risk or frequency of errors, and (c) avoid punitive reactions to honest mistakes (Pelletier & Beaudin, 2018). Awareness of your professional and site-specific responsibilities related to the quality of care, including the prevention and reporting of events, is central to your work as a nursing leader. In a "just" culture, the question asked following a problematic event should be "What went wrong?" rather than "Who is to blame?" Often, these questions are asked, and solutions are identified during root-cause analyses.

Root-Cause Analyses

Root-cause analysis (RCA) in health care is a systematic, retrospective analytic approach to health care improvement. TJC requires hospitals and health systems to conduct RCAs for every sentinel event in an effort to identify the "root causes" so that systemic changes can be implemented to prevent future events. Root causes can be grouped into several categories affecting the micro, meso, and macro levels, such as the following: institutional, organizational, work environment, team environment, staffing, task-related, and patient characteristics. RCAs are designed to review what, how, and why sentinel events occur. RCAs are performed by a small team, generally four to 10 individuals, comprised of members from all levels associated with the event. Although RCAs can help identify areas to improve the quality of care, they have some limitations. The quality of RCA can vary across facilities and is dependent on the accuracy of input data and the capability of the team. RCAs can also be very time-consuming, as teams must gather and organize the data (Shaqdan et al., 2014). As a nursing leader, you may be called upon to take part in an RCA, or even to lead one. Let's consider a sample case of how errors, as well as solutions, can be addressed using reporting and an RCA (see Box 2.5).

BOX 2.5: CASE EXAMPLE

A 3-week-old premature infant in the neonatal unit has an umbilical central venous catheter for multiple IV antibiotic administrations. Following evidence-based guidelines, Nurse A, a nurse with 1 year of experience, flushes the line with 10 units of heparin per protocol to keep the central venous catheter patent. Ten hours into Nurse A's shift, she feeds the infant a bottle of previously frozen breast milk and notices a tinge of pink when the infant spits up. After caring for her other patient, Nurse A returns and changes the infant's diaper, noticing stool mixed with blood. The infant spits up again, this time producing bright red blood. Nurse A immediately notifies the on-call neonatal nurse practitioner (NNP) of this new finding.

The NNP comes to the infant's bedside, performs a thorough assessment, and orders several lab tests and administration of vitamin K while further investigating the cause of the bleeding. During his assessment, the NP notices the vial of heparin that Nurse A used for the flush sitting on the bedside table; on close inspection, he realizes that it is a 10,000 unit/1mL heparin vial, not the 10 unit/1mL heparin vial usually stocked on the unit. As both vials have a dark blue cap and blue lettering, they look very similar.

Having recognized the vial mix-up as the cause of the infant's bleeding, the NNP works with the physician team to reverse the effects of the heparin overdose. The CNS informs the infant's family of the incident and what is being done to correct its effects and offers support. The nursing manager assists the bedside nurse, providing a calming presence; the manager also guides Nurse A in completing an incident report. After several hours and multiple blood transfusions, the bleeding slows, and the infant's vital signs stabilize.

Outcome

Following this incident, the CNS worked with all team members to gather data regarding the event and led an RCA with the nurse, clinical team, unit leadership, pharmacy leadership, and patient safety experts. Upon review of the medication process, several issues were identified, including (a) the manufacturer had nondistinct "look-alike" labels on all heparin vials, making it difficult to tell them apart; (b) similar sizes of heparin vials were available, as both the 10,000-unit and 10-unit doses were in 1mL vials; (c) the pharmacy technician placed the wrong heparin vials in the automated drug-dispensing cabinets in the neonatal unit; (d) the nurse failed to carefully and accurately read the label on the medical vial prior to administering the drug to the patient; and (e) as the drug was used for a line flush, the hospital did not require the use of medication barcode scanning.

The harm to the patient and the potential for a dangerous outcome was serious but temporary, and the infant experienced complete recovery, likely due to rapid care coordination, subsequent interventions, and continued monitoring. Within 1 week, following a review, a second debriefing with leadership occurred, during which evidence was presented to the entire team involved in the event. Based on the issues identified, system-level practice changes were needed. Later that month, in all units within the large health care system, barcode scanning and a second witness were required for all heparin administrations, including flushes. The Institute for Safe Medication Practices (ISMP) also put out an urgent alert to notify other health care systems of the look-alike drug vials, and the manufacturer quickly worked to change the colors of the vial caps and print so that the vials would be more distinct. There have been no known cases of medication errors related to heparin in the neonatal unit since this improvement was made years ago.

Critical Reflection

What comes to your mind when you consider the unintentional occurrences outlined in this example? As we learned in Chapter 1, nursing is not a solo profession; we work as part of a system. Reflecting on this case may help you to think critically about the safety and quality of care you will provide as a nursing leader.

Patient harm resulted from the error in this case. The error was reported in a timely fashion, and ultimately, future harm was likely prevented due to local- and system-level changes resulting from adherence to proper reporting mechanisms. Remember that adopting a systems mind-set, and role-modeling this behavior as a leader, requires thinking beyond blame. As seen in this example, simply blaming Nurse A for not carefully reading the heparin vial would have masked the many other systems- and manufacturer-related failures that led to the medication error. Individual behavior can cause errors; however, viewing health care delivery from a systems perspective enables nurses to identify and respond to threats to safety and find effective, comprehensive, and long-lasting solutions (Pelletier & Beaudin, 2018).

EBPQI

As a nursing leader, you will find no shortage of opportunities to improve the quality of care (often multiple opportunities will present themselves in your clinical area). Once you have identified areas for improvement through benchmark data, incident reports, or your clinical experience, what should be your next steps? First, you will need to *prioritize* the many potential EBPQI initiatives with which you are faced. Next, you will need to work with your team to systematically improve the quality of care. EBPQI is, simply, the use of *evidence in practice* to *improve* the *quality* of care. EBPQI is a problem-solving approach centered on continuous learning and inquiry. As a nursing leader, you will be poised to lead various types of initiatives to improve the quality-of-care provision. Further information on how to prioritize and improve the quality of care is provided in Chapter 9.

WELLNESS IN ACTION: ENVIRONMENTAL HEALTH

Climate change and the environment are public health issues. The ICN position statement on nurses, climate change and health states "leadership from nurses to take immediate action to build climate-resilient health systems is necessary" (ICN, 2018, para. 1). Hospitals are responsible for over 29 pounds of waste per day per hospital bed. There are many different types of hospital waste (e.g., regulated medical waste, pharmaceutical waste, hazardous and universal infectious waste, food and solid waste), and even the waste of water and energy can be reduced. *Source*: https://practicegreenhealth.org/topics/waste/waste-0

Many waste problems, particularly the disposal of single-use plastics, became worse as a result of the COVID-19 pandemic. Green health care encompasses the concept of eco-friendliness and creates economic value by reducing waste and operational costs in a way that balances disease eradiation (public health) and environmental health. The Global Green and Healthy Hospitals Sustainability Agenda provides guidance to support change. For leaders, it provides a list of action items (greenhospitals.org/leadership). As a nurse leader, you may be charged with engaging others to make a difference by reviewing policies, proposing initiatives using a value driven analysis, or just setting a good example and asking questions when you observe wasteful practices. Any situation that results in avoidable waste presents an opportunity for an EBPQI initiative!

WRAPPING UP

As a nurse in an advanced role, you will (a) lead teams that interact with patients and families across health care settings and throughout the care continuum, (b) have significant responsibility for identifying quality and safety issues as well as problem-solving, evidence-based strategies to improve them, and (c) must ensure that EBPQI becomes achievable for patient populations. This chapter provided foundational knowledge about how health care quality and safety metrics are defined and measured in the United States and how to identify problems and evidence/data to lead and drive improvement.

Reflection Questions

1. What is the leading cause of errors in health care?
2. How does your organization define and measure health care quality?
3. A colleague expresses several barriers to implementing an evidence-based practice, one of which is that they do not understand the research supporting the practice. As a nurse in an advanced role, how can you mitigate this barrier?
4. A near-miss event involving four nurses occurs on your unit. As a nursing leader on this unit, you request that the nurses complete an incident report; however, they are hesitant to complete the report for fear of retaliation. How will you discuss the importance of incident reports and their role in improving the quality of care?
5. In what ways have you observed the environment and climate impacting health?

REFERENCES

Agency for Healthcare Research and Quality. (2019). Adverse events, near misses and errors. The PS Net Collection, https://psnet.ahrq.gov/primer/adverse-events-near-misses-and-errors

Allen-Duck, A., Robinson, J. C., & Stewart, M. W. (2017). Healthcare quality: A concept analysis. *Nursing Forum*, *52*(4), 377–386. https://doi.org/10.1111/nuf.12207

Altan, D., Leya, G. A., & Chang, D. C. (2022). Tracking the "end result" and long-term patient outcomes—Failure to rescue and the shrinking denominator. *JAMA Surgery*, *157*(3), 268. https://doi.org/10.1001/jamasurg.2021.6905

American Academy of Nursing. (2015). American Academy of Nursing announced engagement in the national Choosing Wisely campaign. *Nursing Outlook*, *63*(1), 96–98. http://doi.org/10.1016/j.outlook.2014.12.017

American Association of Critical Care Nurses. (2016). *AACN standards for establishing and sustaining healthy work environments: A journey to excellence.*

Bates, D. W., Levine, D. M., Salmasian, H., Syrowatka, A., Shahian, D. M., Lipsitz, S., Zebrowski, J. P., Myers, L. C., ... & Mort, E. (2023). The safety of inpatient health care. *New England Journal of Medicine*, *388*(2), 142–153. https://doi.org/10.1056/NEJMsa2206117

Berwick, D. M. (1991a). Blazing the trail of quality: The HFHS quality management process. *Frontiers of Health Services Management*, *7*(4), 47–50. https://www.ncbi.nlm.nih.gov/pubmed/10110631
Berwick, D. M. (1991b). Controlling variation in health care: A consultation from Walter Shewhart. *Medical Care*, *29*(12), 1212–1225. https://www.ncbi.nlm.nih.gov/pubmed/1745079
Berwick, D. M., Nolan, T. W., & Whittington, J. (2008). The triple aim: Care, health, and cost. *Health Affairs*, *27*(3), 759–769. https://doi.org/10.1377/hlthaff.27.3.759
Bodenheimer, T., & Sinsky, C. (2014). From triple to quadruple aim: Care of the patient requires care of the provider. *Annals of Family Medicine, 12*(6), 573–576. https://doi.org/10.1370/afm.1713
Boysen, P. G., II. (2013). Just culture: A foundation for balanced accountability and patient safety. *Ochsner Journal*, *13*(3), 400–406. https://www.ncbi.nlm.nih.gov/pubmed/24052772
Centers for Disease Control and Prevention. (n.d.). What is Health Equity. *https://www.cdc.gov/health-equity/what-is/index.html*
Chun, J., & Bafford, A. C. (2014). History and background of quality measurement. *Clinics in Colon and Rectal Surgery*, *27*(1), 5–9. https://doi.org/10.1055/s-0034-1366912
D'Sa, J. L., & Varghese, R. (2020). Perceived Barriers to Research Utilization among Surgical Nurses: A Cross-Sectional Survey. *I-Manager's Journal on Nursing*, *10*(1), 11–21. https://doi.org/10.26634/jnur.10.1.16731
Fulop, N., & Robert, G. (2015, October). *Context for successful quality improvement. The Health Foundation.* https://www.health.org.uk/sites/default/files/ContextForSuccessfulQuality-Improvement.pdf
Glickman, S. W., Baggett, K. A., Krubert, C. G., Peterson, E. D., & Schulman, K. A. (2007). Promoting quality: The health-care organization from a management perspective. *International Journal of Quality Health Care*, *19*(6), 341–348.
Institute of Medicine's Committee on Quality of Health Care in America. (2000). *To err is human: Building a safer health system* (L. T. Kohn, J. M. Corrigan, & M. S. Donaldson, Eds.). National Academies Press. http://www.ncbi.nlm.nih.gov/books/NBK225182/
Institute of Medicine's Committee on Quality of Health Care in America. (2001). *Crossing the quality chasm: A new health system for the 21st century.* National Academies Press. http://www.ncbi.nlm.nih.gov/books/NBK222274/
Institute for Healthcare Improvement. (2009, January–February). The triple aim: Optimizing health, care, and cost. *Healthcare Executive*, 64–66.
International Council of Nurses. (2018). *Position statement: Nurses, climate change and health.* https://www.icn.ch/sites/default/files/inline-files/ICN%20PS%20Nurses%252c%20climate%20change%20and%20health%20FINAL%20.pdf
Jarvis, J., Blessing, R., Naglee, C., & Reynolds, S. (2023). Implementation of an early mobility protocol in the neuroscience ICU. *International Journal of Critical Care*, *17*(3), 115–127. https://doi.org/10.29173/ijcc67
The Joint Commission. (2023). *R3 report issue 38: National patient safety goal to improve health equity.* https://www.jointcommission.org/standards/r3-report/r3-report-issue-38-national-patient-safety-goal-to-improve-health-care-equity/#.Y9eyfezMKjA
Kalisch, B. J. (2006). Missed nursing care: A qualitative study. *Journal of Nursing Care Quality*, *21*(4), 306–315. https://doi.org/10.1097/00001786-200610000-00006
Kalisch, B. J., Landstrom, G. L., & Hinshaw, A. S. (2009). Missed nursing care: A concept analysis. *Journal of Advanced Nursing*, *65*(7), 1509–1517. https://doi.org/10.1111/j.1365-2648.2009.05027.x

Marks, C. M., Kasda, E., Pain, L., & Wu, A.W. "That was a close call": Endorsing a broad definition of near misses in health care. *The Joint Commission Journal on Quality and Patient Safety, 39*(10), 475–479. https://doi.org/10.1016/S1553-7250(13)39061-8
Marx D. (2019). Patient Safety and the Just Culture. *Obstetrics and gynecology clinics of North America, 46*(2), 239–245. https://doi.org/10.1016/j.ogc.2019.01.003
Montalvo, I. (2007). The National Database of Nursing Quality Indicators (NDNQI). *OJIN: The Online Journal of Issues in Nursing, 12*(3). https://doi.org/10.3912/OJIN.Vol12No03Man02
National Academies of Sciences, Engineering, Medicine. (n.d.). *About us*. https://www.nationalacademies.org/about
National Academies of Sciences, Engineering, and Medicine. (2021). *The future of nursing 2020-2030: Charting a path to achieve health equity*. National Academies Press. https://doi.org/10.17226/25982
Nightingale, F. (1863). *Notes on hospitals* (R. A. G. Longman, Ed., 3rd ed. London: UK).
Nightingale, F. (1985). *Notes on nursing: What it is and what it is not*. Harrison of Pall Mall, London: UK.
Nunday, S., Cooper, L. A., Mate, K. S. (2022). The quintuple aim for health care improvement: A new imperative to advance health equity. *JAMA, 327*(6), 521–522. https://doi.org/10.1001/jama.2021.25181
Nurse Drawdown. (n.d.). *Home page*. https://www.nursesdrawdown.org/
Pelletier, L. R., & Beaudin, C. L. (2018). *HQ solutions: Resource for the healthcare quality professional* (4th ed.). Wolters Kluwer.
Porter, M. E. (2009). A strategy for health care reform—Toward a value-based system. *The New England journal of medicine, 361*(2), 109-112. https://doi.org/10.1056/NEJMp0904131
Pressley, C. & Garside, J. (2023). Safeguarding the retention of nurses: A systematic review on determinants of nurses' intentions to stay. *Nursing Open, 10*(5), 2842–2858. https://doi.org/10.1002/nop2.1588
Saar, L., Unbeck, M., Bachnick, S., Gehri, B., & Simon, M. (2021). Exploring omissions in nursing cae using retrospective chart review: An observational study. International Journal of Nursing Studies, 122, 104009. https://doi.org/10.1016/j.ijnurstu.2021.104009
Shaqdan, K., Aran, S., Daftari Besheli, L., & Abujudeh, H. (2014). Root-cause analysis and health failure mode and effect analysis: Two leading techniques in health care quality assessment. *Journal of the American College of Radiology, 11*(6), 572–579. https://doi.org/10.1016/j.jacr.2013.10.024
Ulrich, B., & Kear, T. (2014). Patient Safety and Patient Safety Culture: Foundations of Excellent Health Care Delivery. *Nephrology nursing journal : journal of the American Nephrology Nurses' Association, 41*(5), 447–456.
Watts, N., Amann, M., Arnell, N., Ayeb-Karlsson, S., Beagley, J., Belesova, K., Boykoff, M., Byass, P., Cai, W., Campbell-Lendrum, D., Capstick, S., Chambers, J., Coleman, S., Dalin, C., Daly, M., Dasandi, N., Dasgupta, S., Davies, M., Di Napoli, C., Dominguez-Salas, P., ... & Costello, A. (2021). The 2020 report of the *Lancet* countdown on health and climate change: responding to converging crises. *Lancet, 397*(10269), 129–170. https://doi.org/10.1016/S0140-6736(20)32290-X
Yang, Y., & Liu, H. (2021). The effect of patient safety culture on nurses' near-miss reporting intention: the moderating role of perceived severity of near misses. *Journal of research in nursing : JRN, 26*(1-2), 6–16. https://doi.org/10.1177/1744987120979344

IMAGE CREDITS

Fig. 2.1: Jayne Jennings Dunlap and Julee Briscoe Waldrop, *Introduction to Evidence-Based Practice and Quality Improvement for Professional Nursing Practice: A Competency Based Approach*, p. 27. Copyright © 2024 by Cognella, Inc. Reprinted with permission.

Fig. 2.2: Copyright © by Peter Irwin Lachman, Paul B. Batalden, Kris Vanhaecht (CC BY 4.0) at *F1000Research*, vol. 9, no. 1140; https://f1000research.com/articles/9-1140/v3.

Fig. 2.3: Source: https://www.kff.org/report-section/beyond-health-care-the-role-of-social-determinants-in-promoting-health-and-health-equity-issue-brief/.

Fig. 2.4: Jayne Jennings Dunlap and Julee Briscoe Waldrop, *Introduction to Evidence-Based Practice and Quality Improvement for Professional Nursing Practice: A Competency Based Approach*, p. 31. Copyright © 2024 by Cognella, Inc. Reprinted with permission.

CHAPTER 3

Leading the Development of Clinical Questions and Aims

Julee Briscoe Waldrop

KEY CONCEPTS

Questions to guide searching for the evidence

PICO(T)(S)

PPCO

SMART aims

LEARNING OBJECTIVES

1. Develop questions to guide your search for the evidence using a framework-guided approach.
2. Analyze an aim statement using SMART components.

> Science requires training. It is a disciplined method that tries to systematically overcome or bypass our intuitions and cognitive biases and follow the evidence regardless of our prior beliefs, expectations, preferences, or personal investment
>
> —Ralph Lewis

Introduction

Now that you have learned how to identify a clinical or health systems issue (Chapter 2), you are probably eager to solve the problems you identify. Before you can search for research evidence to address any health-related problem, however, you must be certain that you thoroughly understand that problem or issue; this is especially important as a leader. In this chapter, we present frameworks that you can use to build searchable clinical or health issue questions and EBPQI initiative aims. In your ANP role, you know that a responsible approach to finding evidence-based solutions is required to support any proposed practice changes in health care. This is why it is critical that everyone who engages in the EBPQI process understands the step we are about to discuss. Let's get started with some examples.

Example 1: Vaccination Rates

Let's suppose that you are a nurse practitioner in a primary care pediatric practice. You have noticed that your vaccination rates have fallen since the COVID-19 pandemic, and families are increasingly choosing to defer not only COVID-19 vaccines and boosters but even routine vaccinations. How can you find the evidence you need to support clinical decision-making around this issue?

External or Research Evidence on the Problem

In this case, you must first gather more details about the problem. You must develop a question systematically (i.e., not just by Googling) that will help you to find reputable and recent information about the larger health issue of lower vaccination rates; this type of information-seeking question is sometimes called the *background question* (Melnyk & Fineout-Overholt, 2023). Background questions are the foundation for *foreground questions*—questions about solutions to the problem, such as whether or how well previous interventions, programs, or practice changes have worked.

Problems can be multifaceted and hard to pin down. Your problem could pertain to a disease or symptom, behavior, process, or policy. One way to develop a background question is to consider the outcome if the problem or issue remains untreated or if a practice change is not implemented. You can make the problem more specific by adding the affected population. The outcome is what you want to improve; it could be the consequence of a disease or, in this case, of deferring vaccinations.

Moving back to our case study in Example 1, the problem (P) you want to learn more about is lower vaccination rates; the population is children; and the outcome (O) is vaccination rates. You can formulate a background question such as "In children, what are the consequences of not getting vaccinated?" In Chapter 4, you will learn how to use this type of question to search for evidence from the literature (i.e., published research) and other evidence, such as professional publications (e.g., practice guidelines or recommendations).

Example 2: Nurse Turnover

Suppose that as a chief nursing officer you are very concerned about the continued rapid turnover of nurses in your hospital. Your hospital cannot sustain its resources for orienting new nurses and the cost of hiring travel nurses. Moreover, the Bureau of Labor Statistics (2024) projects an estimated 203,200 openings for nurses yearly through 2031, despite an increase in workforce growth, due to retirements and nurses leaving the profession.

External or Research Evidence on the Problem

In this case, the problem is the turnover rate of nursing positions. Nurse turnover significantly drains the financial and other resources of health care organizations. In an American Nurses Foundation (2022) national survey of 12,694 nurses across the entire continuum of care, over 50% of respondents indicated an intent to leave their current position due to insufficient staffing, the inability to deliver quality patient care, and a negative impact on their health and well-being. Evidence like this obtained from research databases such as PubMed and CINAHL constitutes *external evidence*. Table 3.1 presents an example of how you might now write a background question for this problem.

TABLE 3.1 Background Question Examples

Element	Definition	Example 1	Example 2
P (problem/ population)	Who?	Children who are un- or under-vaccinated	Nurses
O (Outcome)	What about the population and the exposure (issue/ problem) do I want to examine?	Health consequences	Turnover costs
Question example	Using just the P and the O of the future PICO question	In children, what are the health consequences of non- or under-vaccination?	What is the cost of nurse turnover to health care organizations?

Example 1: Internal Evidence on the Problem

Let's return to your observation of a decrease in immunization acceptance at your clinic. You are now ready to move from finding external evidence (about the problem in general) to finding *internal evidence* (evidence from your specific setting). In this case, you have observed and noted the problem, and your observation constitutes anecdotal evidence (i.e., evidence based on personal experience). We will discuss anecdotal evidence further in Chapter 7. Your clinic may already track vaccination rates as a quality metric; if so, this data will be readily available to you, and if not, you will have to seek it. You could start by identifying a vaccination (or set of vaccinations) on which to focus, such as the standard ones (DPT, polio, MMR, Hib, HepB by 36 months of life) recommended by the Centers for Disease Control (CDC, 2023), then have the billing department assist you with identifying all 3-year old children seen for the 36-month visit. Subsequently, you could perform a retrospective chart review of a sample of patients using a random strategy, such as by choosing charts to review based on the last digit in the medical record number (e.g., even or odd).

The sample would serve as your denominator (e.g., 50), and the number of patients found to have not received the recommended vaccines would serve as your numerator (e.g., 30), resulting in your rate (60%), which is well below the national average of 76%. Once you have found sufficient data to confirm that there exists a problematic issue in your clinic, you are ready to find solutions or potential ways to address it.

Example 2: Internal Evidence of the Problem

Regarding this case example, it is likely that your human resources department will have data on the hospital's nurse turnover rate and will continue to track it, thereby saving you the effort of tracking it yourself. Let's suppose that you request this information and find that your hospital's nurse turnover rate is 35%. Your critical review of the data reveals that 60% of newly hired nurses stayed for less than 2 years. As the national RN turnover rate in 2023 was 22.5% (Nursing Solutions, Inc. [NSI], 2023), your organization recently calculated that a benchmark turnover rate of 25% would be sustainable given its current financial situation. You know that the average cost of turnover for a bedside RN is $52,350 (NSI, 2023; see Chapters 2 and 9 for more information on benchmarks and metrics), so you need to find a solution to this cost drain. This is when a clinical question on solutions comes in!

Clinical Questions to Guide the Search for Evidence on Solutions to the Problem or Issue

There are many ways to write a clinical question. Most are variations of the traditional PICO (population, intervention, comparison, outcome) question. The PICO question framework was developed for use in the field of medicine, so its focus is on treatments or interventions, making it an excellent way to search for evidence to answer a question about the most effective treatment for a specific patient population with a specific health problem (Huang et al., 2006). Although the traditional PICO question seeks to find the best available research evidence to support EBP, keep in mind that it privileges experimental research and medical interventions (Booth et al., 2023).

In general, the C (comparison) component of the PICO question is often the most difficult to include. In the classic PICO question, the P (population) component can include many options, such as age, gender, disease, symptoms, or current treatment. The I (intervention) and C components can incorporate all therapies (e.g., drugs, procedures, tests, surgeries, usual care, or placebo). The O (outcome) occurs as the result of the I and C; therefore, you should keep in mind that choosing the intervention and comparison before you have completed a search of the evidence could lead to premature bias toward an already-known intervention or practice change. A search that is biased toward a chosen intervention or solution risks overlooking an alternative that might be more effective (Cullen et al., 2023; Waldrop & Dunlap, 2024). An outcome could be whether there was improvement in the disease or symptoms. You can also include other elements in your question, such as a specific timeframe (PICOT) or setting (PICOS). We will revisit the PICO(T)(S) format in Chapter 5.

The best evidence is usually defined through a hierarchical approach, which can be visualized as a pyramid (see Figure 3.1). The top of the pyramid reflects the highest level of evidence and includes systematic reviews and meta-analyses composed of RCTs. As mentioned in Chapter 1, most research studies have excluded minority populations; therefore, depending on your population, the PICO question may reveal significant gaps in evidence for nondominant populations (Booth et al., 2023).

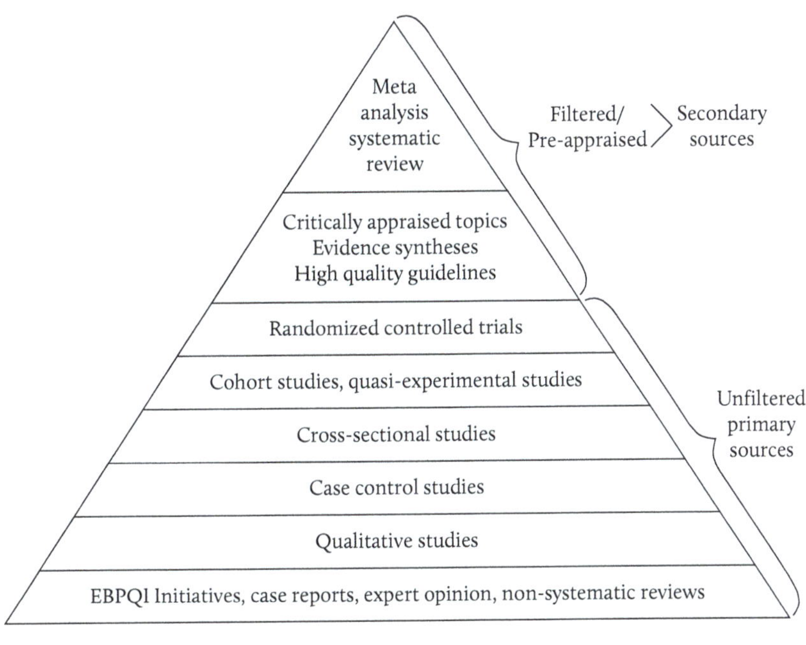

FIGURE 3.1 Evidence pyramid.

Example 1: Vaccination Rate Clinical Question Development

Using the PICO format, your problem/population will be "un- or under-vaccinated children aged 3 and under." You will have already determined your intervention, likely based on your expertise or a recommendation. Your comparison will be "usual care" (in your practice). Your outcome, or the goal of the intervention(s), will be improving your vaccination rate.

Example 2: Nurse Turnover Clinical Question Development

For this example, using the PICO format, your problem/population will be "nurse turnover," and your intervention will be based on your experience and the information you already have. Your comparison will be "no intervention or the usual practice," and your outcome will be "nurse turnover rate." Creating a table (like Table 3.2) will help to ensure that you have included all the components in your clinical question.

TABLE 3.2 PICO(T)(S) Question Examples

Element	Definition	Example 1	Example 2
Population/ problem	Who?	Children 3 years and under who are un- or under-vaccinated	Nurse turnover
Intervention	What is proposed?	Provider recommendation	Nonsalary-related benefits
Comparison	Intervention or no intervention?	Care as usual	Current practice
Outcome	What is the desired outcome?	Vaccination rate	Turnover rate
PICO question for searching example		In children 3 years and under who are un- or under-vaccinated, does provider recommendation or discussion compared to current practice impact vaccination rates?	In nurses who are current employees, does adding benefits compared to the current policies impact nurse turnover rate (i.e., increase retention)?

Ideas are only as good as the evidence that supports them, which is why we go through the systematic process of searching the evidence—every time! Additionally, this process will reveal whether the quantity and quality of evidence are sufficient to change practice. If you haven't found enough evidence to support a change in practice to address the problem, you will need to do more research before you can responsibly make a change. If this is the case, consider participating in the research process! Your recognition of clinical issues or areas of practice that should be investigated through research provides nurse scientists with valuable input. Remember that the PICO framework also works well for writing a research question that focuses on an intervention's effectiveness. If you are passionate about discovering new understanding of issues in health care, we encourage you to volunteer to be part of a research team.

A good research question can include your method (how the problem is investigated) as well as what you want to find out. Because there are many different study designs, there are many different types of questions. We introduced some research study designs in Chapter 1. *Observational studies* aim to explore and describe a problem further and in new ways. *Experimental studies* are designed to determine the effect(s) of introducing an intervention. You will learn more about study designs in Chapters 5 and 6.

The traditional PICO format for a guiding question is less accurate when it concerns ways of "treating" a population/problem. Despite its widespread use, there is limited evidence to support its efficacy, especially in nursing (Eriksen & Frandsen, 2018; Schiavenato & Chu, 2021), so don't feel confined to using this format. There are emerging formats that might be better suited to your needs. Many problems that nurses in advanced roles encounter are unrelated to treatment; they may pertain to personnel management (as in Example 2), systems of care, program effectiveness, policies, or public disaster responses. Moreover, nurse leaders identify problems that impact health not only in the workplace but in every aspect of their lives.

PPCO

An alternative to the PICO question is an evidence-searching question designed by nurses for nurses: the PPCO (problem, population, change, outcomes) statement (Waldrop & Dunlap, 2024). This acronym reflects a combination of the background and the foreground questions, with the first P representing the problem you wish to address. The "problem P" reminds you that you need to ask a background question to make certain that you are well informed on the problem in general as well as in your local context before you look for evidence-based solutions. The second P refers to the population, which should always be specified as you need to know whom the problem is impacting. The C refers to change—in other words, what has been recommended or already done (research evidence) that addresses the problem. Finally, the O refers to the outcome—that is, how you will know that the change made a difference. If we reworded the two example problems using PCCO questions, they would look like Table 3.3.

Another acronym that is overarching and inclusive of additional aspects of an EBP/QI initiative is PURPOSE (Cullen et al., 2022). A PURPOSE question includes components that provide you with more guidance regarding future implementation and evaluation of an EBPQI initiative, such as who will be users of or responsible for the outcomes, where the initiative will take place, and how many resources it will require.

Any of the PURPOSE statement elements can help you search the literature for research to support your EBPQI initiative. An added benefit is that you can easily build on this framework to write specific and measurable aims for the initiative.

TABLE 3.3 PPCO Question

Element	Description	Example 1	Example 2
Problem	What is the problem, both in general and specifically in your local context?	Un- and under-vaccination	High turnover rate
Population	Whom does the problem impact?	Children 3 years and under	Nurses
Change	What has been recommended or done to improve the problem?	Change in practice, protocol, policy, or process	Change in practice, protocol, policy, or process
Outcomes	How is improvement reported (measured)?	Vaccination rates	Turnover rate
PPCO question for searching example		In children 3 and under who are un- or under-vaccinated, what interventions impact vaccination rates?	In organizations with high nurse turnover rates, what policies impact turnover rate (or retention)?

TABLE 3.4 Purpose Statement

Element	Description	Example 1	Example 2
Patient/ population	Who is being affected by the problem, and whom do you want to benefit from the improvement? Always think about whom the problem might disadvantage (i.e., look at it through a health equity lens).	Children 3 and under	Nurses
Users	Who will need to change their behavior, or what process will need to change?	Pediatric providers Nurses	Human resources Administrators Managers Nurses
Responsible team	Who needs to be involved for the initiative to be successful?	Pediatric providers and nurses	Human resources Chief executive officer Chief financial officer Chief nursing officer
Problem	(The first P from the PPCO statement) The specific target (issue) for the EBP change	Un- or under-vaccination rates	Nurse turnover (i.e., nurses are hired, oriented, and then leave the organization)

Element	Description	Example 1	Example 2
Outcome(s)	The measurable goal or aim of the initiative	Vaccination rate	Turnover rate
Setting	Where the EBP/QI initiative will take place (describe it)	Clinic	Hospital
Effort	Can be the time frame for completion and/or resources needed	Provider/RN time resources and workflow changes to incorporate time for practice change will need to be planned and agreed upon prior to the start of the intervention.	Interventions selected may take time and will need to be planned, and policies will need to be written and approved prior to the start of practice change.

Source: Adapted from Cullen et al. (2022).

Introduction to Aims, Goals, and Objectives

You may hear people use the terms aims, goals, and objectives interchangeably (Table 3.5). Sometimes, this is fine, as you may only sometimes need all three to plan an EBPQI initiative. Sometimes, the scope and time frame can overlap. We prefer to keep it simple and just use a broad purpose statement and then SMART aims.

TABLE 3.5 Aims, Goals, and Objectives

Aspect	Aims	Goals	Objectives
Definition	Broad, general intentions or desired outcomes	Specific, measurable targets to achieve aims*	Detailed steps or actions to achieve goals
Scope	Wide-ranging and long-term	Narrower, midterm	Very specific, short-term
Nature	Abstract and qualitative	Concrete and often quantitative	Quantifiable and actionable
Time Frame	Long-term, often indefinite	Midterm, usually within months to years	Short-term, often within days to months
Purpose	To provide a direction or vision	To set a path toward achieving the aim	To outline specific actions to achieve the goal
Example	Improve overall health and well-being	Lose 20 pounds within a year	Exercise for 30 minutes, five times a week

**SMART aims are more like goals because of their specificity and measurability.*

We will talk about AIMS some more in Chapter 10, but you will recall from Chapter 1 that all EBPQI initiatives begin with three questions:

- What are we trying to accomplish?
- How will we know whether a change is an improvement?
- What change can we make that will result in an improvement?

Written aims offer a guide to answering these questions. SMART is a useful acronym developed by George Doran et al. (1981) to help you remember that your aims should be **s**pecific, **m**easurable, **a**ttainable, **r**elevant, and **t**imely. Consider these important criteria as you determine your aims.

TABLE 3.6 SMART Aims

Component	Description
Specific	Be specific about who, what, where, and when: What are you trying to accomplish? What change will be made to produce an improvement? Who is going to be part of the change process? Where will the changes take place? When will the change happen?
Measurable	How will you know that there has been an improvement? How will you measure the improvement?
Attainable	Is your aim attainable? Do you have all the resources or tools you need? If not, can you find a way to get them?
Relevent	Is your aim meaningful and does it align with your priorities and values?
Timely	What timeline is needed to achieve your aim? Is there a deadline? If there is no specific deadline, how can you create a sense of urgency to motivate team members to make the change happen in a timely manner?

Example 1

The vaccination rate for children 3 years and under will increase by 10% by 6 months after the practice change(s) is implemented.

Example 2

Nurse turnover at Universal Hospital will decrease by 5% by 6 months after the practice change(s) is implemented. Let's analyze these aims based on the SMART principles.

TABLE 3.7 Analysis of SMART Aims Examples

Principle	Description	Example 1	Example 2
Specific	Who?	Children 3 years old and under	Nurses
	What changed?	A provider discussion using motivational interviewing was implemented as standard care	Nonsalary benefits
	When and where?	At each clinic visit	For all nurses
Measurable	What is being measured?	The number of each of the seven vaccinations recommended by 36 months of age is divided by the total number of children 3 years old and under in the practice	Monthly/annual turnover rate
Attainable	Resources needed?	Time to conduct the conversation is the resource most needed. Before you begin this project, you must ascertain (a) the length of the proposed discussions and (b) whether the discussions can be conducted without adversely impacting other provider and nurse responsibilities	Additional funding Budget forecasting
Relevent	Is it meaningful?	Illness and possibly death will be prevented in young children	Nurse turnover and costs may decrease
Timely	Over what period of time will the change take place and the outcomes be assessed?	An assessment of immunization status will occur at every visit to identify all possible opportunities for vaccination Vaccination rates will be reported monthly	To all current nurse employees and new hires Each month/year, the hospital reports its retention/turnover rate

These are examples of *outcome-based aims*. In EBPQI initiatives, there are also *process or feasibility aims and measures* (aims that measure whether the intervention or behavior change actually occurred) as well as *balancing aims or measures* (aims intended to ensure awareness of potential unintended consequences of, or processes that might be negatively impacted by, the initiative). For example, in our vaccination example, a process measure or aim could be documentation in the patient record that a discussion about immunizations has occurred. A SMART aim statement might be "For 90% of vaccine-eligible patients, documentation of a discussion will be present at 3 months post-practice change implementation." A balancing measure might be that the providers report that adding a conversation on immunization is feasible in their current practice. This aim could be worded as follows: "Of providers, 90% report the practice change as feasible to implement."

In the nurse turnover example, a process measure or aim could be worded this way: "Of nurses, 50% will participate in one of the noneconomic benefits offered within 3 months of availability." A balancing measure could be worded like this: "Workplace climate survey scores will remain stable" (note that, ideally, the climate should improve, but that will depend on the percentage of nurses who take advantage of the new benefits).

WELLNESS IN ACTION: BRIEF REST

I (Julee) had a coach (for running) who would say, "Rest is a piece of the pie" to remind us that stressed muscles only adapt if given an opportunity to rest. It is during rest that stressors can be incorporated in a functional way (Devantier-Thomas et al., 2024). Rest is an often-overlooked prerequisite for managing stress (regulating the central nervous system), problem solving, and creativity. There is clear evidence that sleep is the foundation of a rested and restored nervous system (Zhang et al., 2023), but there are other means of resetting the nervous system, such as brief rest or respite from sympathetic overstimulation (Bentley et al., 2023; Mandlik et al., 2023). Health care organizations are discovering the important benefits of integrating stress-reducing practices into the workflow. Brief rest practices, including breathwork, meditation, yoga (movement with breath), and restorative yoga (stillness with breath), are evidence-based remedies that everyone can use to decrease stress and increase creativity and problem-solving.

See https://www.youtube.com/@NurseYogisPracticesforCaregive/ for examples of brief practices for rest and stress reduction.

WRAPPING UP

In your ANP role, it is essential to fully understand the problem your team is trying to improve prior to initiating EBPQI. Crafting evidence-searching questions that bring you unbiased and complete results will allow you the confidence you need to support evidence-based decision-making. As the leader, your expertise gives you credibility with the rest of the team and other stakeholders you will need to engage for the success of your practice change initiative. It is equally important to show leadership in developing SMART aims. Without measurable, meaningful aims, you and your team (and your organization) will not be able to determine if your EBPQI initiative made a difference. In Chapter 4, we will discuss advanced literature searching so that you can lead your team through searching the evidence with or without the help of a librarian if one is not available to your team. Right now, let's pause and consider the importance of resting briefly before moving on to the next mountain tier together.

REFLECTION QUESTIONS

1. Have you noticed a problem in your clinical setting or organization that needs improvement? If so, try writing an evidence-searching question to identify changes that research has demonstrated to impact the problem. You can use the PICO or PPCO question, or try both to see which brings you better results!
2. Based on the problem you identified for question 1, can you identify something you could measure that would demonstrate a change or an improvement? Write a SMART outcome aim based on that measure.

REFERENCES

American Nurses Foundation. (2022). *Pulse on the nation's nurses survey series: COVID-19 two-year impact assessment survey.*

Bentley, T. G. K., D'Andrea-Penna, G., Rakic, M., Arce, N., LaFaille, M., Berman, R., Cooley, K., & Sprimont, P. (2023). Breathing practices for stress and anxiety reduction: Conceptual framework of implementation guidelines based on a systematic review of the published literature. *Brain Sciences*, *13*(12), 1612. https://doi.org/10.3390/brainsci13121612

Booth, A., Noyes, J., Flemming, K., Moore, G., Tuncalp, O., Shakibazadeh, E. (2023). Formulating questions to explore complex interventions with qualitative evidence synthesis. *BMJ Global Health*, *4*, e001107. https://doi.org/10.1136/bmjgh-2018-001107

Bureau of Labor Statistics. (2024). *Registered nurses.* Occupational Outlook Handbook. https://www.bls.gov/ooh/healthcare/registered-nurses.htm

Centers for Disease Control and Prevention. (n.d.). *Vaccination coverage among young children (0-35 months).* https://www.cdc.gov/vaccines/imz-managers/coverage/childvaxview/interactive-reports/index.html

Centers for Disease Control and Prevention, National Center for Health Statistics. (2023). *Immunizations.* https://www.cdc.gov/nchs/fastats/immunize.htm#:~:text=Diphtheria%2C%20Tetanus%2C%20Pertussis%20(4,(3%2B%20doses)%3A%2091.4%25)

Cullen, L., Hanrahan, K., Farrington, M. M., Tucker, S. J., & Edmonds, S. (2022). *Evidence-based practice in action* (2nd ed.). Sigma Theta Tau International.

Cullen, L., Hanrahan, K., Tucker, S., Edmonds, S. W., & Laures, E. (2023). The Problem With the PICO Question: Shiny Object Syndrome and the PURPOSE Statement Solution. *Journal of perianesthesia nursing: official journal of the American Society of PeriAnesthesia Nurses*, *38*(3), 516–518. https://doi.org/10.1016/j.jopan.2023.01.024

Devantier-Thomas, B., Deakin, G. B., Crowther, F., Schumann, M., & Doma, K. (2024). The impact of exercise-induced muscle damage on various cycling performance metrics: A systematic review and meta-analysis. *Journal of Strength and Conditioning Research*, *38*(8), 1509–1525. https://doi.org/10.1519/JSC.0000000000004629

Doran, G. (1981). There's a S.M.A.R.T. way to write management's goals and objectives. *Management Review*, *70*, 35–36.

Eriksen, M. B., & Frandsen, T. F. (2018). The impact of patient, intervention, comparison, outcome (PICO) as a search strategy tool on literature search quality: A systematic review. *Journal of the Medical Library Association*, *106*(4), 420–431. https://doi.org/10.5195/jmla.2018.345

Huang, X., Lin, J., & Demner-Fushman, D. (2006). Evaluation of PICO as a knowledge representation for clinical questions. *AMIA Annual Symposium Proceedings*, *2006*, 359–363.

Mandlik, G. V., Siopis, G., Nguyen, B., Ding, D., & Edwards, K. M. (2023). Effect of a single session of yoga and meditation on stress reactivity: A systematic review. *Stress and health: Journal of the International Society for the Investigation of Stress*, 40(3), e3324. https://doi.org/10.1002/smi.3324

Melnyk, B., & Fineout-Overholt, E. (2023). *Evidence-based practice in nursing & healthcare: A guide to best practice* (5th ed.). LWW.

Nursing Solutions, Inc. (2023). *2023 NSI national health care retention & RN staffing report.* https://www.nsinursingsolutions.com/Documents/Library/NSI_National_Health_Care_Retention_Report.pdf

Schiavenato, M., & Chu, F. (2021). PICO: What it is and what it is not. *Nurse Education in Practice, 56*, 103194. https://doi.org/10.1016/j.nepr.2021.103194

Waldrop, J., & Dunlap, J. (2024). Beyond PICO—A new question simplifies the search for evidence. *American Journal of Nursing, 124*(3), 34–37. https://doi.org/10.1097/01.NAJ.0001007676.91191.dd

IMAGE CREDITS

Fig. 3.1: Jayne Jennings Dunlap and Julee Briscoe Waldrop, *Introduction to Evidence-Based Practice and Quality Improvement for Professional Nursing Practice: A Competency Based Approach,* p. 55. Copyright © 2024 by Cognella, Inc. Reprinted with permission.

CHAPTER 4

The Leadership Role of the Advanced Nurse in Searching for Evidence

Heather Carter-Templeton, Niki Cobb, Erin Whitaker, Tracy Brewer, and Julee Briscoe Waldrop

KEY CONCEPTS

Evidence hierarchy
Journal
Credibility
Database
Keyword
Inclusion/exclusion criteria
Limitations/filters

LEARNING OBJECTIVES

1. Examine nurse leadership in accessing evidence-based information to inform clinical decisions.
2. Develop a strategy for searching for evidence and scientific literature.
3. Develop and use an evidence-searching question that guides the literature search.
4. Identify various sources of credible evidence for use in practice.
5. Identify the level of evidence within a hierarchy pyramid.

> Facts are stubborn things; and whatever may be our wishes, our inclinations, or the dictates of our passion, they cannot alter the state of facts and evidence.
>
> —John Adams

Introduction

Nurses in leadership and advanced practice roles must be able to function in ever-evolving, high-tech, and high-touch settings. To deliver the best possible care, you must be able to locate, assess, synthesize, and apply evidence and findings from scientific literature; in other words, you must be information literate. Information literacy skills can be considered a precursor to EBP.

Nurses in advanced roles translate current evidence-based information into best practices and clinical decisions across all health care settings; however, there continues to be an estimated gap of 17 years between research and subsequent practice change (Balas & Boren, 2000; Borsky et al., 2018). As discussed in Chapter 3, as a nurse leader, you play a key role in identifying problems affecting patients, populations, and health-related organizations, but you must also seek and find reliable evidence to solve those problems. In this chapter, we will focus on how to identify evidence sources by type, strength, and placement within the evidence hierarchy. In order to apply what you learned in Chapter 3, you must search for evidence through a systematic process that involves keywords related to a focused evidence-searching question about a specific issue or topic.

Nurses and clinicians cultivate numerous questions at the point of care every day. Surprisingly, only 51% of clinicians seek answers to these questions, although at least one question arises for every two patients seen (Del Fiol et al., 2014). Common barriers or obstacles to the pursuit of solutions to clinical questions include care providers' lack of (a) time, (b) skill at seeking information, (c) access to information, (d) authority to make changes, and (e) guidance. As a nurse leader in an advanced role, it is your obligation to seek answers to clinical questions, regardless of barriers, to ensure health care quality and safety.

Internet search engines often provide less reliable search results. Google, a common search engine, indexes web pages; it can be a great resource for searching websites and web pages but not for locating evidence-based information. The use of Google Scholar in searching for scientific evidence has been debated; it can assist in searching but will likely miss important and relevant information. Google and Google Scholar provide an easy search interface, but both are limited to openly available information found on the web. Additionally, Google searches are often overwhelming in quantity, and their accuracy or truthfulness can be difficult to verify due to search flaws, low quality of site content, and numerous other reasons. Most scientific research relies on scholarly databases, many of which require a subscription.

More sophisticated forms of artificial intelligence (AI), such as generative AI, are rapidly expanding into clinical practice and other areas of health care; Google's Gemini or ChatGPT are examples. Again, these resources are easy to use but may not provide the most credible information. Any information found through these tools must be verified for accuracy, which undermines the convenience and swiftness of the search (Hostetler et al., 2024).

Evidence can be derived from primary, secondary, or tertiary sources. A *primary source* is the report of an original research study written by those who conducted the study. After the original study results have been published, *secondary sources* are written by scholars other than the original authors with the aim of (a) appraising the research, (b) reviewing the research, or (c) developing recommendations. A *tertiary source* (e.g., textbook, organizational report, practice guideline) reports on secondary and primary sources depending on their methods.

Information literacy, a key to providing care based on evidence (Carter-Templeton, 2013), involves finding information and critically appraising, synthesizing, and applying it (the next chapters address this process further). In 2013, the Association of College & Research Libraries (ACRL, 2013) released information literacy competency standards specific to the skills, resources, and language that nurses need to promote and ensure EBP (Adams, 2014). Information-literate nurses must know how to clearly define or describe the subject or concept to be examined, use suitable terminology, and formulate a search strategy to retrieve evidence; this strategy may include using online bibliographic databases and entering a combination of keywords and Boolean operators (AND, OR, NOT) to search for relevant and appropriate resources. Also required are critical thinking skills to (a) assess the information collected for value and suitability, and (b) potentially convert that information into knowledge. **Librarians** are experts in information literacy and can provide vital assistance in searching and retrieving various types of evidence. Consulting a librarian can save you significant time and produce valuable information. If you do not have access to a librarian in your academic or practice setting, you can seek out trusted mentors to help you with this process. We discuss mentorship in detail in Chapter 13.

Hierarchy of Evidence

As discussed in Chapter 1, all evidence is not of equal quality. Characteristics of research studies are evaluated hierarchically to classify or categorize the quality of evidence. There are many examples of evidence pyramids in the literature, with slight differences among them regarding what is included at each level; however, all are similar in their general categories and the increased rigor of levels from the bottom to the top of the pyramid. Consider the hierarchy of evidence pyramid in Figure 4.1. The design of the research study is the primary characteristic included, and there are various types of evidence at each level of the pyramid. Note that the rigor of study design increases as you move up the pyramid; this is only one aspect of the quality of evidence, however. You will learn more about evaluating your evidence's quality in Chapters 5, 6, and 7.

Note that the hierarchy pyramid is divided into two segments: The top segment, or point of the pyramid, refers to filtered or pre-appraised synthesized evidence based on experimental research studies (usually RCTs) known as **systematic reviews**. The pyramid tip includes the highest level of systematic review: a meta-analysis of an outcome from multiple RCTs. Of note, systematic reviews of qualitative studies and studies that are not RCTs are increasing in the nursing literature. Although these systematic reviews offer a synthesis based on the included studies, they describe associations rather than cause and effect (e.g., the review includes cohort studies) or a phenomenon (e.g., the review includes qualitative studies), and their quality reflects the level of the included research studies.

Also included at the top of the pyramid are evidence-based guidelines based on systematic reviews. These types of evidence are described as **secondary sources**. Notice that the pyramid tip is small, signifying that less evidence is available at this high level. The lower segment includes individual research studies based on study design. For example, an RCT (as discussed in Chapter 1) using experimental designs will most likely predict cause and effect between an intervention and outcome; thus, it is higher on the pyramid. A cohort study or a qualitative study intended

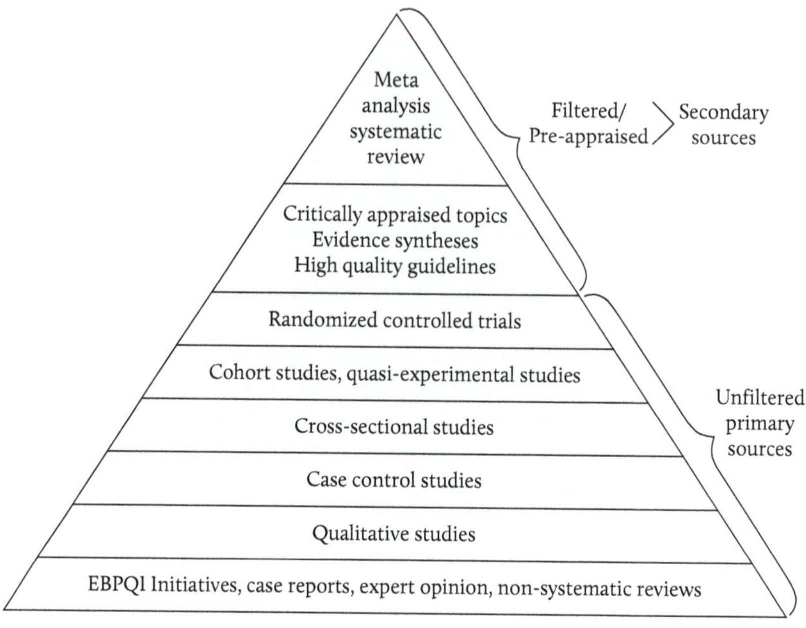

FIGURE 4.1 Hierarchy of evidence pyramid.

to describe the characteristics of a phenomenon or individual variable implies associations but not cause and effect; therefore, these are lower on the pyramid.

Individual studies are considered **primary sources**. You will learn more about how to lead your team in critically appraising systematic reviews and quantitative experimental research studies in Chapter 5, and qualitative research studies in Chapter 6. The bottom tier of the pyramid is considered foundational and includes nonresearch and other types of evidence. Note the broadness at the pyramid's base, signifying how much more of this type of evidence exists. In Chapter 7, we discuss in depth how to explore and lead critical appraisal of various types of nonresearch and other evidence.

Each pyramid level can provide evidence essential to answering a clinical question. Regardless of the tier or level to which a type of research evidence belongs, your team must consider the amount of risk or harm associated with the intervention(s) or practice changes the evidence describes. The level of evidence you are willing to consider for making a practice change will be determined by the potential risk of harm or adverse events associated with the interventions in the evidence (Dang et al., 2022; Melnyk & Fineout-Overhold, 2023). For example, findings based on systematic reviews of RCTs will garner more confidence if the quality of the systematic review is high. Most nursing interventions do not carry a high risk of harm or lend themselves to RCTs, so very few systematic reviews exist on nursing care practices. Although the evidence you find will most likely be from the lower tiers of the pyramid, this evidence will still be valuable to your decision-making as you strive to provide the safest possible patient care.

From Evidence-Searching Question to Searching the Literature

Cultivating inquiry in ANP is critical. In previous chapters, you learned that the purpose of your formatted question is to aid your search for the best external (research) literature. You also learned that it is essential to take time to develop a clear searching question for your clinical issue because your search strategy will use terms from the question to conduct a precise and unbiased search. Let's consider a hypothetical evidence search based on a potential clinical situation that a nurse practitioner might encounter.

Suppose that as a family nurse practitioner, you commonly provide care to older adults with varying levels of cognitive ability. In your practice, you frequently see older adults with mild cognitive impairment, a stage between normal aging and early dementia. You want to provide information and resources to your patients, so exploring ideas to assist them with this aging process may be helpful. Many activities may have been determined to be helpful, but you are specifically interested in the effectiveness of web-based cognitive training activities. However, you want to further explore these activities and their impact on cognitive function before recommending them to patients. You start by carefully structuring a PPCO question:

In older adults with identified mild cognitive impairment, does participation in web-based cognitive training activities impact cognitive function?

In this question, we have identified the following:

- P = mild cognitive impairment
- P = older adults
- C = web-based cognitive training activities
- O = cognitive function and dementia progression

Inclusion and Exclusion Criteria

Before beginning a database search, you must specify which types of evidence to include or exclude from your search. **Inclusion criteria** are the detailed study characteristics that a research report must include to be appropriate for your issue and context (Stern & McArthur, 2014). For example, you may determine inclusion criteria based on the following:

- study design types (e.g., systematic reviews, RCTs, phenomenology)
- participant or population characteristics (e.g., age, sex, race/ethnicity, diagnosis, location)
- intervention types or issues of interest (e.g., specific therapy, exposure, risk behavior)
- outcome measure types (e.g., outcomes expected from the intervention or clinical change, risk of disease, rate of adverse events, types of measurement)

Exclusion criteria must also be identified before you begin your search (Stern & McArthur, 2014). **Exclusion criteria** are those characteristics that will result in a study being excluded from your search because they will not help answer your question. For example, if you are looking for studies on patients 60 years of age or older with mild cognitive impairment, you will exclude studies that focus on those who are younger than age 60.

Filters

Inclusion and exclusion criteria are often confused with database filters, which serve different purposes. **Filters** (also referred to as limiters) are applied to narrow the evidence *returned from your search* to make it more relevant to answering your question. Filters are applied to the database *before* reviewing individual article results. For example, you can use filtering to narrow a search by study design (RCTs, systematic review), publication type (journal article, book), language (English), publication year, population age, or full text–only options (Hartzell et al., 2023). However, be careful not to apply too many filters, or you may exclude relevant information (Dang et al., 2022).

Using the PPCO question that you developed for identifying the impact of web-based cognitive training activities, apply inclusion and exclusion criteria relevant to the search. Broadening initial inclusion/exclusion criteria is recommended to avoid missing important articles or reports. There are several ways to define each element of the PPCO to establish your inclusion/exclusion criteria. Consider the characteristics and criteria choices in Table 4.1.

There are a few other criteria that you may want to consider when determining the best evidence to include. Setting is often a relevant aspect of determining inclusion or exclusion. Other factors may be the publication date and study design.

TABLE 4.1 Inclusion/Exclusion Criteria

PPCO Element	Criteria	Include	Exclude
Problem	Mild cognitive impairment	Mild cognitive impairment	Severe cognitive impairment Alzheimer's disease Other specific forms of dementia
Population	Older patients	Adults (≥ 60 years of age)	Adults (< 60 years of age)
Change	Participation in web-based cognitive training activities	All types of web-based cognitive training activities	Cognitive training activities not offered in a web-based format
Outcome	Cognitive function	Any study that reported cognitive function	No report of cognitive function

To summarize, inclusion and exclusion criteria are used to improve the relevance of the literature you collect. You must define each element of your PPCO question specific to your inquiry before deciding on the criteria that will predetermine the characteristics of studies included or excluded from your search results. Specified study characteristics for inclusion/exclusion are not easily searched with keywords (i.e., filters/limits you would apply for database searching). You will need to read, at a minimum, the title and abstract to decide whether to include or exclude an article. If precise interpretation is required, you may need to screen the full-text article.

Fundamentals of Database Searching

Once you have determined your PPCO question and identified your inclusion and exclusion criteria, the next step is to build your search strategy. Let's discuss the elements and mechanics of database searching.

A term you will frequently encounter during your search is **article**. An article is a publication that gathers and synthesizes information about a specific topic, study, or subject. In terms of the hierarchy of evidence, articles encompass all the types of evidence you seek. As you gather evidence, it is essential to remember that all works contain inherent biases (effects of factors or assumptions that skew viewpoints, findings, or outcomes). For example, an article will include information that the author *wants* us to understand, but the details of the article (the journal in which it appears, who wrote it, who published it, whether any organization funded it) provide clues as to its credibility. **Credibility** is the reliability of a source. To determine a source's credibility, we must ask questions such as "Can this source be trusted?" and "Why should one trust this source?" Both information and disinformation are readily available, and it can be challenging to distinguish credible sources and evidence from suspect ones. Fortunately, we can offer a tip to help you choose wisely: Consider whether an article has been vetted through a peer-review process and published in a respected scholarly journal.

Peer review is a process that ensures integrity in publication. After an article is submitted for publication, the editor sends it to experts (peer reviewers) in the discipline who read it and assess its credibility. Peer reviewers provide comments, questions, and suggestions based on their expertise. This process helps to ensure that an article's information is factual and well represented and adheres to the field's conventions. You will learn more about peer review in Chapter 12.

As you begin searching the literature, you will notice that many articles are published in **journals**. Journals are serial publications comprised of articles and other works by experts in a specific field or fields. There are many nursing-specific journals, such as *The American Journal of Nursing*, as well as specialty-specific journals, such as *The Journal for Nurse Practitioners*. Each journal issue generally includes peer-reviewed articles and some nonpeer-reviewed material relevant to the discipline, such as editorials and commentaries. Unfortunately, some journals do not provide true peer review or editorial services and thus do not meet publishing and editorial standards. Although not foolproof, using reputable databases decreases your chance of finding this type of journal during your search (Oermann et al., 2022).

Some material, referred to as **gray literature**, are published to be shared with a specific disciplinary audience but are not formally peer reviewed or published in scholarly channels such as journals, trade publications, or periodicals. Gray literature includes material such as dissertations, preprints, whitepapers, and conference proceedings; these can be good sources of evidence when you have assessed their credibility.

Selection of Databases

Journals and articles can often be discovered in **databases**. Databases are collections of resources (e.g., journals, trade publications, and periodicals) that are curated, typically electronic, and frequently updated. Databases will likely yield the most relevant, high-quality evidence to answer your clinical question. Typically, databases are subject specific. Database collections are often housed on **platforms**. Platforms allow users to search a single database or several simultaneously, if they are owned by the same companies. Some databases are free to the public; others require a subscription.

PubMed

PubMed is a publicly available government site (pubmed.gov) and a premier biomedical, health, and life sciences literature search system. PubMed was created and is maintained by the National Center for Biotechnology Information (NCBI) at the U.S. National Library of Medicine (NLM), located at the National Institutes of Health (NIH), which serves as an agency under the U.S. Department of Health & Human Services (HHS). PubMed provides over 35 million citations and is an excellent resource for locating research and other evidence (National Library of Medicine, n.d.a.). Full-text content for some articles may be available from PubMed Central (a free public database) or publisher websites; other articles may require subscription access from the publisher or database platform site to view the full content. You can contact your academic, institutional, or public library for assistance with accessing full-text content. A primary component of PubMed is MEDLINE, NLM's premier bibliographic database, which provides nearly 30 million biomedical references indexed using NLM's (n.d.b.) Medical Subject Headings (MeSH as n.d.c.).

Subject headings aid users in locating materials by using a set of terms or phrases known as controlled vocabulary (EBSCO, n.d.). Some advantages of subject headings are that they reveal specific terms used when classifying articles and provide additional headings or subheadings for your search. **MeSH** are subject headings developed and cataloged by a team of reviewers to help users identify related resources within the MEDLINE database. As the MEDLINE database serves as a component of PubMed, MeSH terms can be used to search within the PubMed database along with keywords (NLM, n.d.d.). You will learn more about subject headings and see an example for searching with MeSH terms later in this chapter.

PubMed's interface has several beneficial features, such as the visibility of similar resources for full-text records and the creation of an NCBI account for saving, organizing, and receiving updates about saved searches and citations. Your NCBI account can be used across several NLM databases (NLM, n.d.c.). PubMed and other databases have similarities and specific differences related to their use.

CINAHL Complete

CINAHL Complete is the Cumulative Indexes of Nursing and Allied Health Literature databases. Access is provided through their EBSCO platform. CINHAL is an excellent resource for research and other evidence; it provides an authoritative index of nursing and allied health journals, and content for over 7,000 journals (EBSCO, n.d.). CINAHL Complete also allows access to CINHAL subject headings, which use controlled vocabulary with a hierarchical arrangement of terms for indexing articles and are similar to PubMed's MeSH (ESBCO, n.d.). CINAHL is a subscription-based resource (access to full-text articles requires payment). It can be helpful to consult with your librarian (if you have access to this resource) for assistance in locating articles within this database.

Cochrane Library

The Cochrane Library is an excellent resource for locating systematic reviews and other resources. The Cochrane Library, published by Wiley, consists of multiple databases provided by Cochrane, an international network that provides evidence to support medical and health care decision-making. The Cochrane Library databases include the Cochrane Database of Systematic Reviews (CDSR), Cochrane Central Register of Controlled Trials (CENTRAL), and Cochrane Clinical Answers. These databases provide featured content in special collections on curated topics and allow the user to search for content provided by the McMaster Health Forum's repositories: Health Systems Evidence (HSE) and Social Systems Evidence (SSE) (Cochrane Library, n.d.). Table 4.2 provides links to tutorials for up-to-date training on how to use them.

TABLE 4.2 Resources on How to Search Databases

Database	Defining Characteristics	Link to Training Tutorial
PubMed	Multilanguage, international database A free resource supporting the search and retrieval of biomedical and life science literature Contains 35 million citations and abstracts of biomedical literature PubMed is provided by the NLM, the NCBI, and the NIH	Online Training https://learn.nlm.nih.gov/documentation/training-packets/T0042010P/ PubMed YouTube playlist (English) https://www.youtube.com/playlist?list=PL7dF9e2qSW0YkmxDTsUG6p4hJjYOPT0Uj PubMed YouTube playlist (Spanish) https://www.youtube.com/playlist?list=PL7dF9e2qSW0Y8MqgB0rLnrJH-ypnsj00H

(*Continued*)

TABLE 4.2 *(Continued)*

CINAHL Complete	CINAHL is the acronym for Cumulative Index of Nursing and Allied Health Literature Contains journals in nursing and 17 allied health fields, as well as biomedicine and consumer health Additional topics include exercise science, health administration, nursing education, and public health Contains journal articles, ebooks, evidence-based care sheets, quick lessons, legal cases, clinical trials, gray literature, etc. Audience: nurses, medical personnel, social workers, counselors, occupational therapists, physical therapists, speech therapists, audiologists, etc. Contains literature back to 1937 Provides a search term thesaurus for searching literature in nursing and allied fields	CINAHL YouTube video training https://www.youtube.com/results?search_query=cinahl+database+ebsco+channel Basic Searching PowerPoint and video https://connect.ebsco.com/s/article/CINAHL-Databases-Basic-Searching-Tutorial?language=en_US Advanced Search PowerPoint and video https://connect.ebsco.com/s/article/CINAHL-Databases-Advanced-Searching-Tutorial?language=en_US CINAHL and MeSH Headings PowerPoint and video https://connect.ebsco.com/s/article/Using-the-CINAHL-MeSH-Headings-Feature-in-EBSCOhost-Tutorial?language=en_US
Cochrane Library	Cochrane Library is a collection of databases containing the leading resources for high-quality systematic reviews in health care Cochrane reviews are peer reviewed Contains the *Cochrane Handbook for System Reviews of Interventions* and the *Cochrane Handbook for Diagnostic Test Accuracy Reviews* Contains the Cochrane Central Register of Controlled Trials (CENTRAL) and the Cochrane Clinical Answers for "actionable" point-of-care decision-making	Cochrane Library Users Guide PowerPoint https://www.wiley.com/en-us/customer-success/cochrane/cochrane-library-user-guide How to Use Cochrane PICO search PowerPoint https://www.wiley.com/en-us/customer-success/cochrane/how-to-use-pico-search Cochrane Training: Learning Live https://training.cochrane.org/learning-events/learning-live

Building the Search Strategy

To begin your search, you will use the elements of your clinical question to select keywords and synonyms that align with your search goals. After determining search terms, you will use operators and search strategy enhancers to perform your search in a database or platform. Most databases are configured to run keyword searches. Unlike platforms such as Google, which allow users to phrase searches in the form of questions (natural language to most users), many databases require users to compile searches of essential words or phrases. For example, suppose you wanted to search for sources on the PPCO question we considered earlier. The terms "older adults," "mild cognitive impairment," and "web-based cognitive training activities" would be acceptable keywords to form your search. Synonyms for these keywords could also be included.

Some databases allow users to search sets of predefined words and phrases called subject headings. **Subject headings** are control vocabulary used by a database or platform to index articles relevant to a specific term or specialization, substance, or publication type. Not every article may be indexed by subject headings, so we always use them combined with keywords. The primary function of keywords is to enhance the search in combination with the subject headings. Combining your subject headings with your keywords will increase the possibility of capturing articles related to your topic, which could be missed by your keyword search strategy alone.

You can use words like AND, OR, and NOT to connect your search terms. These terms are called **Boolean operators** and indicate the relationship between your search's keywords, phrases, or subject headings (Figure 4.2). Adding the operator AND to your search will tell the platform or database that you want to include both terms. For example, you might combine the terms "cognitive training activities" AND "web-based" to expand your results. The operator OR indicates to the platform that you want your search to include results that cover two or more terms. For example, you could search for "patient" OR "inpatient" to widen your search net. Finally, the operator NOT tells the platform or database that you want to exclude results. For example, if you searched "elderly," NOT "adults," your results would include items related to persons who are elderly (according to the authors) but not to an adult population alone.

Using our PPCO question from the beginning of this chapter, we could simply search for "mild cognitive impairment," but it is unlikely that this would return relevant results. However, combining terms using Boolean operators would make the results more focused. The more Boolean operators your search contains, the narrower your search becomes.

Finally, **truncation, quotation marks, and parentheses (TQP)** can be used to refine your search strategy, especially in combination with Boolean operators. These concepts are described in more detail in Table 4.3.

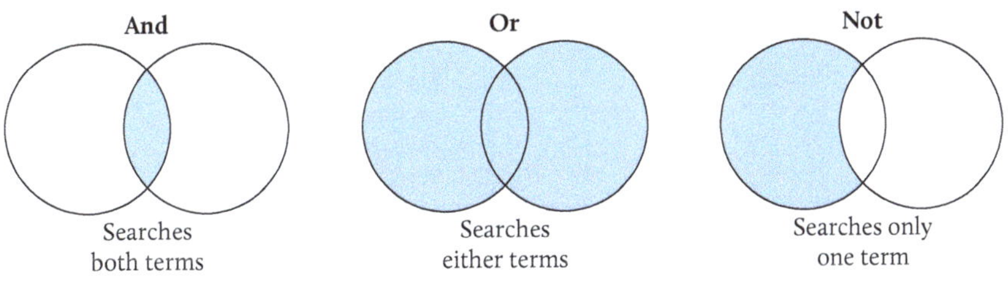

FIGURE 4.2 Boolean operator diagrams.

TABLE 4.3 TQP Functions

Function	Symbol	Example	Purpose
Truncation	*	impair* = impair, impaired, impairment, etc.	Truncating a search term lets a database platform know that you are looking for results that have multiple endings of the key word
Quotation marks	Be sure to use straight quote marks instead of the traditional curly quotes	"mild cognitive impairment"	Using quotation marks around a search term lets the database platform know that you want to search the term as a phrase rather than each of the words individually
Parentheses	( )	cognitive training* AND (web-based* OR electronic*)	Using parentheses around search terms allows you to keep terms together. The database platform looks for the terms "web-based" or "electronic" along with the first term "cognitive"

Searching for Evidence

Using your PPCO search terms, you can begin to arrange your terms using the Boolean operators AND, OR, and NOT. Table 4.4 shows an example of a concept table that you can use to arrange your PPCO keywords.

TABLE 4.4 Example Concept Table for Developing Keywords for Searching

	Concept 1 Problem	Concept 2 Population	Concept 3 Change	Concept 4 Outcome
	Mild cognitive impairment	Elderly	Web-based Strategies	Cognitive ability
Keywords (synonyms)	Mild cognitive impair* Mild dementia	Elderly Older adults	Web-based cognitive training Electronic cognitive training Web-based exercises Web-based strategies	Cognitive ability

If we were to break down our PPCO question into search terms using the methods described, it might look something like this:

Problem: mild cognitive impair*

Population: elderly*

Change: "cognitive training*" AND ("web-based*" OR "electronic*")

Outcome: cognitive ability

Searching a Database Using Your Keywords and Terms

When you perform a search in PubMed or other databases, you will find a search box or boxes in which to insert your keywords. For example, PubMed has a simple search box and an advanced search builder. Usually, you want to use advanced search builders because they allow more options for your search strategy. Depending on the database, you can apply filters and limiters at the onset.

A simple search in PubMed based only on your PPCO question words "elderly AND mild cognitive impairment OR cognitive impairment AND cognitive training" yields 7,099 results. If you use the building blocks approach and PubMed's advanced search builder, your search will look like this: (elderly* AND mild cognitive impairment AND cognitive training). There will be 2,009 article citations retrieved with this more specific search process. Further specification (elderly* AND mild cognitive impairment AND cognitive training AND web-based) yields 19 results. You can add limiters, such as publication dates or types of studies, such as reviews. If your team's results are too narrow, you can always broaden them by eliminating one of the terms or changing a Boolean operator (e.g., AND to OR).

Information Access

During your search, you may come across resources behind **paywalls**. Access to an article behind a paywall requires payment or a subscription. If you have access to a librarian, make sure to consult with them before paying; your institution may have or be able to obtain access to the resource. If not, your librarian can often find an accessible alternative resource.

Conversely, some resources are **open access**. Open access refers to resources that are publicly available at no cost. These resources do not require an institutional affiliation to read or download; access to them does not depend on whether your university, college, hospital, or organization has a subscription. You should be aware, however, that a payment has been made to keep them open to all. Many governmental organizations that fund research with taxpayer dollars now mandate that researchers publish in open-access journals. The rationale is that if the public (taxpayers) have paid for the research, they deserve to be able to read it and know the results.

As you consider sources with paid and open access, it is essential to remember that one is not inherently more authoritative or credible than the other. Just because an article is behind a paywall does not mean that it will be of better quality or more beneficial for your practice than an open-access article. You must lead your team in investigating the reliability and relevance of evidence through critical appraisal (Chapters 5, 6, and 7).

The Librarian as a Resource

Ultimately, your expert librarian is one of your greatest assets during your search process. Just as you will be an expert in your nursing practice, librarians are experts at searching for evidence. As illustrated in this chapter, you and your librarian can create sophisticated search strategies together using the combined knowledge of your fields. Librarians can provide various resources and related materials to grow your search abilities.

Librarians often curate subject-specific lists of resources called **research guides**. These guides (called LibGuides at some institutions) are updated consistently with information about the subjects they cover. Research guides typically also include information about contacting your librarians, tips for research and writing, and database tutorials (many of which are free to access).

Finishing Up the Search Process

After searching select databases for evidence, don't forget to review your list of potential articles with regard to the inclusion/exclusion criteria. Let's say that the following are two of the articles found in your search. You must read the abstract or summary of the article to determine whether it meets your inclusion criteria or should be excluded.

- "Examining Internet and eHealth Practices and Preferences: Survey Study of Australian Older Adults With Subjective Memory Complaints, Mild Cognitive Impairment, or Dementia." https://pubmed.ncbi.nlm.nih.gov/29070481/

  After reading the abstract, you might decide to exclude the article even though it meets the inclusion criteria related to the intervention (web-based cognitive training). However, the population extends to 50-year-olds and up.

- "Web-Based Intervention Effects on Mild Cognitive Impairment Based on Apolipoprotein E Genotype: Quasi-Experimental Study."https://pubmed.ncbi.nlm.nih.gov/32379048/

After reading the abstract, you determine that the article meets all the inclusion criteria established. You will want to read this one not only for evidence but to integrate important aspects of their project with your EBPQI initiative.

You may wonder, "How can I keep track of all the articles I read and review and determine which ones should be included or excluded?" As team leader, you can make this easy for everyone by setting up a Google spreadsheet. Each article you or a team member review should be included on the spreadsheet and sorted by date, with the most recent publications at the top. A final decision column and notes about your rationale for inclusion or exclusion will be necessary for final team decisions. You can even color code the boxes with a drop-down choice. Figure 4.3 is an example.

Next Step: Critical Appraisal

Critical appraisal is the process of evaluating a study or piece of literature for its worth. When we critically appraise a piece of evidence, we always ask the following:

- Can the work be duplicated under similar conditions? (**reliability**)
- Are the results a true reflection of what they are intended to measure? (**validity**)
- Is this work applicable to the issue I am wondering about? (**applicability**)

Critical appraisal is a vital and fundamental skill for making sound recommendations about evidence obtained through an EBP-approach to decision-making. Critically appraising a piece of literature accomplishes several things: It helps you to gain a deeper understanding of the research (particularly of the quality and strength of the evidence), and it helps you to decide whether the evidence provided is needed to answer your question.

Unfortunately, critical appraisal may be skipped or overlooked in real-world settings because nurses often view it as one of the most difficult steps in EBP and feel that they lack the skill or competence to perform it (Melnyk et al., 2014). Omitting critical appraisal from the EBP process creates a dangerous situation in which poorly conducted work (research, literature reviews, some quality improvement and EBP initiatives) or inadequate evidence may be used to inform decisions, thus placing the patients, clinicians, organizations, and communities served at risk for less than best outcomes. As a nurse leader, your abilities in this area can help you to model the necessity of critically appraising all the evidence you use to justify a practice change intended to impact patient outcomes.

The next three chapters will guide you in critically appraising (a) quantitative research evidence (Chapter 5), (b) qualitative research evidence (Chapter 6), and (c) other types of evidence (Chapter 7).

#	**Reference** (APA citation)	**Problem**	**Population** (Target population characteristics (e.g., age, sex/ gender, diagnosis as well, as any other relevant factors)	**Change** (Description of the strategy or practice change being implemented or investigated)	**Date Range** (Use recent publications to support your EBPQI)	**Setting** (The environment and context in which the study was conducted)	**Study Design** (Appropriate study design for the aim of the study)	**Outcome Measures** (Use of validated and reliable measurement tools to obtain and examine measurable outcomes (clinical, behavioral))	**Overall Determination**	**Rationale** (Can provide a brief note about why you included or excluded the article; its particular relevance for your project; or why you included the article if it met exclusion criteria)
	Questions to ask to determine if the article is an include or exclude:	*Does the article focus on the problem you have identified?*	*Does the sample described align with your evidence searching question?*	*Does the practice change address the problem?*	*Publication date (year)*	*Is the setting similar to where you want to conduct your EBPQI*	*Heirarch of Evidence can be include here*	*Are the outcomes relevant for your EBPQI project?*	*Are you going to include or exclude the article?*	*Why did you include or exclude the article?*
1	Tsolaki, A. C., et al.,. (2020). Web-Based Intervention Effects on Mild Cognitive Impairment Based on Apolipoprotein E Genotype: Quasi-Experimental Study. *Journal of medical Internet research, 22* (5), e14617. https://doi.org/10.2196/14617.	Yes	Include	Include	Include	Include	Include	Include	Include	Although a quasi-experimental study, this type of intervention is hard to blind from participants and researchers. Many reliable and valid cognitive outcomes were measured.
2	LaMonica, H. M., et al.. (2017). Examining Internet and eHealth Practices and Preferences: Survey Study of Australian Older Adults With Subjective Memory Complaints, Mild Cognitive Impairment, or Dementia. Journal of medical Internet research, 19(10), e358.	Yes	Exclude	Exclude	Include	Exclude	Exclude	Exclude	Exclude	The sample includes adults > 50 years old. It was conducted in person at a memory focused clinic. There is no intervention or training. This is a descriptive correlational study.
3										
4										

FIGURE 4.3 Inclusion/exclusion table.

WELLNESS IN ACTION: HABITS

Habits are skills and learning that result from repetition and attention. You do many things daily that have become so routine that you don't even think about them. For better or worse, these are your habits. Changing habits can be hard because one's brain resists making the extra effort required to change; it takes far less energy to continue doing things in the same habitual way. Suppose you want to develop a new habit, though. How long it will take to lock in your new habit will depend on the complexity of the new behavior and your individual circumstances? For example, performing regular exercise is considered one of the hardest habits to establish (Buyalskaya et al., 2023).

Habits are a skill set; we can learn or change them, just as we learned to assess vital signs (Duhigg, 2014). One way is to start with mini habits. A **mini habit** refers to a short period (1–5 minutes) of doing whatever it is that you want to become a habit. The most important thing about mini habits is that they build consistency; prioritize consistency over intensity. Over time, consistency will build confidence and self-efficacy—a belief in your ability to influence an outcome. Action, builds motivation, and motivation follows action. So just get started! Our brains don't always like to start healthy habits, but they usually love continuing them (Guise & Penz, 2021). Consider the following three tips for building mini habits:

- Link your new habit to one you already have (i.e., tell yourself that after you perform a current habit or cue, you will add the new one).
- Celebrate progress by rewarding yourself, because you will initially need positive reinforcement.
- Only try to develop two to four mini habits at a time.

WRAPPING UP

After reading and participating in this chapter, we encourage you to review and reflect on your newly acquired literature-searching knowledge and skills. You will learn more in the next chapters about the critical appraisal of various types of evidence that you may have accessed or will access in the future. Remember that although literature searching takes time and practice, your investment in this valuable EBP step constitutes a precious gift to your team and the people for whom you provide care. This skill set will allow you to emerge as a leader in the nursing profession, with hands-on practice experience leading literature searches. As a nurse leader, you must be able to assist your team in finding and appraising the best current evidence to answer new clinical questions as they arise. Moreover, you must model an active involvement and meticulous adherence to high standards that will inspire others to make these values into habits.

REFLECTION QUESTIONS

1. Why must nurse leaders and advanced practice nurses know when to access literature/evidence to answer clinical questions?
2. How can you mentor other nurses in learning about literature/evidence searching to hone the skills discussed in this chapter?
3. When a problem arises, how can you role-model and support other nurses in exploring the evidence to determine whether a practice change is needed?

REFERENCES

Adams, N. E. (2014). A comparison of evidence-based practice and the ACRL information literacy standards: Implications for information literacy practice. *College & Research Libraries, 75*(2), 232–248.

Association of College & Research Libraries. (2013, October). *Information literacy competency standards for nursing.* American Library Association. https://www.ala.org/acrl/standards/nursing

Balas, E. A., & Boren, S. A. (2000). Managing clinical knowledge for health care improvement. *Yearbook of Medical Informatics*, (1), 65–70.

Borsky, A., Zhan, C., Miller, T., Ngo-Metzger, Q., Bierman, A. S., & Meyers, D. (2018). Few Americans receive all high-priority, appropriate clinical preventive services. *Health Affairs, 37*(6), 925–928.

Buyalskaya, A., Ho, H., Milkman, K. L., Li, X., Duckworth, A. & Camerer, C. (2023). What can machine learning teach us about habit formation? Evidence from exercise and hygiene. *Proceedings of the National Academies of Science, 120*(17), e2216115120. https://doi.org/10.1073/pnas.2216115120

Carter-Templeton H. (2013). Nurses' information appraisal within the clinical setting. *Comput Inform Nurs., 31*(4), 167–175. https://doi.org/10.1097/NXN.0b013e31828l2ef6

Cochrane Library. (n.d.). *About.* https://www.cochranelibrary.com/about/about-cochrane-library

Dang, D., Dearholt, S., Bissett, K., Ascenzi, J., & Whalen, M. (2022). *Johns Hopkins evidence-based practice for nurses and healthcare professionals: Models and guidelines* (4th ed.). Sigma Theta Tau International.

Del Fiol, G., Workman, T. E., & Gorman, P. N. (2014). Clinical questions raised by clinicians at the point of care: A systematic review. *JAMA International Medicine, 174*(5), 710–718.

Duhigg, C. (2014). *The Power of Habit.* Random House.

EBSCO. (n.d.). *CINAHL database.* https://www.ebsco.com/products/research-databases/cinahl-database#:~:text=CINAHL%20includes%201%2C314%20journals%20with%20searchable%20cited%20references

Elliott, A. F., Horgas, A. L., & Marsiske, M. (2008). Nurses' role in identifying mild cognitive impairment in older adults. *Geriatric Nursing, 29*(1), 38–47. https://doi.org/10.1016/j.gerinurse.2007.04.015

Guise, S. & Penz, D. (2021). *Mini Habits: Smaller Habits, Bigger Results.* Selective Entertainment LLC.

Hartzell, T. A., Fineout-Overholt, E., & Kelley, C. B. (2023). Finding relevant evidence to answer clinical questions. In Melnyk, B. & Fineout-Overholt, E. (Eds.), *Evidence-based practice in nursing & healthcare: A guide to best practice* (5th ed., p. 89). Wolters Kluwer.

Hillier, M. D. (2020). Using effective hand hygiene practice to prevent and control infection. *Nursing Standard, 35*(5), 45–50. https://doi.org/10.7748/ns.2020.e11552

Hostetler, T., Owens, J. K., Waldrop, J., Oermann, M. H., & Carter-Templeton, H. (2024). Generative artificial intelligence detectors and accuracy: Implications for nurses. *CIN: Computers, Informatics, Nursing 42*(5), 315–319. https://doi.org/10.1097/CIN.0000000000001134

LaMonica, H. M., et al. (2017). Examining internet and eHealth practices and preferences: Survey study of Australian older adults with subjective memory complaints, mild cognitive impairment, or dementia. *Journal of Medical Internet Research, 19*(10), e358. https://doi.org/10.2196/jmir.7981

McClinton, T. D. (2022) A guided search: Formulating a PICOT from assigned areas of inquiry. *Worldviews on Evidence-Based Nursing, 19*, 426–427. https://doi.org/10.1111/wvn.12598

Melnyk, B., & Fineout-Overholt, E. (2023). Making the case for evidence-based practice and cultivating a spirit of Inquiry. In Melnyk, B. & Fineout-Overholt, E. (Eds.), *Evidence-based practice in nursing & healthcare: A guide to best practice* (5th ed., pp. 22–23). Wolters Kluwer.

Melnyk, B. M., Gallagher-Ford, L., Long, L. E., & Fineout-Overholt, E. (2014). The establishment of evidence-based practice competencies for practicing registered nurses and advanced practice nurses in real-world clinical settings: Proficiencies to improve healthcare quality, reliability, patient outcomes, and costs. *Worldviews on Evidence-Based Nursing, 11*(1), 5–15. https://doi.org/10.1111/wvn.12021

National Library of Medicine. (n.d.a.). *Medical subject headings.* https://www.nlm.nih.gov/mesh/meshhome.html

National Library of Medicine. (n.d.b.). *Medline overview.* https://www.nlm.nih.gov/medline/medline_overview.html

National Library of Medicine. (n.d.c.). *My NCBI help.* https://www.ncbi.nlm.nih.gov/books/NBK3842/#MyNCBI.What_Is_My_NCBI

National Library of Medicine. (n.d.d.). *PubMed overview.* https://pubmed.ncbi.nlm.nih.gov/about/

Nelson, R. (2020). Informatics: Evolution of the Nelson data, information, knowledge and wisdom model: Part 2. *The Online Journal of Issues in Nursing, 25(3).* https://doi.org/10.3912/OJIN.Vol25No03InfoCol01

Oermann, M. H., Nicoll, L. H., Carter-Templeton, H., Owens, J. K., Wrigley, J., Ledbetter, L. S., & Chinn, P. L. (2022). How to identify predatory journals in a search: Precautions for nurses. *Nursing*, 52(4), 41–45. https://doi.org/10.1097/01.NURSE.0000823280.93554.1a

Reiner, M., Niermann, C., Jekauc, D. et al. *(2013).* Long-term health benefits of physical activity—A systematic review of longitudinal studies. *BMC Public Health, 13*, 813. https://doi.org/10.1186/1471-2458-13-813

Ruegsegger, G. N., & Booth, F. W. (2018). Health benefits of exercise. *Cold Spring Harbor Perspectives in Medicine, 8*(7), a029694. https://doi.org/10.1101/cshperspect.a029694

Skeith, J. (n.d.). *"I'll just Google it": The case against internet searching for clinical evidence.* EBSCO. https://www.ebsco.com/sites/g/files/nabnos191/files/acquiadam-assets/The-Case-Against-Internet-Searching-for-Cinical-Evidence-White-Paper.pdf

Stern, C. & McArthur, A. (2014). Developing the review question and inclusion criteria. *AJN, 114*(4), 53–56.

Tsolaki, A. C., et al. (2020). Web-based intervention effects on mild cognitive impairment based on apolipoprotein E genotype: Quasi-experimental study. *Journal of Medical Internet Research, 22*(5), e14617. https://doi.org/10.2196/14617
Warburton, D. E., Nicol, C. W., & Bredin, S. S. (2006). Health benefits of physical activity: The evidence. *CMAJ: Canadian Medical Association Journal, 174*(6), 801–809. https://doi.org/10.1503/cmaj.051351
World Health Organization. (2020, July 9). *Transmission of SARS-CoV-2: Implications for infection prevention precautions.* https://www.who.int/news-room/commentaries/detail/transmission-of-sars-cov-2-implications-for-infection-prevention-precautions

IMAGE CREDITS

Fig. 4.1: Jayne Jennings Dunlap and Julee Briscoe Waldrop, *Introduction to Evidence-Based Practice and Quality Improvement for Professional Nursing Practice: A Competency Based Approach,* p. 67. Copyright © 2024 by Cognella, Inc. Reprinted with permission.
Fig. 4.2: Jayne Jennings Dunlap and Julee Briscoe Waldrop, *Introduction to Evidence-Based Practice and Quality Improvement for Professional Nursing Practice: A Competency Based Approach,* p. 76. Copyright © 2024 by Cognella, Inc. Reprinted with permission.

CHAPTER 5

Leading Critical Appraisal of Quantitative Evidence

Julee Briscoe Waldrop, Garry J. Brydges, Ninotchka Brydges, Jayne Jennings Dunlap, Tracy Brewer, and Melissa Hessock

KEY CONCEPTS

Quantitative research
Primary sources
Body of evidence
Evidence synthesis
Critical appraisal

LEARNING OBJECTIVES

1. Describe the role of quantitative research evidence in making EBPQI recommendations.
2. Differentiate between different quantitative research designs.
3. Use a hierarchy of evidence to determine levels of evidence.
4. Explore leadership roles in the critical appraisal of quantitative research evidence.
5. Identify critical appraisal resources for quantitative research studies.
6. Describe the four steps of the critical appraisal process.

A leader is one who knows the way, goes the way and shows the way.

—John C. Maxwell

Introduction

As a leader, it is vital that you understand the value of ensuring use of quality evidence for decision-making and how to connect your team with resources to fully engage in the process of critical appraisal to inform scalable EBPQI initiatives. If you remember from Chapter 1 and the evidence pyramid, quantitative research studies are at the top. Considered as high-level evidence in most cases, these study results often form the backbone of supporting evidence to change practice. It is not enough, however, to find one study and decide to change practice based on that one article; you need to lead your team in searching for the most current highest quality evidence available, as you learned in Chapter 4, and then understand it well enough to critically appraise it and synthesize it to make a recommendation. Then and only then can you feel confident in your proposed practice change.

Let's start with a personal example of quantitative research. A few years ago, I (Julee) was mentoring a nursing student in an honors program. She was interested in why there was not more uptake of the human papillomavirus (HPV) vaccine in adolescents and young adult males. When she reviewed the literature, she found that males and parents of males felt that there was no direct benefit for them (prevention of female cervical cancer was not a good reason apparently). She also wondered what nurses knew about HPV or the HPV vaccine. There were scattered studies done that provided inconsistent information but revealed that in general nurses might need more education on HPV and the vaccines. Given the state of the evidence we designed a cross-sectional study (a type of observational study) with the purpose of identifying knowledge and attitudes of registered nurses and potential barriers to achieving adequate HPV vaccination rates in males. We developed a survey or questionnaire, and the participants' answers were in response to statements on a Likert scale. A Likert scale is one way to transform or order text responses into numbers for statistical analysis. The result is an ordinal scale not an interval scale (e.g., height or weight) and one of the key features that differentiates quantitative from qualitative research designs (Table 5.5).

The conclusions from the data collected from this study revealed that although nurses in our sample had favorable attitudes toward the vaccine, they also had a lack of knowledge about HPV and its associated cancers and the HPV vaccine itself. Recommendations for more education spanned all contexts in which nurses are present—nursing preparation, continuing education, and public health campaigns. Specific content that addresses the HPV vaccine's effectiveness in preventing conditions specifically associated with HPV in males and vaccine safety are essential to these messages. Health promotion and disease prevention are staples of nursing education and practice. Immunizations are a cornerstone of disease prevention, and although HPV is almost exclusively sexually transmitted, the HPV vaccine is unique in that it can also prevent many types of cancer in both females and males. A greater understanding of the power of the HPV vaccine to improve health and prevent disease by all RNs will increase accurate communication between not only nurses and patients, but friends and family as well, hopefully leading to an increased acceptance and improved vaccination rates (White et al., 2016). This study was conducted almost 10 years ago, and we are sure you know that the issue of vaccine hesitancy is still a prevalent one. This is just one of many examples of quantitative research you will see in this chapter and that you will learn how to critically appraise. Let's begin with a clarification of terms.

Critical Appraisal versus Critique of Research

The terms "critique" and "critical appraisal" are often used synonymously, but they are not the same processes. Critical appraisal is the process of carefully and systematically examining research to judge its trustworthiness and its value and relevance in a particular context (Critical Appraisal Skills Programme [CASP], 2024). Critical appraisal applies to all types of evidence. Standardized tools can be helpful in this process, and we recommend using them to foster a systematic approach. It is important to distinguish critical appraisal from the process of research critique.

A critique of research involves comprehensively analyzing the strengths and limitations of the study's design, methods, statistical analysis, and conclusions. When we critique a research article, the focus surrounds researcher aims, methodology, fit of methodology, thorough conduction, and discovery of gaps. A critique typically includes evaluator feedback as well as suggestions for study improvement (Polit & Beck, 2021), and a standardized tool is not used.

Critical appraisal engagement is essential for informed decision-making that directly impacts patient outcomes and health care quality (Tomotaki et al., 2023). By critically appraising research studies, your team can identify evidence-based interventions and practices that contribute to positive patient outcomes while avoiding potential harm (Agency for Healthcare Research and Quality [AHRQ], 2018). Critical appraisal also enables leaders to keep abreast with the latest advancements in health care and tailor care practices to individual patient characteristics in the context of complex patient cases (Tomotaki et al., 2023). Critical appraisal fosters a culture of professional accountability by enabling us to confidently articulate and justify our choices to colleagues, patients, and other health care professionals. We cannot overemphasize this point because as a leader and fellow participant in EBPQI, you must demonstrate sound, evidence-based rationales for decisions.

Interdisciplinary collaboration is enhanced when we, as leaders, engage in meaningful discussions with other health care team members based on a shared understanding of the evidence. In the realm of policy and guideline development, critical appraisal skills are instrumental to inform evidence-based policy analysis. As leaders in health care, we should contribute to developing and implementing policies and guidelines within and beyond practice settings. Critical appraisal skills enable us to assess the robustness of existing evidence, influencing the creation of policies that reflect the best available knowledge and promote evidence-based standards of care. Critical appraisal is significant in creating and sustaining a culture of EBP, enhancing the quality of decision-making processes, driving positive outcomes within organizations, and contributing to continuous improvement in health care.

The Leader's Role in Critical Appraisal Engagement

We recognize the dynamic nature of health care and the continuous evolution of research methodologies. As leaders, we must stay abreast of emerging trends and advancements in research design and synthesis methods, fostering a culture of lifelong learning within EBPQI. Leaders set the tone for the organization's commitment to EBPQI and establish expectations for incorporating the outputs of critical appraisal into decision-making processes. We must allocate resources effectively to support these endeavors, including providing access to training, databases, tools, and technology. Leadership involvement extends to promoting interdisciplinary collaboration and advocating for a feedback loop in which critical appraisal of bodies of evidence inform organizational decision-making and policy development. You can also serve as a bridge between EBPQI appraisal efforts and the broader organizational goals by advocating for resources and dissemination (you will learn more about dissemination in Chapter 12). This approach ensures that the benefits of critical appraisal are realized through improved practices, enhanced patient care, and strengthened quality and safety measures.

The ability to critically appraise research evidence is a critical skill for you as an EBPQI leader, and this comprehensive overview offers a roadmap for mastering research methodology and synthesis. In this chapter the research designs will focus on quantitative research, and all types of research (including qualitative research; see Chapter 6), even other evidence (Chapter 7), can be incorporated into your final synthesis of the evidence and inform your ultimate recommendations. Leaders in ANP must understand the nuances of various research designs, including quantitative, qualitative, and mixed-methods approaches; appraise research findings critically; and apply them to their clinical practice (Takona, 2024). As you proceed through this chapter, you will be following the four steps of leading the critical appraisal process as outlined in Table 5.1. We reviewed the first step, selection of relevant studies, in Chapter 4, so let's move on to assessment of study quality.

TABLE 5.1 Key Steps in Evidence Appraisal

Step	Process	Appraisal
Selection of Relevant Studies	Identify studies using databases, journals, reputable sources.	Ensure studies align with clinical question.
Assessment of Study Quality	Use established appraisal tools or criteria.	Evaluate clarity of questions, appropriateness of design, adequacy of sample size/randomization, validity of measurements, and potential bias.

Step	Process	Appraisal
Data Extraction	Systematically extract relevant data (characteristics, interventions, outcomes, statistics).	Critically assess consistency/ variability of results across studies.
Synthesis and Recommendations	Synthesize data/results based on quality, quantity, and consistency.	Evaluate appropriateness for your context and make recommendations

Assessment of Study Quality: Levels of Evidence and the Evidence Hierarchy

As you learned in Chapter 4 and visualized in Figure 4.1, evidence hierarchies are typically illustrated with a pyramid that ranks evidence based on the research study design. Generally, studies at the top levels of the pyramid provide the most reliable and robust evidence. In contrast, studies at the bottom of the pyramid may be subject to bias and provide weaker evidence. Numerous evidence hierarchies exist to guide clinicians as they search for evidence to answer clinical questions. The scientific community considers randomized controlled trials (RCTs) the most rigorous study design as they have the highest probability of establishing causality between variables while minimizing bias. Although research studies using qualitative, descriptive, or nonresearch designs were not included in original evidence pyramids, they can now be found in several modifications of the pyramid used in health care settings (Polit & Beck, 2021; Whalen & Dang, 2021). There is no consensus on what constitutes "best evidence" in EBP, yet there is general agreement that findings from well-designed research studies are essential to best practice (Polit & Beck, 2021).

Hierarchy pyramids can offer a visual representation of the *levels* of different types of evidence used in clinical decision-making, but they do not signify the *quality* (validity and reliability) of evidence. Quality of evidence can be determined only by conducting a thorough critical appraisal using a systematic approach. Remember, a study situated higher on the pyramid is not necessarily of higher quality than a well-conducted descriptive study situated closer to the pyramid base (Murad et al., 2016).

Levels of Evidence

Assigning an evidence level refers to making an objective hierarchical rating of a research study or other source of evidence according to its design and methodology. This is the initial step in the critical appraisal process. Evidence levels are often assigned based on established guidelines or frameworks, such as an evidence hierarchy pyramid. Numerous guides and scales exist for assigning levels of evidence, with variations in the ranking of research and other evidence designs. For example, in some level ratings, Roman numerals are used to rank evidence from I to VII (Melnyk & Fineout-Overholt, 2023). In contrast, the Johns Hopkins evidence-based practice model provides a five-level evidence hierarchy for research (levels I, II, and III) and other evidence (levels IV, and V; Whalen & Dang, 2022). As a leader of an EBPQI team, you can guide your team to choose a single rating scale and use it consistently throughout the critical appraisal process. You will find some examples of levels-of-evidence rating guides to add to your EBP resources in Table 5.2.

TABLE 5.2 Level of Evidence Guides

Sources for Level Guides	Website Access	Access and Fee
Oxford Centre for Evidence-Based Medicine Levels of Evidence	https://www.cebm.ox.ac.uk/resources/levels-of-evidence/ocebm-levels-of-evidence	Free A downloadable version is available.
Johns Hopkins Evidence-Based Practice Model for Nursing and Healthcare Professionals Appendix D: Hierarchy of Evidence Guide	https://www.hopkinsmedicine.org/evidence-based-practice/model-tools	Free Must complete a copyright permission form for access. A zipped file with all model appendices is sent via email and made available for download and use.
Evidence-Based Practice Step by Step: Critical Appraisal of the Evidence: Part I (Fineout-Overholt et al., 2010) Hierarchy of Evidence for Intervention Studies	https://journals.lww.com/ajnonline/Fulltext/2010/07000/Evidence_Based_Practice_Step_by_Step__Critical.26.aspx	Free The article is available as open access through the *American Journal of Nursing* (*AJN*). Hierarchy of evidence table is in the article.

Key Components of Quantitative Research Design

As a leader, understanding different types of research designs is integral to your ability to critically appraise the evidence and apply it to practice. Several key components shape the structure and rigor of a quantitative research study, such as hypothesis testing, choice of variables and their measurement, the sampling process, how the data is collected and analyzed statistically, and the interpretation and conclusion drawn from that data. The choice of a research design influences the internal validity of the study and the extent to which causal relationships can be established (see Table 5.3).

TABLE 5.3 Key Components of Quantitative Research Design

Aspect	Description	Importance for ANP
Hypothesis testing	Enables testing of specific predictions through numerical data	Evaluates validity of findings and alignment with research question
Variables	The characteristics or phenomena observed, measured, or manipulated in a study	Should align with the practice issue or problem, population, and setting of proposed EBPQI
Statistical analysis	Assesses the appropriateness of analytical methods (e.g., regression, t-tests)	Critically appraises significance and generalizability of findings for informed decision-making
Sampling techniques	Ensure representativeness of study samples (e.g., random, stratified)	Evaluates external validity and relevance to specific patient populations
Bias, confounding variables, validity threats	Recognize potential limitations and control methods employed	Ensures reliability and applicability of evidence to clinical practice

Hypothesis Formulation

One of the fundamental components of quantitative research design is the research hypothesis. It is a clear and testable statement that guides the investigation. It guides designing the study, selecting variables, and determining the appropriate statistical analyses. The systematic nature of hypothesis testing contributes to the robustness of quantitative research, making it one of the most reliable research methodologies in health care. In the realm of ANP and quality and safety, hypotheses often pertain to the effectiveness of specific interventions, the impact of practices on patient outcomes, or the association between particular variables and health care quality indicators. You may find that some studies make a purpose statement instead of a hypothesis. See Table 5.4, which includes hypotheses and purposes from the examples presented in this chapter.

TABLE 5.4 Hypothesis or Purpose Statement Examples

Study	Hypothesis/Purpose
Khalili, S., Shirinkam, F., Ghadimi, R., & Karimi, H. (2022). The effect of group walking program on social physique anxiety and the risk of eating disorders in aged women: A randomized clinical trial study. *Applied Nursing Research*, *64*, 151555. https://doi.org/10.1016/j.apnr.2021.151555	A group walking program will have a positive effect on the risk of EDs and SPA in aged women (hypothesis).

(Continued)

TABLE 5.4 *(Continued)*

Study	Hypothesis/Purpose
Farrow, K. A., & Neff, F. (2024). Bereavement care team: Improving ICU nurses' professional bereavement and patient family experience. *Nursing Administration Quarterly, 48*(2), 97–106.	The purpose of this study was to determine if the implementation of a bereavement care team (BCT) could decrease RNs' professional bereavement over a 6-week period (purpose statement).
White, L., Waldrop, J., & Waldrop, C. (2016). Human papillomavirus and vaccination of males: Knowledge and attitudes of registered nurses. *Pediatric Nursing, 42*(1), 21–30, 35.	The purpose of this research study is to identify knowledge and attitudes of registered nurses and potential barriers to achieving adequate HPV vaccination rates in males (purpose statement).

Variables

Variables are another critical component of quantitative research design. They are the characteristics or phenomena observed, measured, or manipulated in a study, and understanding their selection and operationalization is crucial for ANP leaders to assess the precision and validity of research findings. Operationalization involves specifying how a variable will be observed, measured, or manipulated in the study. Without proper identification and operationalization of variables, studies cannot produce reliable results, and evidence-based decision-making is compromised (Polit & Beck, 2021).

There are many different types of variables. However, the two main types are the independent variable and the dependent variable. The independent variable is the one that the researcher believes (or hypothesizes) influences the dependent variable. The independent variable is the one that is manipulated (the intervention) by the researcher (tip for remembering which is which: think I = independent and goes with I = intervention). The dependent variable is what is being measured or the outcome variable of interest. See Table 5.5 for more variable descriptions and their practice relevance.

TABLE 5.5 Variables in Quantitative Research

Variable Type	Description	Relevance in Practice
Independent	Factor (or intervention) manipulated or assessed to observe impact on other variables	Guides intervention design and identifies potential predictors of outcomes
Dependent	Outcome or effect measured to determine impact of independent variable	Represents desired changes in patient care or practice
Moderating	Influences strength or direction of independent–dependent variable relationship	Helps understand factors affecting intervention effectiveness or outcome variations

Variable Type	Description	Relevance in Practice
Mediating	Explains how the independent variable affects the dependent variable	Provides deeper insights into intervention mechanisms and pathways
Extraneous/ Confounding	May affect the independent-dependent variable relationship but is not the focus	Requires control to ensure internal validity and isolate true intervention effects

The accurate determination of potential causality is pivotal in understanding the relationship between independent and dependent variables. However, confounding variables can distort this relationship, resulting in inaccurate and misleading conclusions, especially in observational studies. It is important to note that confounding variables, while not causing the studied outcome, can significantly influence both the independent and the dependent variable, leading to the false suggestion of a relationship, diminishing the validity and reliability (certainty) of research findings.

Sampling

Sampling techniques play a crucial role in quantitative research design. Sampling, or selecting a representative subset from a larger population, influences the generalizability and validity of research findings. Effective sampling ensures the study findings accurately reflect the larger population of interest, like nurses, patients, or health care teams. The external validity of research findings depends on the appropriateness of the sampling method. ANP leaders must be vigilant in assessing its relevance to their patient population. The sampling method and size directly impact the generalizability of findings. It is critically important that you as a leader assess the appropriateness of sampling strategies to ensure that the study's results can be extrapolated to the broader population (see Table 5.6, page 94).

Randomization and Blinding

Random sample selection and blinding contribute significantly to the robustness of studies by minimizing biases and enhancing the reliability of causal inferences. Randomization is a crucial method in experimental research that involves randomly assigning participants to either the experimental or control group (Capili & Anastasi, 2023). This method ensures that each participant has an equal chance of being assigned to either group, minimizing selection bias and creating comparable groups at baseline. Similarly, blinding, or masking, is crucial to minimizing bias in research studies. It involves keeping participants, researchers, or outcome assessors unaware of group assignments during the study. Blinding is particularly important when subjective outcomes, such as patient-reported measures or clinical assessments, are involved. Expectations or

TABLE 5.6 Types of Sampling Methods

Sampling Method	Description	Advantages	Disadvantages	Applicability
Random Sampling	Each member of the population has an equal chance of being selected	Ensures representativeness. Minimizes selection bias Allows generalizability to the entire population	Time-consuming and impractical for large populations May require specialized tools or techniques	Research requiring representative samples for generalizability Studies with well-defined populations
Stratified Sampling	Population is divided into subgroups (strata) based on shared characteristics. Sample is then drawn proportionally from each stratum	Ensures each stratum is represented in the sample Enhances precision by capturing variability within strata	Requires prior knowledge of strata and their characteristics Can be complex to implement if strata are numerous or overlapping	Research whereby specific subgroups are of interest Studies investigating differences or interactions between strata
Convenience Sampling	Selecting readily available subjects, often those easiest to access	Fast and cost-effective Easy to implement	May not be representative of the entire population High risk of selection bias Limits generalizability of findings	Exploratory research or pilot studies Research on readily available populations when generalizability is not a major concern
Snowball Sampling	Identifying initial participants who then refer others in their network who share relevant characteristics	Useful for accessing hard-to-reach populations Explores hidden knowledge and experiences within networks	Can lead to biased samples influenced by initial participants' networks Difficult to assess representativeness and generalizability	Researching hidden or difficult-to-reach populations Studies exploring knowledge, attitudes, or behaviors within specific networks

Source: Adapted from Polit and Beck (2021).

behaviors that may unintentionally influence the reported outcomes are minimized by keeping participants and researchers unaware of the treatment group assignment. The placebo effect or the Hawthorne effect in participants or the observer effect in researchers can reduce the credibility of a study if it is impossible to blind participants to an intervention. This happens more than you think. For example, if you were a participant in a research study on the effect of regular walking on blood pressure, you would know if you were in the walking group. You really can't be blinded in this type of study. However, being blinded may or may not make any difference on the results (e.g., blood pressure as an outcome measure or dependent variable).

Bias

There are different types of bias related to the sampling process, the group allocation, attrition, and blinding (Table 5.7). There are two other types of bias not related to the sample, reporting bias and other sources of bias. Reporting bias occurs when researchers choose not to report some of the results—selecting the outcomes that support a particular conclusion. An example of another source of bias might be a conflict of interest by the funder of the research or one of the researchers (Cochrane Risk of Bias Assessment Tool; Epstein et al., 2015).

TABLE 5.7 Types of Bias Related to Sample

Type of Bias	Reduces Bias	Increases Bias
Selection (or Allocation) Bias	Random sample Sampling plan was followed appropriate sample size (powered)	The selection of the sample is not representative of the target population Participants are not randomly selected Exclusion criteria exclude certain groups more than others
Detection Bias	Blinding investigators and/or participants to who is receiving the intervention Blinding assignment to groups	Investigators and/or participants are not blinded so they know what intervention they are receiving
Attrition Bias	Offer incentives or reminders to keep participants engaged	Participants drop out or are lost to follow up

Source: Adapted from Polit and Beck (2021).

Experimental and Control Groups

Depending on the study design, the sample may be divided into groups such as experimental and control groups. The experimental group, also known as the treatment group, is exposed to the intervention or manipulation of the independent variable, while the control group serves as a baseline or comparison group that does not receive the experimental intervention. Groups should be well matched or not significantly different to ensure that any observed effects can be attributed to the intervention rather than external factors (confounders; see Table 5.8).

TABLE 5.8 Experimental and Control Groups

Aspect	Description	Importance for ANP Leaders
Purpose	Enables determination of intervention effectiveness and causal relationships	Informs evidence-based decisions about practices and interventions
Experimental Group	Receives the intervention/ manipulation	Represents the group experiencing the intervention's potential effects
Control Group	Serves as a baseline comparison	Helps isolate the intervention's effect and control for other influences
Control Group Adequacy	Assesses if groups are well matched and differences are due to intervention	Avoids misinterpretations and misleading conclusions
Randomization	Minimizes bias and strengthens causal inferences	Enhances internal validity and generalizability of findings
Blinding	Reduces bias from knowledge of group assignments	Improves study credibility and minimizes potential confounding factors
Double-Blind Studies	Both participants and researchers are unaware of group assignments	Highest level of bias control and strengthens study validity

Sources: Adapted from Capili and Anastasi (2023); Melnyk and Fineout-Overholt (2023); Polit and Beck (2021).

Enrollment

The researchers should tell you how they recruited and enrolled their participants. Sometimes this is done with a flow chart. The flow chart easily demonstrates the allocation to a group, follow-up, and how the group's data was analyzed. The CONSORT diagram is a standard way you will see this presented in a research study (Figure 5.1).

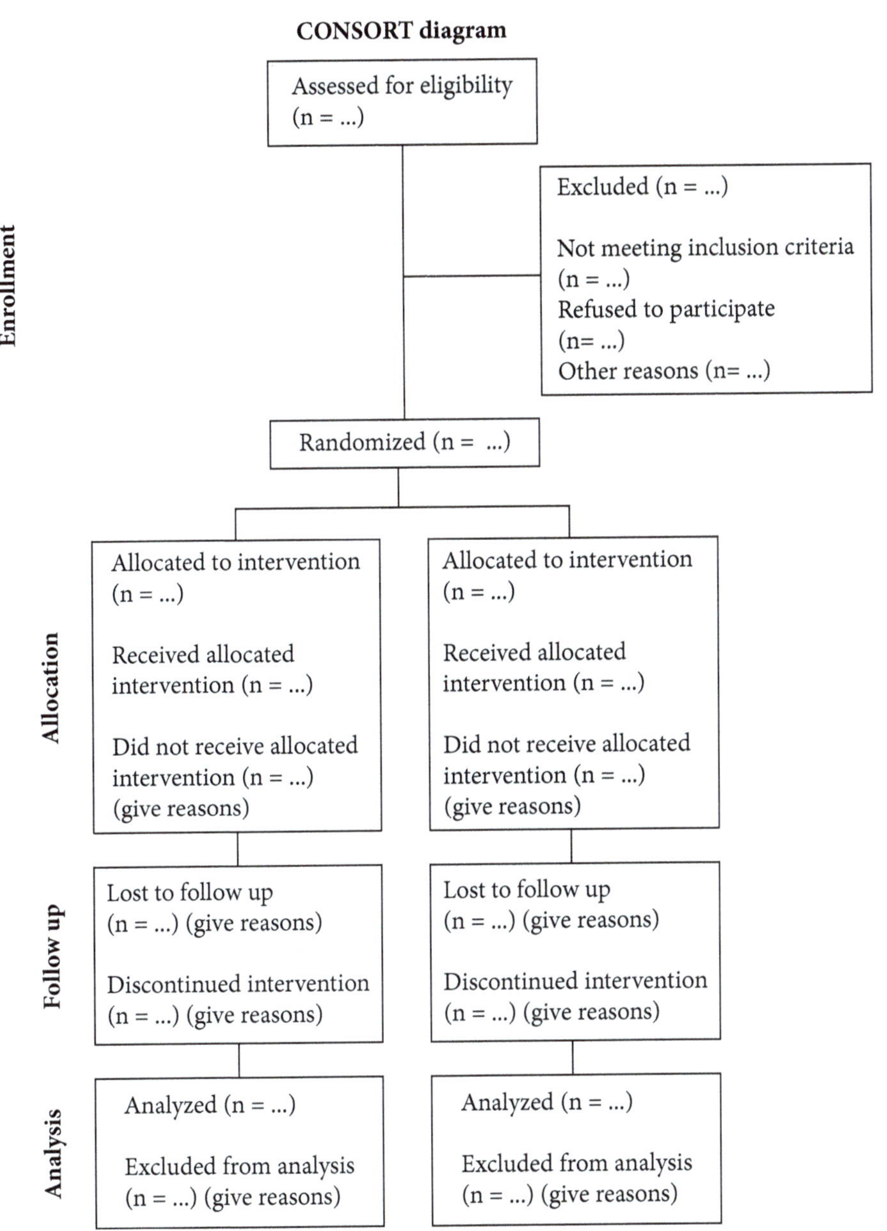

FIGURE 5.1 CONSORT diagram. Source: www.equator-network.org/reporting-guidelines/consort/.

Types of Quantitative Studies

Different designs, such as experimental, quasi-experimental, or observational, offer distinct advantages and disadvantages. Randomized controlled trials (RCTs) are considered the gold standard for establishing cause-and-effect relationships (Baldi et al., 2017; Weber & Prouse, 2018). Observational studies, on the other hand, offer valuable insights into real-world scenarios. While quasi-experimental studies can offer a practical alternative in specific healthcare settings, they lack randomization and intervention-control conditions. ANP leaders must carefully analyze the study design, methods, and potential for selection bias to understand the limitations in inferring causality. Let's begin at the top of the pyramid!

Systematic Reviews and Meta-Analyses

A systematic review is a rigorous synthesis of multiple research studies' findings that address a specific question. A team of experts conducts a systematic review using a stringent protocol, including predetermined inclusion and exclusion criteria to reduce biases and errors in reporting; these criteria may be specific to the study's design, population, or setting. The preferred reporting items for systematic reviews and meta-analyses (PRISMA) diagram visually represents a clear and concise summary of the selection of studies for inclusion in a systematic review and/or meta-analysis (Page, 2021; see example PRISMA in Figure 5.2). The research team can use a standard tool to critically appraise each study's quality by determining the risk of bias (RoB; e.g. Cochrane risk of bias) and display the findings in a chart or graph (Figure 5.2). In this example, you can see that for all potential risks of bias but one (they did not describe whether blinding of participants and personnel occurred) were reported. In fact, in addition to being unclear, common sense tells you that if the studies in this review that used yoga as an intervention, would make it very difficult to blind participants and personnel to the intervention.

Next, the outcomes from all the findings are synthesized and interpreted, accounting for each study's quality and applicability to your proposed EBPQI initiative (Rochwerg, 2022). PRISMA provides a standard guideline and checklist for authors, reviewers, and editors to ensure that the systematic review or meta-analysis is transparent, comprehensive, and reproducible for publication (Page, 2021). The newest version includes a separate flow chart for records identified outside of systematic searches in databases (Figure 5.3).

In a systematic review, the study results will be reported narratively. However, if there is enough similarity in the interventions and the data collected among the studies, it is possible for the researchers to combine results using statistical analysis to perform a "meta-analysis" (Rochwerg, 2022). The addition of a meta-analysis allows the team to report an overall summary of the treatment effect (i.e., the strength of the relationship between the intervention and its outcomes). The effect size assesses the difference between the means in a study group. The higher the effect size (see Table 5.9), the more confident you can be that the intervention caused the effect found in the outcomes (results) of the combined studies (Whalen

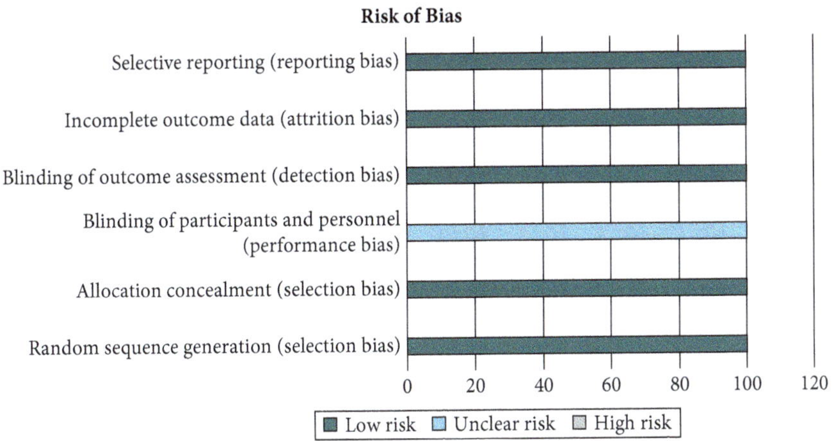

FIGURE 5.2 Risk of bias chart.

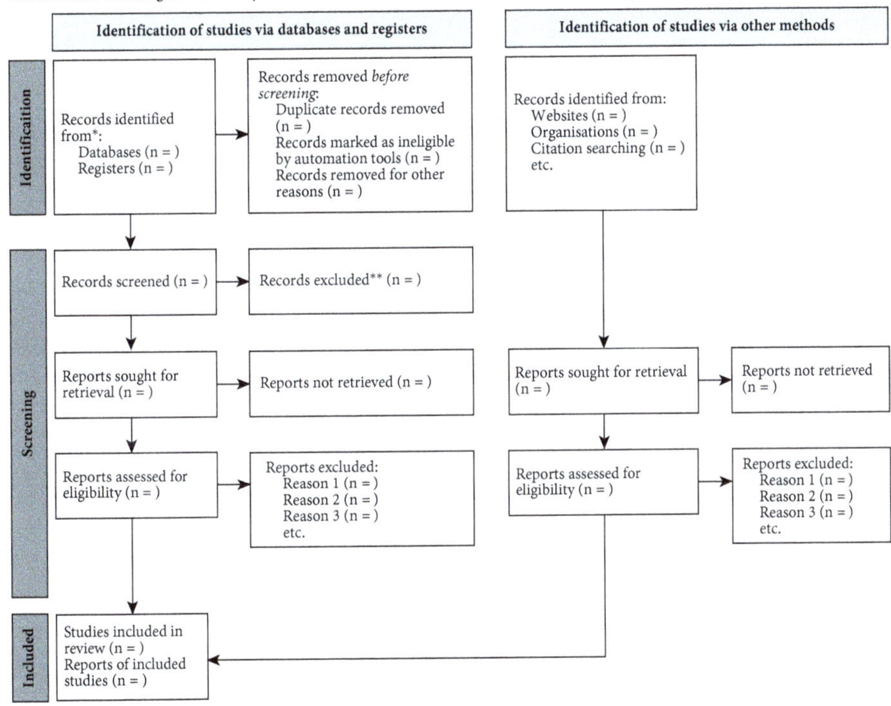

FIGURE 5.3 PRISMA flow diagram for systematic reviews.

TABLE 5.9 Interpretation of an Effect Size

Effect Size	Cohen's d
Small	0.2
Medium	0.5
Large	0.8 or greater

& Dang, 2022). For example, an effect size of 0.9 would instill confidence that the intervention(s) affected the outcome(s).

Another way of displaying the grand or overall mean effect size is with a forest plot. A forest plot is a useful and often beautiful visual summary of all the effect sizes and their confidence intervals that includes the weight of the studies from a meta-analysis based on sample size and the resulting point estimate of the true effect in the included population. A vertical reference line is usually plotted at the null hypothesis (or no difference between groups). The statistical significance of each point and whisker (the lines coming out from the sides of the shape (box, circle, or diamond) is compared to this line. For example, a wide horizontal line that crosses the null effect line with a black box to the right of the line may indicate a small-scale study with few participants. A large diamond at the bottom of the forest plot represents the overall pooled effect from all the included studies. The width of the diamond shows the confidence interval for the overall effect. Other statistics that can be displayed in a forest plot include standard deviation, number of participants, and mean difference (Chang et al., 2022), as you can see in Figure 5.4.

A well-conducted systematic review of randomized controlled trials with a meta-analysis is considered the highest level of evidence to answer specific clinical questions for making practice recommendations (Rochwerg, 2022). The *Cochrane Database of Systematic Reviews* (*CDSR*) is the leading journal and database for accessing systematic reviews and meta-analyses in health care. When searching for systematic reviews, a good place to begin your search is the Cochrane database, which is also indexed in PubMed, Web of Science, and Scopus.

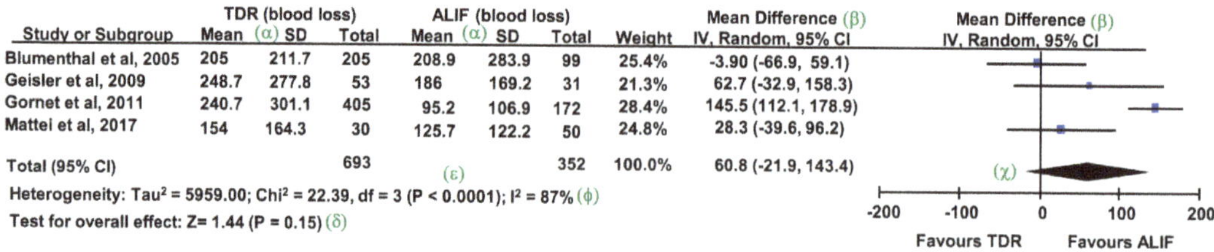

(α) Group mean, sd, and sample size
(β) Mean difference in numeric and graphical presentation
(χ) Pooled effect and 95% CI crosses the line of no effect
(δ) P = 0.15 (test for overall effect) confirms no statistical difference illustrated by the diamond crossing the line of effect
(ε) P <0.001, we reject the hypothesis of no heterogeneity
(ϕ) Amount of heterogeneity (I² = 87%) is considerable

FIGURE 5.4 Forest plot example.

There are many articles published with the word "review" in the title (Carter-Templeton et al., 2022). In a general search you may see that there is an overabundance of these types of reviews compared to the availability of systematic reviews and meta-analyses. Although these reviews may be useful in answering your clinical question, they lack the rigor and quality assessment performed in the systematic review process (more on these types of reviews in Chapter 7).

BOX 5.1: EXAMPLE SYSTEMATIC REVIEW WITH META-ANALYSIS

The purpose of this systematic review with meta-analysis (SRMA) was to quantitatively analyze the outcomes of pain, anxiety, depression, stress, blood pressure, and heart rate in experimental studies on animal-assisted therapy (AAT) with hospitalized children and adolescents (Feng et al., 2021; note that SRMAs do not necessarily have a hypothesis). Inclusion and exclusion criteria for the studies were established. The review was conducted using the methods in the *Cochrane Handbook for Systematic Reviews of Interventions* (Higgins & Thompson, 2002) and reported using the PRISMA (Page & Moher, 2017). Four Chinese and nine English databases were searched with key words. Ultimately eight studies met inclusion criteria. Studies were assessed for risk of bias and evaluated using the GRADE criteria (www.gradeworking-group.org/). Mean differences, or standardized mean differences (SMD) with 95% confidence intervals, were calculated for the pooled effect of outcomes. Results demonstrated statistically significant improvement in pain (SMD = -0.49, 95% CI -0.77 to -0.22) and BP (SMD = -0.19, 95% CI -0.44 to 0.06) but not HR, anxiety, depression, or stress. There were two recommendations based on the results: (a) ATT may be a feasible, nonpharmacological approach to reducing pain in children and adolescents and (b) nurses should take the lead in developing and implementing evidence-based AAT programs.

Quantitative Research Study Designs: Randomized Controlled Trials

Randomized controlled trials are considered the gold standard for evaluating the effectiveness of interventions because the researcher uses randomization and blinding to minimize risk of bias and to control for confounding variables (Polit & Beck, 2021). The participants are informed before the study begins that they will not know whether they have been assigned to the intervention or the control group (i.e., blind to which group they are in). (See Chapter 10 for more information on consent to participate in research.)

BOX 5.2: EXAMPLE RCT

Social physique anxiety (SPA) is common in women ages 60–80 (~ 27%). While physical exercise has a positive effect on SPA, there is also an associated risk of eating disorders (ED). EDs occur in approximately 3.5% of aged women. In Iran there is very limited literature on SPA and ED, but a pilot study revealed a risk of 60%. The hypothesis of this RCT was that a group walking program would have a positive effect on the risk of EDs and SPA in older women as the primary outcomes (Khalili et al., 2022). The sample population was women 60–74 years old without chronic illness and with scores of > 15 on the EPAS (social physique anxiety scale) and 20 or more on the EAT-26 (eating attitude test-26) and no regular program of exercise in the last 6 months. The needed sample size was determined to be 70 participants (35 in each group). The sampling process was done in two stages (stratified sampling). First, each of the 12 health centers participating in the study was considered as a cluster (see Table 5.6 for a definition of stratified sampling). Then six of these centers were randomly selected. Within those centers, women who met the inclusion criteria were randomly assigned to the experimental (intervention) group or the control group and matched in terms of age and body mass index. All instruments used for measurement were presented as valid and reliable. The intervention group walked for 30 minutes three times week for 8 weeks. The control group received nothing during this period. The participant flow chart documents that 31 participants in each group completed the study. The results demonstrated that participants in the experimental group reduced their mean SPA and ED scores ($p < 0.008$; $p < 0.001$, respectively) compared to the control group. The results support that walking is an effective means of improving risk of SPA and ED in older women.

Quasi-Experimental

Although considered a type of experimental design, quasi-experimental studies lack randomization and usually do not include a separate control group; therefore, they are considered much less rigorous than RCTs. However, keep in mind that the use of a control group is not always possible or ethical; in such cases, a comparison group is typically created by selecting subjects who are like the experimental group but will not receive the treatment or intervention being studied. Another way to create a comparison group is to evaluate the same participants prior to and after the intervention is implemented (i.e., a "before and after" comparison). Although quasi-experimental studies can be useful for evaluating interventions when randomization is not feasible or ethical, they are more susceptible to bias and confounding variables than RCTs. As a result, the conclusions drawn from quasi-experimental studies are generally considered less certain than those from RCTs, but they may still be transferable to clinical practice (Whalen & Dang, 2022).

BOX 5.3: EXAMPLE QUASI-EXPERIMENTAL STUDY

The purpose of this study was to determine if the implementation of a bereavement care team (BCT) could decrease RNs' professional bereavement over a 6-week period (not a hypothesis, but you could probably write one based on this purpose statement). The design was a pre–post quasi-experimental one, and the sample was RNs whose primary responsibilities were in the intensive care unit. A BCT composed of nurse managers, assistant nurse managers, chaplains, and nurse educators cover the ICU 24 hours/day. The BCT's role was to develop the environment abiding by the principles of a "good death" to support the nurse in caring for the family of the dying patient. To measure the impact of the BCT on the nurses' experience of the death, an adapted version of the Professional Bereavement Scale and a five-question Likert scale on how beneficial specific interventions were was used. Results revealed that the BCT reduced the nurses' professional bereavement scores significantly (a good thing). Feelings related to exhaustion ($P = 0.03$), frustration ($P = 0.03$), nervousness ($P = 0.04$) and fatigue ($P = 0.02$) were reduced postintervention. There were many meaningful comments also reported that added depth to the quantitative results (Farrow & Neff, 2024).

Observational Research Designs

Observational research aims to describe or understand a phenomenon, behavior, or situation in its natural setting. An observational design is a research method in which the researcher observes and records what is being studied as it occurs (prospective) or occurred (retrospective) naturally, without manipulating any variables or interventions. Cohort, case-control, and cross-sectional studies are observational studies that investigate the relationship between an exposure or risk factor and a health outcome or other variable of interest.

Cohort Study

Cohort studies can be either prospective or retrospective, depending on whether the study follows the cohort forward in time (prospective) or looks back at data that has already been collected (retrospective). Prospective cohort studies are considered more reliable because they follow the individuals over time, and the researcher can observe changes in exposure and health outcomes. A classic example of a prospective cohort study is the nurses' health study (https://nurseshealthstudy.org). It began with the purpose of finding risk factors for major chronic diseases in women; however, it now also includes men, given the increasing numbers of men in nursing (Barrett & Noble, 2019). Another example is the Swiss HIV cohort study. It began in 1988, and to date almost 22,000 participants have been enrolled. The aim of the study is to improve the health of persons living with HIV. Data is collected on participants every 6 months, including many biological samples. The resulting database is used by researchers all over the world and has resulted in over 1,400 publications (www.shcs.ch/157-about-shcs).

Case-Control Study

A case-control study compares individuals with a particular health outcome (cases) to those without the health outcome (controls). The researcher looks back in time (retrospective) and identifies potential exposures or risk factors that may have contributed to the outcome being investigated, then compares the frequency of these exposures in cases and controls to determine whether there is a relationship between exposure and the health outcome (Tenny et al., 2022).

BOX 5.4: EXAMPLE CASE CONTROL STUDY

A case control study design was used in one of the first studies to identify the importance of wearing a mask to prevent the spread of SARS-CoV-2 among health care workers (Rodriguez-Lopez et al., 2021). In this study, 110 health care workers with a positive COVID-19 test and 113 health care workers with negative tests were randomly selected and interviewed about their infection-control behaviors. Results demonstrated a strong association between wearing a high-performance filtering mask or double masking and negative COVID test results.

Cross-Sectional Study

Cross sectional studies aim to describe, explain, or summarize a particular phenomenon or behavior without manipulating variables. In this type of study, the researchers collect data from a sample of individuals at a single point in time to describe the prevalence of a phenomenon or characteristics of a specific population. Cross-sectional studies have limitations, such as their inability to establish cause-and-effect relationships between variables or control for confounding factors (Polit & Beck, 2021), although there are many statistical analysis methods attempt to address these limitations. The study described at the beginning of this chapter on nurses' knowledge and attitudes about HPV and the HPV vaccine for males is an example of a cross-sectional study.

TABLE 5.10 Types of Quantitative Studies: Key Considerations

Study Type	Description	Strengths	Limitations
RCTs	Participants randomly assigned to intervention or control groups	Strongest evidence for causal relationships. High internal validity	Can be expensive and time-consuming. Ethical limitations may exist
Observational Studies	**Cohort studies:** Follow a group of individuals over time	Explore risk factors and long-term outcomes. Can study rare diseases	Cannot establish causation due to lack of randomization but may identify correlations between variables
	Cross-sectional studies: Occur at one point in time like a snapshot	Explore a topic of interest	Cannot establish causation but may identify correlations between variables
	Case-control studies: Compare a group with a defining characteristic to a similar group without that characteristic	Identifies variables that are different between the groups	May establish associations between variables but not causation

Study Type	Description	Strengths	Limitations
Quasi-experimental:	Use existing groups without randomization to simulate intervention	Can be practical in health care settings. Offer insights into real-world scenarios	Cannot establish causation due to lack of randomization and a control group. However, it may identify associations and real-world relevance. Selection bias and confounding variables may be present

Sources: Melnyk and Fineout-Overholt (2023); Polit and Beck (2021); Takona (2024).

Statistical Analysis in Quantitative Research

Quantitative evidence (research studies) collect data that can be reported numerically. Statistical analyses are used to draw meaningful conclusions about the data collected. To be a proficient appraiser of quantitative evidence, you must possess a solid understanding of statistical concepts and data analysis techniques. You will likely take other courses or pursue other training that familiarize you with statistical analyses in more detail, but some important aspects are reviewed here.

The variable features affect the type of data and therefore how it can be analyzed. Numerical data can take on any number on a finite or infinite scale. The numbers on the scale can be discrete, like the number of participants in a study, or continuous, like how long something lasted (time). Categorical variables take on a limited number of values. These values can be nominal like blood type or ordinal (ordered; e.g., Likert scale). Nominal variables can be either/or or yes/no; for example, patient education was documented in the patient's chart or not (Figure 5.5). This is labeled a dichotomous variable, as there are only two options. A polytomous variable would have more options, like blood types. An example of ordinal variables are Likert scales. Likert scales are commonly used in questionnaires, like the cross-sectional study example at the beginning of the chapter. An example question from that study was posed as this statement: HPV causes too few cancers among males to make it worthwhile to vaccinate them. Response options ranged from strongly disagree, disagree, neither disagree or agree, agree, and strongly agree. Responses were then ordered with the numerals 1, 2, 3, 4, and 5, with the researcher deciding the order (White et al., 2016).

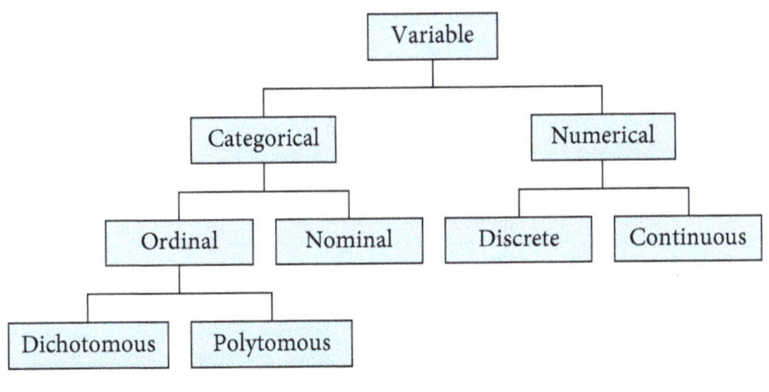

FIGURE 5.5 Types of variables in quantitative studies.

Quantitative research design relies heavily on statistical analysis. Your ability to interpret complex data and understanding effect sizes, confidence intervals, p-values, and statistical power is a vital component of this. For example, when reviewing a study on a new medication, you must consider the effect size, which indicates the magnitude of the drug's impact. If this is large, it may be a promising sign. However, the confidence interval, which is a range of potential actual values, may be broad. This means that the results could vary, and the leader must interpret the findings cautiously.

Similarly, p-values are often misinterpreted as guarantees of truth. However, they must be considered alongside the effect size, as a low p-value suggests that the results are unlikely due to chance. But it does not reveal the size of the effect or its clinical relevance. ANP leaders must carefully assess the study's statistical power, which reflects the probability of detecting an actual effect if one exists. A high power suggests that the study is equipped to identify meaningful changes, while a low power raises concerns about potentially missing essential findings. Finally, the sample size and the number of participants is scrutinized. Larger samples generally lead to more precise estimates and broader applicability of results. However, a small sample might limit the generalizability of the findings to the EBPQI initiatives specific to the patient population (Wasserstein et al., 2019). This aspect of critical appraisal ensures that the evidence used to guide patient care is statistically sound, clinically relevant, and applicable to your specific setting and patient population (see Table 5.11).

TABLE 5.11 Statistic Elements for Evidence Appraisal

Statistic Element	Definition	Importance for ANP Leaders	Limitations
Effect size	Magnitude of observed difference or relationship	Gauges clinical significance and relevance to practice. Larger effect sizes suggest greater impact	May not be directly applicable to different populations or settings
Confidence intervals (CIs)	Range likely to contain the true population parameter	Measures precision and uncertainty of estimates. Narrower CIs indicate higher precision	Wider CIs indicate greater uncertainty, making conclusions less definitive
P-values	Probability of observing similar results if no true effect exists	Assesses statistical significance. Low p-values suggest unlikely chance occurrence	Can be influenced by sample size and effect size, leading to misinterpretations. Not a measure of effect size or clinical importance
Statistical power	Probability of detecting a true effect when it exists	Determines ability to detect clinically relevant findings. Adequate power enhances credibility; low power raises concerns	Difficult to determine precisely, often estimated based on assumptions
Sample size	Number of participants included in the study	Affects precision of estimates and generalizability of findings. Larger samples generally lead to more precise estimates and broader generalizability	Smaller samples may lead to unreliable estimates and conclusions not generalizable to larger populations

Source: Polit and Beck (2021).

You should also be aware that in quantitative research study designs statistical significance is not always meaningful clinically or practically. An important question to ask is if the study's finding(s) will help you to determine whether the effects will have a sufficient influence on practice or your patient outcomes. Stop and consider this question carefully. You and your team should determine whether the study's findings were statistically, practically, and/or clinically significant. A study that does not have statistical significance can still be clinically or practically significant (see Table 5.12). For example, clinical significance occurs when a patient's experience or health parameters are improved (Carpenter et al., 2021). EBPQI teams should closely and thoughtfully assess significance types. It is important to know (a) whether study results were likely (or not) to occur due to chance (the statistical significance); (b) whether patients, families, and/or communities are likely to benefit from the noted effect or change (the clinical significance); and (c) the quantifiable (actual) magnitude (how much change is estimated to occur) of the effect (practical significance).

TABLE 5.12 Brief Descriptions of Significance Types

Significance Type	Description	Questions Asked of the Findings
Statistical	Results due to chance	• Were the results of the intervention due to chance?
		• What is the probability that these results occurred by chance alone?
Practical	Quantifies the impact of a treatment Estimates the magnitude of effect	• How effective was the intervention/treatment?
		• How much change does the intervention/treatment cause?
Clinical	The practical or applied importance of effect, and does it make a difference to clients/subjects/patients in everyday life	• Was the intervention/treatment effective enough to improve the patient's experience (e.g., of their health or provision of care)?
		• Was the intervention/treatment enough to improve or eliminate a diagnostic criterion for a condition?

Source: Carpenter et al. (2021)

Foundations of Critical Appraisal

There are four primary components of critical appraisal: validity, reliability, generalizability and applicability. Without a systematic approach to assessing the quality and relevance of research, you and your team risk making decisions based on flawed or biased information. As a leader, it is essential to have a strong grasp of key concepts, quantitative study design, and critical questions integral to determining the trustworthiness of the research evidence (see Table 5.13).

TABLE 5.13 Key Concepts in Critical Appraisal

Concept	Definition	Importance for ANP Leaders
Validity	Does the study measure what it claims to?	Ensures accurate and trustworthy findings that inform decision-making
Reliability	Can the findings be consistently replicated?	Enhances the dependability and credibility of research results
Generalizability	Can findings be applied to other populations or settings?	Determines the broader impact and relevance of research to diverse contexts
Applicability	Can findings be applied to real-world clinical practice?	Ensures the relevance and usefulness of evidence for ANP leaders

Sources: Chair et al., (2023); JBI (2023); Polit and Beck (2021).

Validity

The term "validity" has been used many times in this chapter to generally indicate aspects of a quantitative research study that help determine how credibly the research study measured the outcomes as intended. This includes the need for the study, based on identified gaps in knowledge, the congruence between the purpose/hypothesis and the methods, the sampling, the measures and measurement/data collected, the analysis (statistics used), results, discussion, and conclusion—all of which are standard parts of a research report.

Internal validity represents *how* the study was conducted. Did the researchers do everything they could to control for bias that might influence the outcome? Table 5.7 lists types of bias that can affect a study's internal validity and how they can be controlled. External validity is the extent to which a study's findings can be generalized to other people, settings, situations, and measures. It helps ensure that the results of a study are not limited to the specific context or people in which it was conducted (Whalen & Dang, 2022).

You also want to determine whether the instruments used were valid and reliable. Does the instrument, survey, or other measurement actually measure the concept or outcome it was intended to (instrument validity), and if it did, did it do so consistently in all the participants (reliability)? Reliability also addresses how likely it is that the findings of the study will be generalizable to other settings (beyond that of the study). In EBPQI, you must know whether the study's findings apply to your patient population before you make recommendations based on the research evidence. Remember that experimental studies, such as RCTs, usually have high internal validity due to the rigorous nature of their methods for controlling confounding variables. However, nonexperimental (quasi-experimental) and observational studies may have lower internal validity yet be more transferable to the clinical setting. You will recall that the level of the study cannot predict its quality; therefore, a high-quality observational study that applies to your setting and patient needs may be of more value to your EBPQI team than an RCT that is not as applicable outside the confines of its study setting (Whalen & Dang, 2022).

Finally, beyond interpreting the study results, you must determine whether the researcher provided clinical implications and addressed study limitations. This is important information to explore as you lead the appraisal of each study with your team.

Critical Appraisal Tools for Quantitative Research Studies

Various critical appraisal tools are available to help you and your team appraise research evidence. The tool you select is based on the study design, so to be accurate they must match. Table 5.14 includes valuable resources to help your team with tool selection. The table contains each tool's copyright owner, website URL, coverage of research designs, download accessibility, and cost, as well as an overview of available instructions. In Appendix C you will find examples of a completed critical appraisal tool for a systematic review with a meta-analysis, an RCT, and a cross-sectional study.

TABLE 5.14 Critical Appraisal Tools and Resources

Critical Appraisal Tool	Website	Research Study Designs	Overview
Critical Appraisal Skills Programme Checklists (CASP)	https://casp-uk.net/casp-tools-checklists/	Systematic review RCT Cohort study Case-control study Diagnostic study	Includes instructions and embedded hints throughout the checklists No level or quality rating guide Free access Full-text PDF, Word, or print and fill
Centre for Evidence-Based Medicine	https://www.cebm.ox.ac.uk/resources/ebm-tools/critical-appraisal-tools	Systematic review RCT Cohort (prognostic) study Diagnostic accuracy study	Embedded hints throughout the form Associated level and quality rating guide (different URL) Free access Full-text downloadable form
JBI Global	https://jbi.global/critical-appraisal-tools	Systematic review RCT Quasi-experimental Cohort study Case-control study Diagnostic test Accuracy studies Analytical cross-sectional Case reports Case series Prevalence studies	Includes instructions with the form No level or quality rating guide Free access Full-text Word document

(Continued)

TABLE 5.14 *(Continued)*

Critical Appraisal Tool	Website	Research Study Designs	Overview
Johns Hopkins EBP model and tools	https://www.hopkinsmedicine.org/evidence-based-practice/model-tools	Quantitative research (RCT, quasi, descriptive) Systematic review	Includes instructions and embedded hints throughout all forms Level and quality guide for ratings Strength of recommendation rating Free access Request permission for use and receive a zip file with all forms
National Heart, Lung and Blood Institute	https://www.nhlbi.nih.gov/health-topics/study-quality-assessment-tools	RCTs Systematic reviews (with meta-analyses) Observational cohort and cross-sectional Quasi-experimental Case series	Free access Includes instructions on how to evaluate criteria

After you have completed the critical appraisal tool or checklist for each of the studies you included to answer your PICOT or PPCO question, you and your team must next conduct an evaluation of the body of evidence.

Evaluation

The next step in the critical appraisal process is evaluation. During the evaluation phase, you will take the information from each study and your critical appraisal and place them into an evidence table or matrix template. At this point, you can discard any evidence that you or your team found to be of low quality or inapplicable to your PICOT or PPCO question, patient population, or setting. There is no magic number of research articles to add to your evaluation tables. The quality and consistency of your research evidence will support your confidence to make practice recommendations (Fineout-Overholt et al., 2010).

An evidence table or matrix is a tool used to summarize and organize the key information from appraising research studies to answer your clinical question (see Table 5.15). As you add each systematic review or study to an evaluation table row, you will observe similarities and differences across the study variables, outcome measures, data analyses, and findings that aid in answering your question. Depending on your question you may need to add columns—such as the

TABLE 5.15 Example Matrix Evaluation Table

Citation	Purpose of Study	Design/ Method	Sample/ Setting	Intervention (if Applicable)	Major Variables Studied and Their Definitions	Measurement of Major Variables	Data Analysis	Study Findings/ Results	Level of Evidence	Worth to Practice

intervention column in this example. You could also consider a column with your critical appraisal summary. Once each study or systematic review has been added to an evaluation table, you will begin to synthesize the evidence for its value to your practice setting (O'Mathuna et al., 2023).

Strength or Recommendation Rating

At this point, you are not ready to make a definitive recommendation for a practice change because other types of evidence remain to be appraised (Chapters 6 and 7), but as you view the key information you have placed into your evaluation and synthesis tables so far, you can begin to evaluate whether consistency in quality and outcomes across studies might support a case for making a change in practice (Newhouse, 2022). The decision loop at the base of the EBPQI mountain (Waldrop & Dunlap, 2024) reflects the possibilities that at this point you may begin to determine whether there is enough evidence to change practice or whether more research is needed before you can pursue change safely (see Figure 5.6). This is an example of how movement within the mountain model can be bidirectional.

Evaluating the body of evidence you have gathered is all about weighing the quality, quantity, and consistency. You have critically appraised each study for quality. However, now also consider the quantity of studies or the total sample size of all the studies combined. How many studies on the topic/outcome are there? Are there only one or two or many? Were the sample sizes small or large? Consider the consistency of the findings across studies. How consistent are their results? Figure 5.7 provides you with a visual to help your team make informed recommendations.

Johns Hopkins uses the following categories for describing the strength of recommendation based on your synthesis:

- **Strong and compelling evidence, consistent results** > Recommendations are reliable; evaluate for organizational translation.
- **Good evidence and consistent results** > Recommendations may be reliable; evaluate for risk and organizational translation.

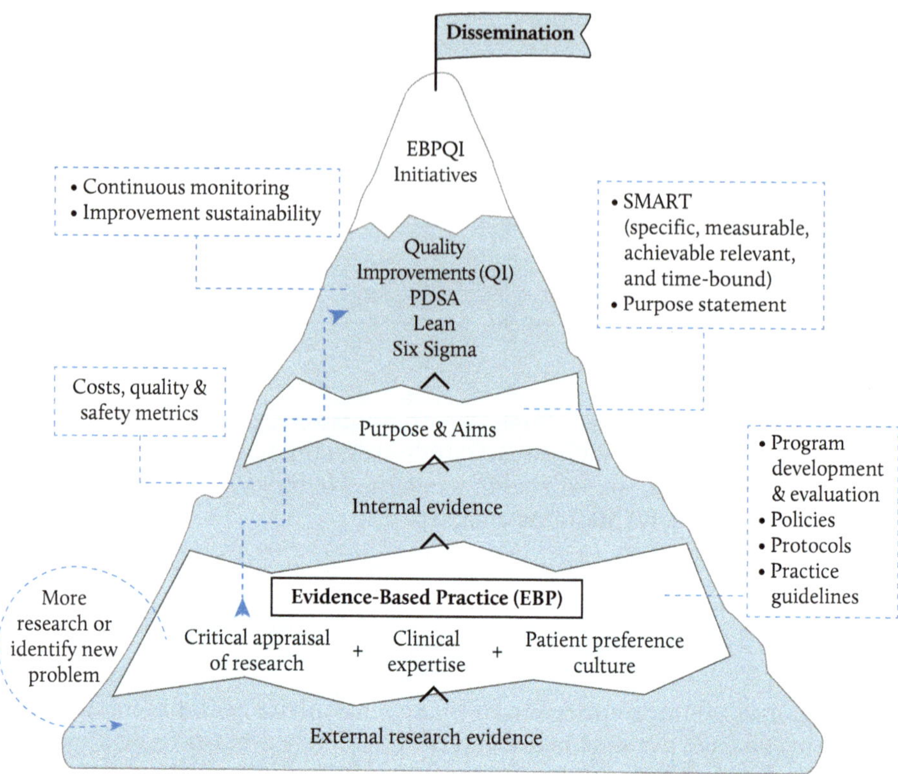

FIGURE 5.6 EBP within the mountain model.

- **Good evidence but conflicting results** > Unable to establish best practice based on current evidence; *evaluate risk*, consider further investigation for new evidence, develop a research study, or discontinue the project.
- **Little or no evidence** > Unable to establish best practice based on current evidence; consider further investigation for new evidence, develop a research study, or discontinue the project. (Newhouse, 2022, p. 321)

Notice that the strength of the recommendation rating "good evidence but conflicting results" allows you to evaluate the risk for patient harm. If the likelihood of harm is low, using a quality improvement approach of manageable plan-do-study-act (PDSA) cycles to pilot a small change may be reasonable (see Chapters 9–11). Always remember that you must determine whether the intervention is feasible in your setting. Consideration of patient preferences and values is an important component of EBP, and it is critical to determine the applicability of the evidence to your practice setting and population (see Chapter 8).

The Grading of Recommendations, Assessment, Development and Evaluations (GRADE) workgroup developed a strong systematic framework for presenting summaries of evidence to make clinical practice recommendations. It begins with rating the quality of a body of evidence for a particular outcome. In the GRADE system there are four levels of evidence based on the certainty of the evidence:

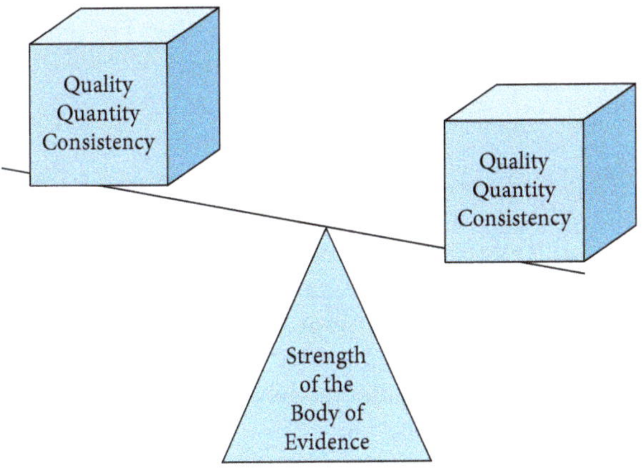

FIGURE 5.7 Weighing the body of evidence.

very low, low, moderate, and high (Table 5.16). An interesting aspect about the GRADE is that all studies start out as equal in certainty but are downgraded or upgraded based on *domains*. You are now familiar with these: risk of bias, the preciseness of the effect, inconsistency, the directness of the effect or application to your patient population, and publication bias.

TABLE 5.16 Grade Certainty Ratings

Criteria	Description	Notes
Rating of Evidence Quality	**High:** The authors have a lot of confidence that the true effect is similar to the estimated effect.	Based on systematic reviews or well-designed RCTs. Strong methodological rigor, low risk of bias, consistent findings
	Moderate: The authors believe that the true effect is probably close to the estimated effect.	Based on well-designed observational studies or RCTs with limitations. Moderate methodological rigor, some risk of bias, somewhat consistent findings
	Low: The true effect might be markedly different from the estimated effect.	Based on poorly designed studies, case reports, or expert opinions. Weak methodological rigor, high risk of bias, inconsistent findings
	Very low: The true effect is probably markedly different from the estimated effect.	Limited or no relevant studies available. Insufficient evidence to draw reliable conclusions

Source: Guyatt et al. (2011).

In health care, synthesized evidence refers to integrating findings from multiple sources, including quantitative and qualitative studies, as well as other evidence. Synthesized evidence is crucial in informing decision-making by offering a comprehensive and evidence-based approach to health care practices. By promoting use of synthesized evidence that has been critically appraised, we can ensure that health care practices are grounded in the latest research and knowledge, leading to better patient outcomes.

Leadership Strategies for Effective Critical Appraisal

Fostering a culture of clinical inquiry is vital for effective critical appraisal within a team. Strategies include empowering team members to ask questions, challenge assumptions, and share their diverse perspectives. As a leader, you should facilitate discussions about current research and EBPs within the team and aim for shared understanding and agreement on the interpretation of the evidence and its application to practice. As an ANP leader, you may be responsible for evaluating synthesized evidence collected by others and their recommendations. You will need to be able to assess the coherence of the synthesized findings and if the findings truly support the proposed EBPQI initiative in your specific context and within the population your organization serves. You will also need to assess how the integrated findings align with the organization's goals, priorities, and the specific context of health care delivery. The leadership team should identify the most relevant and actionable findings from the synthesized evidence and their potential impact on clinical practices, patient outcomes, and organizational policies.

Clear and concise communication is essential for effectively sharing appraisal findings with stakeholders, including other health care professionals, patients, and administrators. Be sure to use language and explanations appropriate for each group's level of understanding. Highlight the most relevant and actionable findings or key points from the appraisal and synthesis (see Box 5.5). Translate findings into concrete recommendations for improving quality and safety.

BOX 5.5: CALL TO ACTION FOR EVIDENCE-BASED DECISION-MAKING

- *Embrace critical appraisal skills.* Invest in learning and refining appraisal skills for yourself and all nurses. This will empower nurses to confidently navigate the complexities of health care research and translate findings into practice.
- *Advocate for EBPQI.* Actively advocate for the integration of research findings into clinical decision-making processes within health care institutions to ensure EBPs gain traction.
- *Collaborate with researchers.* Build bridges between clinical practice and research to faster ongoing exploration and generation of high-quality evidence relevant to the needs of the health care system and the patients it serves.
- *Seek out learning opportunities.* Actively participate in workshops, conferences, and online resources dedicated to enhancing appraisal skills (see Chapter 13).
- *Engage in reflective practice.* Critically reflect on your personal appraisal experiences and seek feedback from colleagues to identify areas for improvement.
- *Contribute to the advancement of appraisal methodologies.* Share feedback and perspectives on existing tools and advocate for the development of novel appraisal frameworks that can shape the future of EBP in advanced nursing.

WELLNESS IN ACTION: SOCIAL WELL-BEING

As an ANP leader, it is important for you to feel comfortable being authentic and professional during social situations. It can be draining to yourself and others if you are unable to disconnect from digital devices and engage in the present. We encourage you to use your time with others to seek to belong rather than fit in. This is an important distinction. Fitting in involves changing who you are inauthentically for some purpose such as fear and is not healthy and may have negative consequences for you and your team. Diverse teams (in race, gender, work experience, age, neurodivergence, etc.) are the strongest groups, and as a leader, you can role-model embracing differences naturally and with respect. This will likely help create social environments where others feel intellectually and emotionally safe, which fosters creativity. Active social engagement has been linked to healthy outcomes; however, it is important to acknowledge healthy lifestyles should be encouraged through positive social engagement (Luo et al., 2020) as well. Reducing screen time has been suggested to establish a better work–life balance through healthy technology use (Thomas et al., 2022). We welcome your consideration of the following steps aimed at increasing your social well-being:

1. Increase authentic engagement with those around you.
2. Treat others with respect always.
3. Welcome diverse viewpoints and engage people who may not share your own opinions in a collegial manner.
4. Seek to understand the perspectives of others with a spirit of curiosity rather than judgment.
5. Maintain and develop new friendships and networks with colleagues and others.
6. Prioritize in-person social interactions when possible.
7. Engage in digital social interactions to supplement (not replace) in-person social engagement.
8. Allow yourself healthy time to disconnect from digital distractions. One way to help you do this is to give digital engagement less visual appeal. For example, you can change your phone to grayscale. (For iPhone users as of 2024, follow these simple steps: Open your settings app, navigate to the accessibility menu, tap on "display & text size menu," turn on color filters, and select the grayscale filter.)
9. Be mindful and present in the moment by noticing social engagements that supply you with peace, calm, or excitement and continue pursuing these.

WRAPPING UP

In conclusion, before you can implement any recommended practice changes, be mindful that various sources of research evidence are acceptable for clinical decision-making. Due to the complexities of health care delivery, several sources of evidence may be needed to answer a clinical question. This chapter has focused on quantitative evidence as it relates to EBP, but you will remember from Chapter 1 that EBP decisions are not based on research evidence alone. Patient preferences and clinical expertise are of equal importance on the second tier of the EBPQI mountain. For example, as a nurse leader or CNM working on the mother/baby unit, you might want to implement evidence-based interventions to support mother/infant breastfeeding, but if you are unaware of how the mothers perceive breastfeeding support, what component of EBP will you focus on to gather information to offer them the types of support they desire? For that you will need to understand patient preferences and values, like the example in the beginning of this chapter and a topic we cover in Chapter 8. We covered significant ground in this chapter and invite you to consider the wellness and reflection information before moving on to the next chapter on qualitative research evidence.

REFLECTION QUESTIONS

1. In what type of study would you expect to find a forest plot?
   a. What information can a forest plot provide?
   b. How might you interpret this information from a clinical perspective instead of a statistically significant one?
2. What challenges do you foresee in leading teams in critical appraisal of quantitative evidence?
3. How can you educate your team in construction of a synthesis table(s)?

REFERENCES

Agency for Healthcare Research and Quality. (2018). *Evidence-based decision-making.* https://www.ahrq.gov/prevention/chronic-care/decision/index.html

Baldi, I., Soriani, N., Lorenzoni, G., Azzolina, D., Dal Lago, E., De Bardi, S., ... & Gregori, D. (2017). Research in nursing and nutrition: Is randomized clinical trial the actual gold standard? *Gastroenterology Nursing, 40*(1), 63–70.

Capili, B., & Anastasi, J. K. (2023). Efficacy randomized controlled trials. *AJN The American Journal of Nursing, 123*(3), 47–51.

Carpenter, R., Waldrop, J., & Carter-Templeton, H. (2021). Statistical, practical and clinical significance and Doctor of Nursing practice projects. *Nurse Author & Editor, 31*(3–4), 50–53.

Chair, S. Y., Wong, F. K. Y., Bryant-Lukosius, D., Liu, T., & Jokiniemi, K. (2023). Construct validity of advanced practice nurse core competence scale: an exploratory factor analysis. *BMC Nursing, 22*(1), 57.

Chang, Y., Phillips, M. R., Guymer, R. H., Thabane, L., Bhandari, M., & Chaudhary, V. (2022). The 5min meta-analysis: Understanding how to read and interpret a forest plot. *Eye, 36*(4), 673–675. https://doi.org/10.1038/s41433-021-01867-6

Critical Appraisal Skills Programme. (n.d.). *Home page.* https://casp-uk.net/

Dang, D., Dearholt, S., Bissett, K., Ascenzi, J., & Whalen, M. (2021). *Johns Hopkins evidence-based practice for nurses and healthcare professionals: model and guidelines.*

Epstein, R., Fonnesbeck, C., Williamson, E., Kuhn, T., Lindegren, M. L., Rizzone, K., Krishnaswami, S., Sathe, N., Ficzere, C. H., Ness, G. L., Wright, G. W., Raj, M., Potter, S., &

McPheeters, M. (2015). *Psychosocial and Pharmacologic Interventions for Disruptive Behavior in Children and Adolescents*. Agency for Healthcare Research and Quality (US). edition. Indianapolis, IN, Sigma Theta Tau International.

Farrow, K. A., & Neff, F. (2024). Bereavement care team: Improving ICU nurses' professional bereavement and patient family experience. *Nursing Administration Quarterly, 48*(2), 97–106. https://doi.org/10.1097/NAQ.0000000000000634

Feng, Y., Lin, Y., Zhang, N., Jiang, X. & Zhang, L. (2021). Effects of animal-assisted therapy on hospitalized children and teenagers: A systematic review and meta-analysis. *Journal of Pediatric Nursing, 60*, 11–23. https://doi.org/10.1016/j.pedn2021.01.020

Fineout-Overholt, E., Melnyk, B. M., Stillwell, S. B., & Williamson, K. M. (2010). Evidence-based practice step by step: Critical appraisal of the evidence: part I. *The American journal of nursing, 110*(7), 47–52. https://doi.org/10.1097/01.NAJ.0000383935.22721.9c

Guyatt, G. H., Oxman, A. D., Kunz, R., Brozek, J., Alonso-Coello, P., Rind, D., et al. (2011). GRADE guidelines 6. Rating the quality of evidence—Imprecision. *Journal of Clinical Epidemiology*, 64(12), 1283–1293.

Joanna Briggs Institute. (2023). *JBI critical appraisal tools.* https://jbi.global/critical-appraisal-tools

Khalili, S. Shirinkam, F., Ghadimi, R., & Karimi, H. (2022). The effect of group walking program on social physique anxiety and the risk of eating disorders in aged women: A randomized clinical trial study. *Applied Nursing Research, 64*, 1–7.

Luo, M., Ding, D., Bauman, A. *et al. (2020).* Social engagement pattern, health behaviors and subjective well-being of older adults: An international perspective using WHO-SAGE survey data. *BMC Public Health, 20*, 99. https://doi.org/10.1186/s12889-019-7841-7

Melnyk, B. M., & Fineout-Overholt, E. (2023). *Evidence-based practice in nursing & healthcare: A guide to best practice*. Lippincott Williams & Wilkins.

Murad, M. H., Asi, N., Alsawas, M., & Alahdab, F. (2016). New evidence pyramid. *Evidence-based medicine, 21*(4), 125–127. https://doi.org/10.1136/ebmed-2016-110401

Polit, D. F., & Beck, C. T. (2021). *Nursing research: Generating and assessing evidence for nursing practice* (11th ed.). Wolters Kluwer.

Rodriguez-Lopez, M., Parra, B., Vergara, E., Rey, L., Salcedo, M., Arturo, G., Alarcon, L., Holguin, J., & Osorio, L. (2021). A case-control study of factors associated with SARS-CoV-2 infection among healthcare workers in Colombia. *BMC infectious diseases, 21*(1), 878. https://doi.org/10.1186/s12879-021-06581-y

Takona, J. P. (2024). Research design: Qualitative, quantitative, and mixed methods approaches. *Quality & Quantity, 58*(1), 1011–1013.

Thomas, N. M., Choudhari, S. G., Gaidhane, A. M., & Quazi Syed, Z. (2022). 'Digital Wellbeing': The Need of the Hour in Today's Digitalized and Technology Driven World! *Cureus, 14*(8), e27743. https://doi.org/10.7759/cureus.27743

Tomotaki, A., Sakai, I., Fukahori, H., Tsuda, Y., & Okumura-Hiroshige, A. (2023). Factors affecting the critical appraisal of research articles in Evidence-Based practices by advanced practice nurses: A descriptive qualitative study. *Nursing Open, 10*(6), 3719–3727. https://doi.org/10.1002/nop2.1628

Waldrop, J., & Dunlap, J. J. (2024). The mountain model for evidence-based practice quality improvement initiatives. *American Journal of Nursing, 124*(5), 32–37. https://doi.org/10.1097/01.NAJ.0001014540.57079.72

Wasserstein, R. L., Schirm, A. L., & Lazar, N. A. (2019). Moving to a world beyond "$p<0.05$." *The American Statistician, 73*(1), 1–19. https://doi.org/10.1080/00031305.2019.1583913

White, L., Waldrop, J., & Waldrop, C. (2016). Human papillomavirus and vaccination of males: Knowledge and attitudes of registered nurses. *Pediatric Nursing, 42*(1), 21–30, 35.

IMAGE CREDITS

Fig. 5.2: Copyright © by MJ Page et al. (CC BY 4.0) at https://www.prisma-statement.org/prisma-2020-flow-diagram.

Fig. 5.4: Joseph R. Dettori, Daniel C. Norvell, and Jens R. Chapman, "Seeing the Forest by Looking at the Trees: How to Interpret a Meta-Analysis Forest Plot," *Global Spine Journal*, vol. 11, no. 4, p. 615. Copyright © 2021 by SAGE Publications.

Fig. 5.6: Jayne Jennings Dunlap and Julee Briscoe Waldrop, *Introduction to Evidence-Based Practice and Quality Improvement for Professional Nursing Practice: A Competency Based Approach,* p. 102. Copyright © 2024 by Cognella, Inc. Reprinted with permission.

CHAPTER 6

Leading Critical Appraisal of Qualitative Evidence

Suzy Lockwood, Kathy A. Baker, and Julee Briscoe Waldrop

KEY CONCEPTS

Critical appraisal
Qualitative methodology
Trustworthiness

LEARNING OBJECTIVES

1. Recognize the value of qualitative methodology for informing advanced nursing practice.
2. Explore the philosophies, paradigms, and assumptions underlying qualitative research methodology.
3. Identify the various qualitative research study designs used in research.
4. Describe the steps involved in leading a critical appraisal of qualitative evidence, including framing the evidence searching question, searching for relevant studies, and selecting appropriate appraisal tools.
5. Understand the role of critical appraisal in evaluating the quality and trustworthiness of qualitative evidence.
6. Collaborate effectively with health care teams to lead critical appraisal discussions and integrate qualitative evidence into leadership and practice.

> Keep your thoughts positive because your thoughts become your words. Keep your words positive because your words become your behavior. Keep your behavior positive because your behavior becomes your habits. Keep your habits positive because your habits become your values. Keep your values positive because your values become your destiny.
>
> —Mahatma Gandhi, *Words of Gandhi*

Introduction

While quantitative studies (Chapter 5) help to establish statistical significance of research findings, qualitative studies provide the personal context of patient experiences, preferences, and priorities crucial to providing holistic care. For example, earlier in my (Julee) career as a NP leading a team of health care providers in caring for newborns, I observed in our hospital that most mothers with Latinx heritage began supplementing breastfeeding with formula before they left the hospital. This supplementation was a contributing factor to the obesity later seen in our clinic. We were a baby-friendly hospital with lactation consultants and nurses supporting exclusive breastfeeding, but all our structures and processes were not having an impact on the behavior of these mothers. I was curious about this phenomenon, so I designed a qualitative research study to explore the mother's experience and what this feeding practice meant to her (Waldrop, 2013). I used qualitative methods and found four themes that described the reasons mothers gave for feeding "los dos": (a) previous experience; (b) "no llora con hambre" (no crying for hunger); (c) "para salud" (for health); and (d) to prevent suffering that might occur when the mother and infant were separated while the mother worked ("no quiero que sufra mientras trabajo"). This information helped providers and staff better understand these mothers and their decisions and frame their communication differently around breastfeeding.

In addition to providing the patient's personal context relative to health care experiences, beliefs, and priorities, qualitative research also provides critical contributions to health care policy (Williams et al., 2020). Understanding more about individual, community, and population beliefs, preferences, and priorities, for instance, can help us to begin to understand behaviors and responses to recommendations for care that may be problematic or burdensome despite the distinction of being "best evidence." Identifying these perspectives and the meaning behind them can then help you contribute to a more sensitive and accurate implementation plan for health initiatives that can ultimately enhance a broader uptake of these evidence-based recommendations.

For example, you might recall that during the COVID-19 pandemic, national recommendations for obtaining the vaccine were questioned by the public. Hu et al. (2021) analyzed the contents of 300,000 tweets in the United States over a 12-month period (March 2020 to February 2021) to investigate public emotions, attitudes, and opinions about the vaccines across time. The researchers described how their ability to explore the keywords and major topics of tweets about COVID-19 provided valuable insights into the public perception and trending attitudes toward vaccine recommendations. Vaccine-averse conspiracy theories contributed to misleading messages. The researchers' recommendations stated that government officials should also use these social media platforms to communicate evidence-based findings, even considering tailoring messages to geographic areas where public sentiments were negative toward COVID-19 vaccinations based on their analysis. They also noted different states reflected different trends in sentiment and emotion toward the vaccine and recommended implementation of government and public health campaigns to address people's fears and concerns in those areas with high negative beliefs and perceptions. Their findings demonstrated that public figures, especially politicians, played a crucial role in swaying public opinion and highlighted the responsibility public figures have to share accurate, evidence-based health information over personal opinion.

Research analysis of qualitative data from conversations such as these not only impact public health and policy but can also be informative to guide NPs and nurse leaders such as yourselves when working with patients who demonstrate diverse opinions and perspectives about important health care recommendations.

Understanding the purpose and contributions of this methodology to knowledge development in nursing and health care will maximize the evidence base for care that you deliver as an APRN or a leader of other direct care providers. In this chapter, you will find an overview of qualitative research methodology; explore the philosophies, paradigms, and assumptions embedded in qualitative methods; identify the primary qualitative study designs; and describe the steps in critical appraisal of qualitative studies. Our goal is for you to be able to evaluate qualitative research studies for their trustworthiness. Additionally, when working with interprofessional and interdisciplinary health care teams, you will be able to lead discussions of qualitative evidence and advocate for its value in care delivery.

Overview of Qualitative Research Methodology

In the late 1800s, German psychologist and historian Dilthey argued that the study of the external world (natural science) is different from the internal world (human science) and that both, while philosophically different, contribute to knowledge development (Feest, 2006). Dilthey argues that the underlying assumptions (objective in natural science versus subjective in human science) allows for different, yet valuable, contributions from both quantitative and qualitative methods. Dilthey's focus was on the importance of understanding human beings alongside positivism's commitment to pure explanatory approaches to science. Dilthey's commitment to understanding human beings became known as qualitative research methodology. Qualitative research focuses on non-numerical data. Therefore, it cannot be collected, measured or analyzed in the same way.

There are multiple approaches to data collection in qualitative methodology, including personal or group interviews, audio recordings, observations, videos, or written text or other documents. A common strategy is to conduct an interview. In a structured interview, every participant is asked the same questions, and no deviation occurs, whereas in a semi-structured interview, the researcher can ask questions to further explore a participant's answer and better understand their experience. Focus group interviews place participants in small groups to respond to questions and discuss answers. Interviews are frequently audio recorded and transcribed into text for analysis. Written words from any source (e.g., open-ended questions, journals, blogs, Twitter feeds) can be analyzed, and observations (either video recorded or in the form of notes taken in real time) can be transcribed, reviewed, and analyzed. While quantitative methods analyze objective data, qualitative methods look at subjective data.

As in all science, the approach to qualitative research is systematic and rigorous. But because the underlying philosophies and goals are different from quantitative methodology, the qualitative approach to research designs, methods, and application is also different. For instance, the ultimate objective of quantitative research findings is generalizability to other subjects and populations. In qualitative research, the objective is to transfer insights from patterns in human experience that can inform how people experience a phenomenon or prioritize their response to a phenomenon. Because human experience is individualized, qualitative methods are more fluid than a priori quantitative methods, often emerging or adapting as a study is conducted in response to the data provided by participants. Instead of a highly controlled setting, data is often collected in the natural setting, where the participant lives and works (see Figure 6.1).

Qualitative research is not intended to determine cause and effect, though qualitative research findings often contribute to the development of theory or hypotheses. Qualitative research is exploratory in nature. Accordingly, the level of evidence attributed to qualitative research is lower on the evidence hierarchy than most quantitative designs. Lower, however, does not mean less valuable. As we have discussed, qualitative methods differ from quantitative approaches, and therefore the intent of qualitative findings differ from quantitative. Both are of value to knowledge development and meaningful understanding in health care. As a nurse in an advanced role, understanding the value and appropriate application of qualitative research studies in supporting patients through their health experiences elevates your contributions and aligns with the holistic approach of nursing.

Philosophies and Paradigms Underlying Qualitative Methods

The philosophy of qualitative methodology provides the researcher's framework or context for designing a qualitative research study and therefore is important to our understanding of qualitative research designs. There are three primary philosophical perspectives for qualitative methodology: postpositivism, interpretivism (social constructionism), and critical theory.

Postpositivism

Postpositivists do not believe in strict cause and effect; all cause and effect are a probability that may or may not occur. They believe subjectivity and objectivity are socially constructed and that knowledge is embedded in our experiences and being (Ryan, 2005). From a qualitative lens, postpositivism states that inquiry is a series of logical related steps. Multiple perspectives rather than a single reality exist. Data collection and analysis embrace rigorous methods such as multiple levels, use of computer programs for data analysis, establishment of validity, and results of studies are still reported in a structure similar to quantitative articles (Creswell & Poth, 2018).

Interpretivism

The philosophical basis for interpretivism is that all understanding and knowledge is socially or culturally constructed. That is, we create our own realities through our social interactions, relationships, and experiences. Because of this, many realities can exist simultaneously (i.e., multiple realities). From this philosophical perspective, the researcher expects complexity of views and does not attempt to narrow the meanings embedded in the data into a few categories or ideas. The researcher inductively develops a theory or pattern of meaning from the discussions and interactions experienced with the research informants/participants. Open-ended questions are embraced. The goal of the research is to understand the historical and cultural settings of the participants and to capture the contexts in which people live and work. When working from this philosophy, the researcher recognizes and acknowledges that their own experience inherently influences how they "interpret" what they find in the research data (Creswell & Poth, 2018; Ryan, 2018).

Critical Theory

Critical theory philosophy emphasizes that reality is shaped by social, political, cultural, economic, ethic, and gender-based forces that are often reflected as social structures. In critical theory, our subjective experiences and values are impacted by social and historical influences. The goal of critical theory philosophy is to ultimately change the world by understanding experiences and empowering participants in a local context to shed restrictions and biases placed on them according to their race, gender, or social class (Creswell & Poth, 2018; Ryan, 2018). Researchers embracing this philosophy recognize that they also bring a power persona to the relationship with the participants and carefully acknowledge this as they interact with participants and study data (DePoy & Gitlin, 2016).

TABLE 6.1 Comparison of the Quantitative and Qualitative Methodologies From a Philosophical Perspective

Quantitative Methods	Qualitative Methods
• Strive for objectivity, replicability, and control with the aim of explanation and generalizability. • Experimental research designs are the ideal. • Large, representative samples are the ideal. • Data must be collected and analyzed in numerical form (reliably measured and statistically analyzed). • The aim is to test a hypothesis derived from theory.	• The emphasis is on intersubjectivity, uniqueness, unrepeatability, and participation. • Phenomena are ideally studied in their naturally occurring context. • Samples are usually small, even single cased. • Data are collected in textual format and analyzed in an active and transaction engagement with the text. • The aim is contextually and critically understanding subjective perspectives and experiences by reconstructing the personal meaning and/or experiences conveyed by participants.

Source: Gelo (2012).

Paradigms

Scientific paradigms provide the *why* of scientific inquiry, providing it with its basic philosophical foundations. A paradigm is a distinct set of concepts or thought patterns that determines the approach to a study. Paradigms include the assumptions and beliefs about what science is and how it should be applied (Kuhn, 2012). In research, the paradigm determines which data about a phenomenon should be collected and analyzed, as well as how it can be applied to extend knowledge. The assumptions for qualitative methodology differ from those for quantitative methods and are based on four general paradigms in research: ontology, epistemology, axiology, and methodology (Table 6.2; Creswell, 2018).

TABLE 6.2 Assumptions for Qualitative Methodology

Ontology	The ontological perspective addresses the nature of being. Because your experience is different from mine, there can be multiple realities versus a single, universal truth.
Epistemology	The assumption of how we know what we know in qualitative methodology stresses that knowledge is actively constructed by the researcher and participant, who exert mutual influence on one another. Knowledge is known through the subjective experience of the informants/participants. In qualitative research, the goal is not to eliminate bias, but to capture the dynamic interaction between the contextualized experiences of the participants; this is known as establishing the trustworthiness of the findings.
Axiology	A third assumption addresses how the researcher's values and assumptions influence the scientific process (axiology). In qualitative research, the assumption is that the researcher is a change agent as they interact with the study participants to gain understanding.
Methodology	Finally, the methodological assumptions for qualitative methodology specify a generally inductive approach, studied within the context of the experience under investigation, and allowing for an emerging (instead of a priori) design.

Sources: Alele and Malau-Aduli (2023); Creswell and Poth (2018).

Qualitative Research Study Designs

In this section, we will explore commonly used qualitative research study designs in nursing and health care: narrative research, phenomenology, grounded theory, ethnography, and case studies. For each one there are considerations for sampling, data collection, and data analysis.

Narrative Research

In narrative research, the researcher studies the lives of individuals through collected stories that are shared either individually or in small groups. The data collected is from participants' "life storytelling" or field notes collected during sessions. Data might also be collected in the form of biographical evidence and the sharing of artifacts (i.e., pictures or documents) that further explore the personal experiences, historical context, or culture. Key to this qualitative design is that the process is an interactive dialogue with the researcher and participant(s) and the contextual details are essential. Data analysis is done thematically (what was said), structurally (telling), verbally, and visually, looking for similarities, differences, or change. Conclusions or findings are established through reflection on the data collected and identification of patterns of meaning.

BOX 6.1: EXAMPLE OF NARRATIVE RESEARCH

Inspired by the 2013 National Patient Safety Foundation roundtable report on joy, mining in work, and workforce safety (Lucien Leape Institute at the National Patient Safety Foundation, 2013), and the IHI whitepaper on a framework to improve joy in work (Perlo et al., 2017), nurse researchers wanted to better understand nurses' experiences of meaning and joy and what factors contributed to these experiences (Galuska et al., 2018). This study addressed this question through narrative analyses of nurse stories that describe their experiences across settings and roles. One interesting aspect of the interviews was that the nurse's stories were recorded through StoryCorps®, which makes the data transparent! Anyone can listen to the stories of these nurses describing meaning and joy in the practice (www.storycorps.org). The 20 participants were very diverse in age, gender, experience, practice specialty, role, setting, and location. Analysis of the interviews revealed four themes: (a) fulfilling purpose: "I am a nurse"; (b) meaningful connection; (c) impact; (d) practice environment. In qualitative study reports you will find the themes are supported by quotes from the participants that reflect the theme. The researchers then use what they learned from the stories to present recommendations for nurse leaders to support and promote more meaning and joy in nursing practice.

Phenomenology

Phenomenology is a unique philosophical approach that seeks to describe the different ways that a group perceives and understands similar experiences. It focuses on the conscious experience of a phenomenon and the collective meaning after reflection (Bayuo et al., 2023). The emphasis is on describing and analyzing the phenomena without making assumptions about underlying causes or preexisting concepts. Sampling requires the identification and recruitment of individuals who have direct experience with the phenomena being examined. This purposeful sampling requires the use of the bracketing principle; the researcher must set aside preconceived ideas (bracket them) and experiences in an effort to understand the experience or phenomena (Creswell & Poth, 2018; Fischer, 2009).

Using in-depth interviewing guided by a few selected broad open-ended questions, participants are asked to reflect on their experience, leading to a conversation from which the researcher is able to do additional clarification and probing. Transcripts and notes from the interviews can then be read and reread with a focus on categorizing and describing the phenomena (Bayuo et al., 2023). Phenomenology requires the researcher to immerse themselves in the data. Systematic data analysis requires interpreting and making sense of the all the data collected. To ensure validity and credibility, researchers may also engage in member checking, sharing the findings and soliciting feedback from the participants, which then allows them to confirm their experiences are accurately represented and also provide an opportunity for them to offer additional insight or corrections. Uncovering the underlying structures and meanings of experiences will then lead to the development of themes that will provide insight into the phenomenon.

BOX 6.2: EXAMPLE OF PHENOMENOLOGY RESEARCH

Traditionally in Korea, when a patient was hospitalized, a family member or other caregiver was required to stay with them to provide daily care. In 2016, an integrated model of nursing care, similar to that in the United States and other countries, was introduced, whereby the nurses provide whole-person care and the burden to the families is therefore reduced. This study aimed to explore the experiences of nurses working in this model to provide formative data for developing measures related to the quality of care being provided (Cho & Kim, 2024). The participants were recruited using a "snowball" method. Seventeen nurses were interviewed using semi-structured interviews before data saturation was achieved. Meaning was interpreted by the researchers through multiple readings of the transcripts in an ongoing manner, and emerging questions were added to the next interview. The transcripts (words, data) were analyzed using the phenomenological approach (Colaizzi, 1978). This approach involves seven steps (see Figure 6.1). Member checking of the transcripts was performed to increase the rigor of the research. Nurse experts in qualitative research were used to verify the reliability of the research processes. There was a total of six theme clusters identified: (a) distorted perceptions of others in the integrated nursing care ward; (b) challenges owing to the distorted perceptions; (c) loneliness and fighting; (d) humiliation and harassment by patients; (e) practicing textbook holistic care; and (f) the pride felt only in the integrated nursing care ward. Per qualitative results, participant quotes were presented to support the themes. This study provided insights into the nurses' experiences that can be used to enhance operational systems and improve work satisfaction in the integrated care ward.

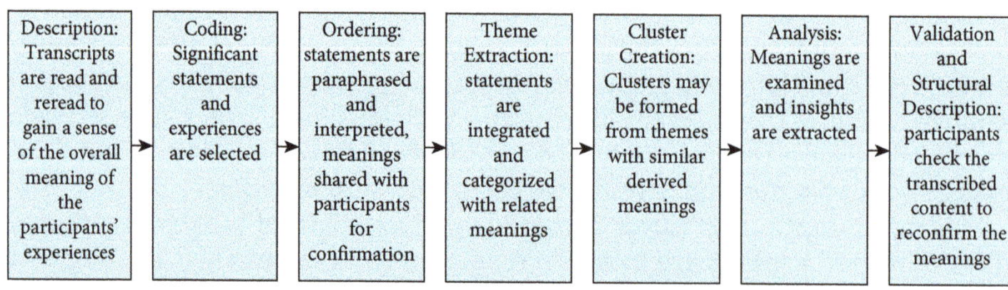

FIGURE 6.1 Example of a phenomenological analysis process.

Ethnography

Ethnography is an approach used to study and understand people and cultures through immersive examination of shared patterns of behavior, language, and actions in a natural setting, ideally over a prolonged period of time (Curtis & Keeler, 2022). "Fieldwork" is the term used when the researchers observe and interact with a community or group over an extended period of time. This can include active engagement in daily activities that then allows for the observation and documentation of behaviors, rituals, and social interactions. Selection of participants or sites, most frequently using criterion or snowball sampling, is based on their relevancy to the research question. The hallmark method for data collection in ethnography is participant observation while actively participating in all aspects of the situation (life) and taking field notes of behaviors, interactions, and cultural practices encountered (Reeves et al., 2013). To gather more detailed information or understanding, the researcher may also conduct interviews either individually or in focus groups with members of the community.

Data organization in a systematic, consistent way is key to management of interviews, field notes, and other raw data. Transcription of interviews or recordings may also require researcher involvement to ensure that nuances of tone and even nonverbal communication is included (Creswell & Poth, 2018). Once organized the analysis of data in ethnography involves the identification and interpretation of patterns or themes within the data. Content analysis and interpretive analysis are frequently used to understand the context, perspective, and subjective interpretations of participants experiences, leading to themes and theory development.

BOX 6.3: EXAMPLE OF ETHNOGRAPHIC RESEARCH

In this example, researchers identified a gap in knowledge related to the use of human-like manikins in student learning (Handeland et al., 2022). The purpose of this study was to gain new insight into the influence of human-like manikins on nursing student learning. This study took place at four different sites and thematic observation forms were used (and turned into text) along with interviews that were conducted using a semi-structured thematic guide. The researchers report using self-reflection during data collection to increase transparency, dependability, and credibility, which you will remember are important components of the trustworthiness of qualitative study results. Results were analyzed using code as well as ethnographic writing. Ethnographic writing is produced by the researcher and reflects what the interpreted data is "really" about (Madden, 2017). These ethnographic writings were combined with the transcripts of the interviews and field notes on each event (or session with the manikins). The data was then coded, resulting in 19 descriptive categories and ultimately five analytic categories: (a) manikin as an object; (b) manikin as a subject; (c) the interplay between the object and the subject; (d) the individual learning space; and (e) the collective learning space. The authors present these results as a visual model (Figure 6.2). The conclusion sheds light on the interplay between the manikin as object and subject and reflects the manikins' dual nature as a mediator of the technical and interpersonal aspects of nursing.

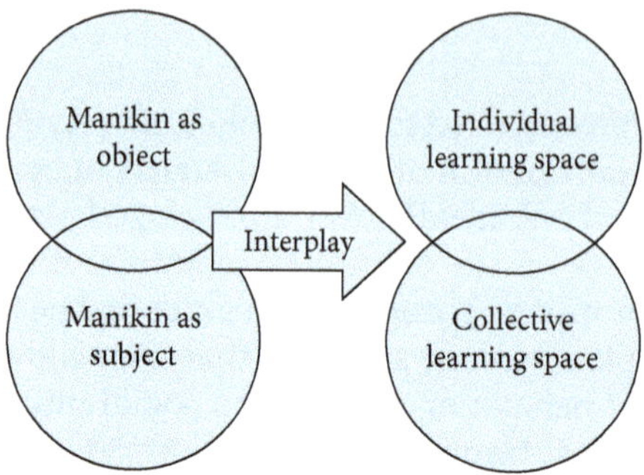

FIGURE 6.2 Interplay between object, subject, and learning space.

Grounded Theory

Grounded theory as a qualitative methodology developed in sociology and is used to develop theories that are based on data collected from participants instead of starting with an established or assumed theory or hypothesis (Creswell & Poth, 2018). It seeks to generate new theories or explanations for observed patterns or phenomena using an iterative process that allows concurrent and constant comparison of codes, categories, and concepts (Curtis & Keeler, 2022). Sampling is purposeful with the goal to select participants or cases that will facilitate acquisition of rich data to explore the question and develop theory. Theoretical sampling, which means the researcher is continually sampling new participants based on the evolution of an emerging theory, is common in grounded theory (Sosa-Diaz & Valverde-Berrocoso, 2022). Overall, data collection must be flexible and iterative based on an evolving understanding. Interviews and observations are the most common method for collecting data in grounded theory. As is typical to qualitative designs, a systematic approach to organizing the data collected that is easy for retrieval and analysis must occur.

BOX 6.4: GROUNDED THEORY RESEARCH EXAMPLE

Despite recommendations involving patients with end-stage heart failure in their care because it leads to better outcomes for patients and families as well as lower cost of care, there has been less progress in making this happen in the real world (Higginbotham et al., 2021). This study aimed to explore how health care professionals in acute settings make decisions when managing patients diagnosed with New York Heart Association (NYHA) III and NYHA IV heart failure and how this impacts the patient's end-of-life experience. The design used was a constructivist grounded theory (Charmaz, 2006). The study took place in England, and the sample was purposefully recruited. The sample included RNs, physicians, and patients. The researchers participated in activities of the wards, such as clinical meetings, rounding, and training (fieldwork, field notes, and diaries for reflection) over a 12-month period. They also conducted semi-structured interviews.

In keeping with grounded theory, the interview questions became more focused based on iterative coding (first stage) as the study progressed. Strategies used to enhance credibility and trustworthiness of the findings were member checking and triangulation of the different types of data. Summative analysis compared transcripts with all other notes, and concepts and categories were developed. The core category was "negotiating the vicious cycle of care": The decision-making within the vicious cycle of care disabled the patient in shared decision-making and led to delays in transitioning to palliative care. Four theoretical categories emerged that patients used to negotiate this cycle: (a) recognized dying, (b) being informed, (c) organizing care, and (d) signposting symptoms. This study resulted in the development of a theory of care—the vicious cycle of care—which was found to be a result of health care systems and rules that neglect the patient's preferences (remember patient preference is one of the cornerstones of EBP!). Patient preferences related to how and where they wish to spend the end of life and how they hope to die must be integrated into the cycle of care, ideally beginning in primary care and transitioning with the patient throughout each level of care.

Case Study

Case study as a qualitative research design is an in-depth exploration of a particular instance, phenomenon, or individual within its real-life context. It involves an intensive examination of a single case or a small number of cases to understand complexities, dynamics, and unique characteristics (Curtis & Keeler, 2022). In qualitative research, case studies are often used to gain insights into specific social, cultural, organizational, or psychological phenomena. Researchers typically collect data through various methods such as interviews, observations, documents, and artifacts, aiming to provide rich, detailed descriptions and interpretations of the case under study. The emphasis is on understanding the case in its entirety, often within its natural setting, rather than testing specific hypotheses or generalizing findings to a larger population.

BOX 6.5: EXAMPLE CASE STUDY

This example is useful because the design is a case study, but the framework used is an evaluation framework. Based on evidence from the United States and the success of the nurse practitioner (NP) role there, the role of the NP was envisioned by the Scottish government as a way of better meeting the primary care needs of the people of Scotland (Strachan et al., 2022). The Scottish School of Primary Care (SSPC) was commissioned by the government to undertake a national evaluation of new models of primary care that included ANPs (advanced nurse practitioner) roles. This case study is one of seven models of care evaluated. The aim of this case study was to evaluate ANP role implementation in primary care across Scotland in contributing to primary care transformation, not just provider substitution. A case in this study was defined as a health board that oversaw primary care services.

Semi-structured telephone interviews were conducted with key informants from each case, and key documents were assessed. The realist evaluation framework was used because it recognizes that there will be differences in program implementation depending on the context (real world). The components of the realist evaluation for the program were context, mechanisms, and outcomes (Pawson & Tilley, 1997). Deductive thematic analysis was performed using the ANP program theory components as the framework. These themes then informed phase 2. Snowballing was used to identify the sample of health care professionals interviewed in this phase. Ultimately, framework analysis was used. In this type of analysis, the data is sifted and sorted according to the program theory components to develop a framework matrix plan. Then the data was synthesized within the realist concepts of mechanisms, context and outcomes. Rigor was established by including health boards from across Scotland, using verbatim transcripts and semi-structured interview templates. Informants were given the opportunity to review the summaries and the final report. Three in-depth CMOs were developed based on the realist evaluation, APN role, APN education, and governance and sustainability. This case study using a comprehensive program evaluation method is a great model for any country wishing to increase health care access by advancing the role of nurses.

Sample Size in Qualitative Research

As you can see from the examples in the boxes, qualitative research designs are not as precisely scripted as quantitative designs. Instead, ongoing evaluation of the study methods occurs and is adapted by the researcher in response to the ongoing analysis of data (Malterud et al., 2016). Evaluating the adequacy of the sample size in qualitative methods is one area where this ongoing evaluation and flexibility from the original plan is manifest. For qualitative studies, instead of statistical predictions of needed sample size, the targeted number of informants is determined based on data adequacy specific to the study at hand (Vasileiou et al., 2018) and consistent with the philosophy, purpose, and methods of the study. Richness or quality of the data contribute to establishing adequacy of sample size (Morse, 1995; Sandelowski, 1995).

Sample sizes in qualitative research are typically small because of the complexity of the data and verbatim analysis of participant responses. The larger the data set, the more likely important themes and codes might be overlooked by researchers because of the sheer volume of data to be managed during analysis (Sandelowski, 1996). Vasileiou et al. (2018) suggest specific aspects of analyzing the sample size in qualitative data, including factors such as the richness and volume of the data, research design requirements and nature of the study, and consistency of findings across the collected data. They point out the fallacy of using quantitative specifications (i.e., "small" or "large" sample sizes, often inappropriately cited by researchers as a study limitation) in that a small sample might still achieve adequate saturation of data or a large sample size might extend beyond the focus of the study, resulting in inefficient use of researchers' time and findings that go beyond the boundaries of the study, possibly diluting the data relative to the actual specified purpose of the study. Two primary approaches for establishing adequacy of sample size are generally referred to in qualitative studies, saturation and information power.

Saturation

Saturation suggests that sample size is considered appropriate once the researcher(s) have reached a point in their data collection that they are gaining no new insight, codes, or themes and when there is enough information provided that a study can be replicated, new information has been obtained, and there is no ability to further code the data for new themes (Fusch & Ness, 2015; Lincoln & Guba, 1985). In fact, if a sample is too diverse in qualitative work, saturation may never be achieved, and the "story" may never emerge (Morse, 1995).

Information Power

Information power is a second approach, more recently embraced for analyzing the sufficiency of sample size in qualitative studies. Malterud et al. (2016) suggest that if a qualitative sample has sufficient information power, fewer participants are required. Like saturation, the study purpose, specifics of the sample, existing theoretical suggestions, quality of the data, and the analysis approach are all considered in evaluating information power. A narrow study aim requires a smaller sample than one with a broader aim. A sample of informants who have been chosen based on tight criteria will typically have higher information power than a sample meeting more diverse inclusion criterion. Malterud et al. note that a convenience sample would, therefore, have less specificity than a purposeful sample.

If a specific theoretical framework is used to guide data collection, a smaller sample would most likely achieve information power sooner than a study in which there is little theoretical perspective. In evaluating the quality of the data, high information power often exists when new perspectives emerge from the data instead of simply a validation of what is already known. And finally, in data analysis, a study that stays true to the study purpose, with rich data that lends itself to codes and themes that align with the study's identified focus, will generally lend higher information power with a smaller sample than will a study seeking to analyze diverse perspectives about a phenomenon. More subjects will be required to establish credibility for the diverse reported experiences and perspectives (Malterud et al., 2016). Remember, methodological specifications are more important than numerical guidelines, norms, and standards when evaluating sample size in qualitative research (Vasileiou et al., 2018).

Mixed-Methods Research

Studies that incorporate both quantitative and qualitative research methods are called mixed methods, although there are separate and clearly defined means of data collection and analysis for each approach. There are three ways that these studies can be designed depending on the purpose: (a) the qualitative component can come first, then the qualitative; (b) the qualitative and quantitative aspects can run simultaneously; and (c) the quantitative part can come first with the qualitative part afterward (Moorley & Cathala, 2019). An example of mixed-method research would be a study of NPs working in acute care settings that has a cross-sectional component requiring the NPs to first complete a questionnaire. After analyzing the data from the questionnaire, the researchers might use a qualitative method such as focus groups to further explore key concepts identified from the NPs' answers in the questionnaire. This study would apply both quantitative and qualitative methods in its design; however, analyzing the written responses to an open-ended question from a questionnaire used in a cross-sectional study does not, in itself, constitute a mixed-methods study (Creswell, 2007; Denzin & Lincoln, 2018; Meadows-Oliver & Kapaale, 2023).

Mixed-method studies provide researchers with a deeper understanding of the topic by applying both strategies. In appraising these studies, the level of evidence will usually align with the qualitative strategies. The quality, however, will be determined by the strength of both methods used for the study (Creswell, 2007; Denzin & Lincoln, 2018; Meadows-Oliver & Kapaale, 2023; Moorley & Cathala, 2019).

Meta-Synthesis

Meta-synthesis is a systematic review that provides a synthesis of evidence. A meta-synthesis may include only qualitative studies or a mix of quantitative, qualitative, or mixed-methods studies. Researchers use a rigorous approach to identify, appraise, and synthesize all studies that address a specific research question. Studies are only included if they meet predetermined inclusion criteria. As with meta-analyses, the authors must assess qualitative studies for quality and risk of bias. A rigorous analytic process of thematic analysis is completed to interpret meaning from the results of all the studies' data (Creswell, 2007; Denzin & Lincoln, 2018; Meadows-Oliver & Kapaale, 2023; Sandolowski & Barroso, 2003).

BOX 6.6: EXAMPLE META-SYNTHESIS RESEARCH STUDY

The issue of psychiatric admissions without patient consent (compulsory) engenders much debate around policies and services for those with mental health and safety needs (Bartl et al., 2024). For legal and policy issues to be informed by evidence, the researchers in this study aimed to provide a synthesis of qualitative studies on both the patients'/families' and the caregivers' experiences. They searched five databases and found 24 studies that had been published since the last synthesis of this evidence. Studies were evaluated for confidence using the GRADE-CERQual (a critical appraisal tool for qualitative syntheses). The research team included a diverse group of authors, including practitioners, those with personal experience with the system, and senior and junior researchers as a method for critical reflection to acknowledge the researcher's values, biases, and experiences, which might influence the research process. They analyzed the results of these studies using a thematic synthesis approach. This resulted in five final themes: (a) emotional impact, (b) availability of support for carers, (c) carer involvement in decision-making and provision of care, (d) carer relationships, and (e) quality care. Many sub-themes were also identified with these larger themes. Their findings reveled that views on compulsory admissions were varied but provided implications for future policy, practice and research.

Critical Appraisal

As you saw in Chapter 5, validated tools provide a template of questions that are used to systematically conduct a critical appraisal. Use of a critical appraisal tool helps ensure that evaluations are systematic, comprehensive, transparent, and based on best practices and helps users of qualitative evidence understand the strength of the evidence and make informed decisions about its use in practice, policy, or further research, ultimately leading to more reliable and valid judgments about the quality of the research or information provided as a result of a study (see Table 6.3).

TABLE 6.3 Comparison of Concepts of Critical Appraisal in Quantitative versus Qualitative Research

Quantitative Terminology	Qualitative Terminology
Validity	Credibility
Reliability	Dependability and confirmability
Generalizability	Transferability
Applicability	

Trustworthiness

Trustworthiness addresses the quality of a qualitative research study based on dependability, credibility, and transferability (Ellis, 2018; Lincoln & Guba, 1985). Trustworthiness reflects that a reader has confidence in a study's findings as being true and therefore meaningful in the contributions to the establishment of scientific knowledge. Because a researcher chooses from multiple philosophies to guide a study's methodology in qualitative research, there is no standard structure to which a qualitative study generally follows as in quantitative methods (Stahl & King, 2020). The point of trustworthiness is for the researcher to be clear about what they are doing and why they are doing it (Nowell et al., 2017).

Dependability

Similar to reliability in quantitative methods, dependability addresses the context in which the study was conducted. Dependability, for example, is supported when the researcher describes how changes in the setting might have impacted the data collection or clarifies how changes were necessary as the setting became more understood by the researcher (Ellis, 2019). These detailed descriptions of methods and the rationale for these methods within the context of the study provide a clear audit trail (Nowell et al., 2017). Using two different people to analyze the data separately and see if they identify the same codes and findings is another common approach to establish the dependability of findings (Ellis, 2019). Researchers' attention to "bracketing" what is observation and what is interpretation is another way to establish dependability. The focus is on being transparent to the reader as to how the researcher's participation in the research could introduce bias (Stahl & King, 2020). While bias is present in all research, quantitative or qualitative, you want to be aware of these possibilities in the study under review and fully consider these implications when critiquing the value of a study for application to practice. The researcher's attention to transparency and detail is an important way to establish dependability.

Credibility

Credibility in qualitative methods addresses how well the reported study findings reflect reality. In other words, how believable are the findings? When critiquing credibility, you question the study methods and processes to assess if the findings are likely to be truthful and accurate (Ellis, 2018; Polit & Beck, 2017; Stahl & King, 2020).

Often, to establish credibility, qualitative researchers will use triangulation. Triangulation means using more than a single approach for data collection or analysis, for example, interviewing more than a single source (i.e., different people, or same person at different time points; Stahl & King, 2020). Member checking is another approach for establishing credibility. In member checking, the researcher goes back to a few of the study informants to have them review the researcher's interpretation of the study data. The informants are asked to evaluate if they see themselves reflected in some aspect of the data and if their experience is accurately reflected by the researcher. If observation was part of the data collection process, establishing that the researcher spent sufficient time with the participants and that the observation was natural (i.e., the researcher's presence was not distracting or impacting the phenomenon under observation), is another way credibility can be established in a qualitative study (Stahl & King, 2020).

Transferability

Transferability is similar to the external validity reflecting generalizability that is sought in quantitative research. While generalizability is not appropriate for qualitative methods, in essence, transferability addresses whether the findings from a qualitative study apply to similar situations and whether findings are meaningful to other individuals or populations (Nowell et al., 2017). To establish transferability, the researcher must have a well-described sample, methods, and findings (Ellis, 2018, 2019; Stahl & King, 2020). The researcher must provide rich (thick) descriptions of the findings so that others can recognize the experience when they see it in practice (Nowell et al., 2017).

Confirmability

Confirmability is established when the researcher's findings and interpretation clearly emerge from the data. In assessing for confirmability, you would expect to see how the researcher arrived at their conclusions through examples of direct quotes with codes and themes that are linked to the quotes, and you would note whether those codes and themes appeared to accurately reflect what was stated by the informant or participant (Nowell et al., 2017). Lincoln and Guba (1989) argue that confirmability is supported when dependability, credibility, and transferability are met.

Critical Appraisal Tools

The Joanna Briggs Institute (JBI) tool for Qualitative Assessment and Review Instrument (QARI) provides a framework for appraising qualitative research studies. QARI assists researchers in the evaluation of the methodological quality, relevance, and trustworthiness of qualitative research. It provides a structured approach to critically analyze various aspects of qualitative studies, such as research design, data collection methods, analysis procedures, and interpretations. This tool helps ensure that qualitative research is rigorously conducted and reported, thereby enhancing the reliability and validity of findings.

The Critical Appraisal Skills Programme's (CASP, 2019) qualitative checklist is often used to assess the quality of qualitative research studies, including those that involve interviews (see example in Appendix C). The CASP qualitative checklist is also endorsed by Cochrane and the World Health Organization (Long et al., 2020), and it appraises the rigor of qualitative studies. The CASP tool consists of 10 main questions and several sub-questions that examine the clarity and appropriateness of the study aim, research design (sampling, data collection, data analysis), and presentation of results. It helps researchers and reviewers critically appraise qualitative studies to determine their trustworthiness and relevance for informing practice and policy.

GRADE-CERTQual (Confidence in the Evidence from Reviews of Qualitative Research) is an approach used to assess the confidence in the evidence generated from qualitative research systematic reviews or meta-syntheses (Lewin et al., 2018). It's a part of the broader GRADE approach, which is commonly used to evaluate the quality of evidence in systematic reviews and guideline development. CERTQual involves an assessment of each individual review finding in terms of four components: (a) methodological limitations, (b) coherence, (c) adequacy of data, and (d) relevance. The assessments of the four components collectively contribute to an overall assessment of whether findings from a qualitative evidence synthesis provide a reasonable representation of the health or social care issue, intervention, or program (phenomenon) of interest, resulting in a confidence assessment from very low confidence to high confidence.

Overall, critical appraisal plays a crucial role in advancing the quality, credibility, and relevance of qualitative research, ultimately contributing to the generation of robust evidence and informed decision-making in diverse fields. Critical appraisal of qualitative research guides the evaluation of trustworthiness, credibility, and relevance of the findings. While qualitative research differs from quantitative research in its methods and focus, it still requires a systematic approach to assessing its quality. Table 6.4 provides information on where to find qualitative research critical appraisal tools.

TABLE 6.4 Qualitative Critical Appraisal Tools

Critical Appraisal Tool	Website	Research Study Designs	Overview
CASP checklists	https://casp-uk.net/casp-tools-checklists/	Qualitative studies checklist	Includes instructions and embedded hints throughout the checklists Free access Full-text PDF, Word, or print and fill
JBI Global	https://jbi.global/critical-appraisal-tools	Qualitative research Qualitative synthesis	Includes instructions with the form Free access Full-text Word document
Johns Hopkins EBP model and tools	https://www.hopkinsmedicine.org/evidence-based-practice/model-tools	Critical appraisal toolkit for all study types, including qualitative	Includes instructions and embedded hints throughout all forms Level and quality guide for ratings Strength of recommendation rating Free access
GRADE-CERTQual	https://www.cerqual.org/	Qualitative research synthesis	Very rigorous process Free access Confidence assessment

As you continue to evaluate the research evidence from all types of research studies, be sure to add them to your synthesis table, keeping in mind the quality of the study design and the strength and consistency of the results. At this point you may be beginning to see what specific practice changes are supported with evidence for your particular problem, population, and context.

WELLNESS IN ACTION: JOURNALING

Journaling can be an important aspect of maintaining your health and wellness. Journaling helps you to develop more self-awareness regarding your thoughts and experiences (Forsyth & Eifert, 2016). Dimitroff (2018) suggests journaling can also help you develop self-compassion and understanding. Writing down your emotions, feelings, thoughts, and experiences allows you to let go of stressors and frustrations, identify opportunities for gratitude, and provide a physical, mental, and spiritual outlet for dealing with day-to-day life experiences, both personal and professional. Research has shown that journaling contributes to health and wellness (Baikie & Wilhelm, 2005), including lowered blood pressure, improved respiratory and hepatic function, more positive emotions, and less work absenteeism, among others.

Consider trialing journaling as a personal action toward wellness. Don't worry about how long you journal; just try to be consistent in your practice. You can journal on your phone at lunch, sit down at your computer and type after finishing your workday, or perhaps write in a bound journal before turning in for bed or first thing in the morning with a cup of coffee. If writing does not come easily to you, you might want to use some of these prompts for getting started:

- What was the best part of your day or week?
- Name two things that frustrate you about your current situation.
- What would your ideal life look like?
- What are your strongest leadership skills? How have you manifested one of these strengths this week in your daily life?
- What aspects of leadership would you like to further develop?
- What is the most fulfilling aspect of being a nurse leader? If you had an opportunity to do it all over, would you? If not, what would you consider instead?

One of the authors (Julee) believes in the power of journaling as a reflective practice and a writing practice, so she and a partner developed and self-published journals to share with others (Maxson & Waldrop, 2023; 2024). It can be fun to regularly review your journal entries and reflect again on your experiences. Contemplate if journaling has been helpful to your health and wellness. What themes emerged in your writing? Are there topics that recur over and over again? How do you feel after each journaling experience? Remember that you do not have to journal every day, but success in use of any exercise targeting health and wellness requires consistency and dedication to see optimum benefits. And one more thing: Consider recommending journaling as a health and wellness exercise for your patients and coworkers as well.

WRAPPING UP

By now you realize how qualitative research studies make an important contribution to scientific knowledge in nursing, helping to provide a holistic perspective to the complex aspects of health. As an APRN or nurse leader, you must be skilled and comfortable in identifying and critiquing qualitative studies as part of evidence-based care to inform your practice. Williams et al. (2019) emphasize that a clear understanding of the methods and related trustworthiness of qualitative studies is critical for applying meaningful research findings to practice. Learning to apply critical appraisal tools to enhance your judgment of a research study's quality contributes to your informed evaluation of the varied philosophies and methodologies underlying qualitative methods. Accordingly, your evaluation will be based on considering the important differences in philosophy and design versus attempting to apply a single standardized approach.

REFLECTION QUESTIONS

1. As a future EBPQI leader, how can you incorporate qualitative research findings to expand a more holistic approach to patient care?
2. How can you continue to enhance your appraisal skills for use of qualitative research in your role?
3. What insights have you gained into the value of qualitative research for informing EBPQI?

REFERENCES

Alele, F., & Maau-Aduli, B. (2023). Chapter 1.3: Research paradigms and philosophical assumptions. *An introduction to research methods for undergraduate health profession students.* Pressbooks. Creative Commons Attribution NonCommercial.

Baikie, K., & Wilhelm, K. (2005). Emotional and physical health benefits of expressive writing. *Advances in Psychiatric Treatment, 11*(5), 338–346.

Bartl, G., Stuart, R., Ahmed, N., Saunders, K., Loizou, S., Brady, G., Gray, H., Grundy, A., Jeynes, T., Nyikavaranda, P., Persaud, K., Raad, A., Foye, U., Simpson, A., Johnson, S., & Lloyd-Evans, B. (2024). A qualitative meta-synthesis of service users' and carers' experiences of assessment and involuntary hospital admissions under mental health legislations: A five-year update. *BMC Psychiatry, 24*(1), 476. https://doi.org/10.1186/s12888-024-05914-w

Bayuo. J., Aziato, L., Wong, K. C. A., Su, J., Abu-Odah, H., & Wong, F. K. Y. (2024). Phemomenography: An emerging qualitative research design for nursing. *J Adv Nurs, 80*, 821–834. https://doi.org/10.1111/jan.15874

Cho, Y., & Kim, S. (2024). A phenomenological study of the experiences of nurses working in integrated nursing care wards in Korea. *BMJ Nursing, 23*(136). https://doi.org/10.1186/s12912-024-01798-z

Colaizzi, P. F. (1978). Psychological research as the phenomenologist views it. In R. S. Valle, M. King (Eds.), *Existential-phenomenological alternatives for psychology*, p. 6. Oxford University Press.

Creswell, J. W., & Guetterman, T. C. (2018). *Educational research: Planning, conducting, and evaluating quantitative and qualitative research* (6th ed.). Pearson.

Creswell, J. W., & Poth, C. N., (2018). *Qualitative inquiry and research design: Choosing among five approaches* (4th ed.). SAGE.

Critical Appraisal Skills Programme. (2018). *CASP qualitative checklist.* https://casp-uk.net/casp-tools-checklists/

Curtis, A. C., & Keeler, C. (2022). Interpretive methodologies in qualitative nursing research. *AJN*, 122(10), 45–49.

DePoy, E., & Gitlin, L. N. (2016). Naturalistic designs (pp. 158-172. In E. Depoy & L. N. Gitlin (Eds.), *Introduction to research* (5th ed., pp. 158–172). Mosby. https://doi.org/10.1016/B978-0-323-26171-5.00011-2

Dimitroff, L. J. (2018). Journaling: A valuable tool for registered nurses. *American Nurse Today, 13*(11), 27–28.

Ellis, P. (2018). The language of research (part 19): Understanding the quality of a qualitative paper (1). *Wounds UK, 14*(5), 134–135.

Ellis, P. (2019). The language of research (part 20): Understanding the quality of a qualitative paper (2). *Wounds UK, 15*(1), 110–111.

Fischer, C. T. (2009). Bracketing in qualitative research: Conceptual and practical matters. *Psychotherapy*, 19(4–5), 583–590. https://doi.org/10.1080/10503300902798375

Forsyth, J. P., & Eifert, G. H. (2016). *The mindfulness & acceptance workbook for anxiety: A guide to breaking free from anxiety, phobias & worry using acceptance & commitment therapy.* New Harbinger.

Fusch, P. I., & Ness, L. R. (2015). Are we there yet? Data saturation in qualitative research. *The Qualitative Report, 20*(9), 1408–1416.

Galuska, L., Hahn, J., Polifroni, E. C., & Crow, G. (2018). A narrative analysis of nurses' experiences with meaning and joy in nursing practice. *Nursing Administration Quarterly, 42*(2), 154–163. https://doi.org/10.1097/NAQ.0000000000000280

Gelo, O. G. C. (2012). On research methods and their philosophical assumptions: "Raising the consciousness of researchers" again. *Psychotherapie & Sozialwissenschaft: Zeitschrift für Qualitative Forschung und Klinische Praxis, 14*(2), 111–130.

Guba, E. G., & Lincoln, Y. (1989). *Fourth generation evaluation.* SAGE.

Handeland J., Prinz, A., Ekra, E. M. R., & Fossum, M. (2022), The sense of a patient: An ethnographic multi-site field study exploring the influence of manikins on nursing students' learning. *International Journal of Educational Research Open, 3*.

Hennink, M. M., Kaiser, B. N., & Marconi, V. C. (2017). Code saturation versus meaning saturation: How many interviews are enough? *Qualitative Health Research, 27*(4), 591–608. https://doi.org/10.1177/1049732316665344

Hennink, M. M., Kaiser, B. N., & Weber, M. B. (2019). What influences saturation? Estimating sample sizes in focus group research. *Qualitative Health Research, 29*(10), 1483–1496. https://doi.org/10.1177/1049732318821692

Higginbotham, K., Jones, I., & Johnson, M. (2021). A grounded theory study: Exploring health care professionals decision making when managing end stage heart failure care. *Journal of Advanced Nursing, 77*, 3142–3155. https://doi.org/10.1111/jan.14852

Hu, T., Wang, S., Luo, W., Zhang, M., Huang, X., Yan, Y., Liu, E., Ly, K., Kacker, V., She, B., & Li, Z., (2021). Revealing public opinion towards COVID-19 vaccines with Twitter data in the United States: Spatiotemporal perspective. *Journal of Medical Internet Research, 23*(9), e30854. https://doi.org/10.2196/30854

Kuhn, T. S. (2012). *The structure of scientific revolutions* (4th ed.). The University of Chicago Press.

Leonidaki, V. (2015). Critical appraisal in the context of integrations of qualitative evidence in applied psychology: The introduction of a new appraisal tool for interview studies. *Qualitative Research in Psychology, 12*, 435–452. https://doi.org/10.1080/14780887.2015.1053643

Lewin, S., Glenton, C., Munthe-Kaas, H., Carlsen, B., Colvin, C. J., Gülmezoglu, M., Noyes, J., Booth, A., Garside, R., & Rashidian, A. (2015). Using qualitative evidence in decision making for health and social interventions: An approach to assess confidence in findings from qualitative evidence syntheses (GRADE-CERQual). *PLoS Medicine, 12*(10), e1001895.

Lincoln, Y., & Guba, E. G. (1985). *Naturalistic inquiry.* SAGE.

Lockwood, C., Porritt, K., Munn, Z., Rittenmeyer, L., Salmond, S., Bjerrum, M., Loveday, H., Carrier, J., & Stannard, D. (2020). Systematic reviews of qualitative evidence. In E. Aromataris & Z. Munn (Eds.), *JBI manual for evidence synthesis* (pp. 23–45). JBI. https://doi.org/10.46658/JBIMES-20-03

Lucien Leape Institute at the National Patient Safety Foundation. (2013). *Through the eyes of the workforce: Creating joy, meaning, and safer health care.* National Patient Safety Foundation.

Madden, R. (2017). *Being ethnographic: A guide to the theory and practice of ethnography* (2nd ed.). SAGE.

Malterud, K., Siersma, V. D., & Guassora, A. D. (2016). Sample size in qualitative interview studies: Guided by information power. *Qualitative Health Research, 26*(13), 1753–1760. https://doi.org/10.1177/1049732315617444

Maxson, P., & Waldrop, J. (2023). *Every woman every day.* Solstice Press.

Maxson, P., & Waldrop, J. (2024). Every Woman Every Day, Volume 2. Soltice Press.

Moorley, C., & Cathala, X. (2019). How to appraise mixed methods research. *Evidence-Based Nursing, 22*(2), 38–41. https://doi.org/10.1136/ebnurs-2019-103076

Morse, J. M. (1995). The significance of saturation. *Qualitative Health Research, 5*(2), 147–149.

Nowell, L. S., Norris, J. M., White, D. E., & Moules, N. J. (2017). Thematic analysis: Striving to meet the trustworthiness criteria. *International Journal of Qualitative Methods, 16*, 1–13. https://doi.org/10.1177/1609406917733847

Pawson, R., & Tilley, N. (1997). *Realistic evaluation*. SAGE.

Perlo, J., Balik, B., Swensen, S., Kabcenell, A., Landsman, J., & Feeley, D. (2017). *IHI framework for improving joy in work* [Whitepaper]. Institute for Healthcare Improvement.

Polit, D. F., & Beck, C. T. (2017) *Essentials of nursing research: Appraising evidence for nursing practice* (9th ed.). Williams and Wilkins.

Reeves, S., Peller, J., Goldman, J., & Kitto, S. (2013). Ethnography in qualitative educational research: AMEE Guide No. 80. *Medical Teacher, 35*(8), e1365–e1379. https://doi.org/10.3109/0142159X.2013.804977

Ryan, A. B. (2006). Post-positivist approaches to research. In *Researching and writing your thesis: A guide for postgraduate students* (pp. 12–26). Maynooth Adult and Community Education.

Ryan, G. (2018). Introduction to positivism, interpretivism and critical theory. *Nurse Researcher, 25*(4), 41–49. https://doi.org/10.7748/nr.2018.e1466

Sandelowski, M. (1995). Sample size in qualitative research. *Research in Nursing & Health, 18*(2), 179–183.

Sandelowski, M. (1996). One is the liveliest number: The case orientation of qualitative research. *Research in Nursing & Health, 19*(6), 525–529.

Sosa-Diaz, M. J., & Valverde-Berrocoso, J. (2022). Grounded theory as a research methodology in educational technology. *International Journal of Qualitative Methods, 21*, 1–13.

Stahl, N. A., & King, J. R. (2020). Expanding approaches for research: Understanding and using trustworthiness in qualitative research. *Journal of Developmental Education*, *44*(1), 26–28.
Strachan, H., Hoskins, G., Wells, M., & Maxwell, M. (2022). A realist evaluation case study of the implementation of advanced nurse practitioner roles in primary care in Scotland. *Journal of Advanced Nursing*, *78*(9), 2916–1932.
Vasileiou, K., Barnett, J., Thorpe, S., & Young, T. (2018). Characterizing and justifying sample size sufficiency in interview-based studies: Systematic analysis of qualitative health research over a 15-year period. *BMC Medical Research Methodology*, *18*, 148. https://doi.org/10.1186/s12874-018-0594-7
Waldrop J. (2013). Exploration of reasons for feeding choices in Hispanic mothers. *MCN: The American Journal of Maternal Child Nursing*, *38*(5), 282–288. https://doi.org/10.1097/NMC.0b013e31829a5625

IMAGE CREDITS

Fig. 6.2: Jorunn Aas Handeland, Andreas Prinz, Else Mari Ruberg Ekra, and Mariann Fossum, "The Sense of a Patient: An Ethnographic Multi-site Field Study Exploring the Influence of Manikins on Nursing Students' Learning," *International Journal of Educational Research Open*, vol. 3, p. 7. Copyright © by Jorunn Aas Handeland, Andreas Prinz, Else Mari Ruberg Ekra, and Mariann Fossum (CC BY 4.0) at *International Journal of Educational Research Open*, vol. 3; https://www.sciencedirect.com/science/article/pii/S2666374021000807#fig0002.

CHAPTER 7

Leading the Appraisal of Other Types of Evidence to Inform Best Practices

Julee Briscoe Waldrop, Jayne Jennings Dunlap, Jennifer Woo, Melissa Hassock, and Tracy Brewer

KEY CONCEPTS

Clinical practice guideline
Consensus statement
Economic evaluation
Expert opinion
Literature reviews
Nonresearch evidence
Position statement

LEARNING OBJECTIVES

1. Describe other types of evidence that can contribute to EBPQI initiatives and improvement in health care.
2. Identify resources and tools that nurse leaders may use to search for and appraise other types of evidence used in EBPQI.
3. Discuss the rationale for critical appraisal of other types of evidence.

> There are three essentials to leadership: humility, clarity and courage.
>
> —Fuchan Yuan

Introduction

In Chapter 4, you learned how to lead the formation or development of your team's clinical question to search for the best available evidence. In Chapters 5 and 6, you learned about levels of quantitative and qualitative research study designs and leading the systematic process of critical appraisal. In this chapter, we will focus on the role and critical appraisal of non-research-based types of contributions to the body (compilation) of evidence that you can use to answer clinical questions.

As you know, research evidence is not the only type of evidence. For example, when you observe or hear about someone else's experience and consider it information that you might use, you are encountering *anecdotal evidence*. Because anecdotal evidence is based on personal accounts or opinions rather than on research, it may not be reliable or factual, and its quality is generally not considered equal to that of research-based evidence, but it is still evidence. Let's begin with an actual example of a nurse practitioner's (NP) use of non-research-based evidence to augment an EBP change within an area of rapid research expansion.

I (Jayne) noticed in my primary care clinical practice that many children diagnosed with autism spectrum disorder (ASD) had not been screened for autism as currently recommended by the Centers for Disease Control and Prevention (CDC) and American Academy of Pediatrics (AAP). Current recommendations are adherence to universal autism-specific screening for all children at 18 and 24 months of age, with special attention to red flags such as lack of eye contact, communication delay, and/or social impairments (CDC, 2022; Hyman et al., 2020; Reece et al., 2023). Although parental concerns had been noted in the primary care medical records of several of these children, there had been no screening, evaluation, or specialist referral completed, and there was no documentation of anticipatory guidance or a follow-up plan. I checked the literature and found that lack of developmental screening was common across health care settings (Hirai et al., 2018). Motivated by the increasing number of individuals diagnosed with ASD (one in 36 children at the time of this writing) (Maenner et al., 2023), I decided to explore how nurses and NPs could use evidence to support this vulnerable group.

Although strong research evidence supports that early detection and treatment for ASD is associated with the best outcomes, and that prompt diagnosis allows earlier access to evidence-based treatments, these practices are not commonplace (Zucherman et al., 2017). After appraising the current literature (research evidence), I contacted Dr. Temple Grandin, an ASD ambassador and early intervention recipient and advocate, as well as one of the first individuals to widely verbalize her experience as a person on the autism spectrum. Her riveting journey was documented in an award-winning film titled *Temple Grandin* based on her life (Jackson, 2010).

During our telephone discussion about the limitations of research and the importance of early ASD detection, she said, "Jayne, at some point, anecdotal becomes evidence!" (personal communication, May 15, 2020). She also stated that if a 2-year-old child is not talking, "Don't wait. Get help immediately."

Dr. Grandin's anecdotal evidence led me to partner with a leading neurologist and ASD expert to build evidence-based continuing education focused on screening and early action recommendations (Dunlap & Filipek, 2020). In our work, we used clinical practice guidelines (CPGs) and expert opinion to complement the research evidence for making evidence-based actionable recommendations for nurses and NPs when ASD is suspected. One practical piece of information highlighted in this work, which incorporated other (nonresearch) sources of evidence, was the critical importance of not dismissing parental concerns for ASD.

Best Available Evidence and the Hierarchy of Evidence

You have learned that EBP is informed by three primary components: the best available (highest quality and most current) evidence, clinical expertise, and patient preferences and values. One strength of EBP is that it incorporates various types of evidence and knowledge (Dang et al., 2022); therefore, your search is incomplete until you have explored all relevant evidence that can inform practice recommendations for the best quality of care. In some discussions of EBP, you may find "best scientific evidence" used synonymously with "best available evidence"; however, the best evidence may comprise both research (scientific) evidence and other evidence (Dang et al., 2022). Although neither type of evidence is necessarily more important, some types of evidence do offer a higher level of reliability and support for EBP recommendations.

Pre-Appraised Evidence

Pre-appraised evidence includes summaries based on high-quality evidence sources such as single RCTs of a specific clinical topic. Authors of this type of evidence appraise the quality of research studies and include a narrative report of their findings. As a nurse in an advanced role, you are likely to use pre-appraised sources of evidence in your daily practice because they offer a time-saving benefit. CPGs and professional consensus or position statements are examples of pre-appraised evidence. Clinical practice guidelines contain practice recommendations based on research evidence, including the benefits and harms of interventions to optimize patient care and outcomes (Grinspun et al., 2023). CPGs are often based on the best available evidence (high-quality, current research). For example, the AAP has several CPGs available with open access, including one for the screening and management of autism (Hyman et al., 2020).

As you learned in previous chapters, specific types of evidence are assigned different levels on the evidence pyramid based on their study design (see Figure 7.1). Let's consider the lower segment of the pyramid (which includes individual research studies of various types of design) and, more specifically, the bottom tier of the pyramid (which includes nonresearch and other types of evidence). Note the broadness of the pyramid's base compared to its top tier; this broadness signifies the large amount of various types of evidence you may find there, depending on your topic of EBPQI interest.

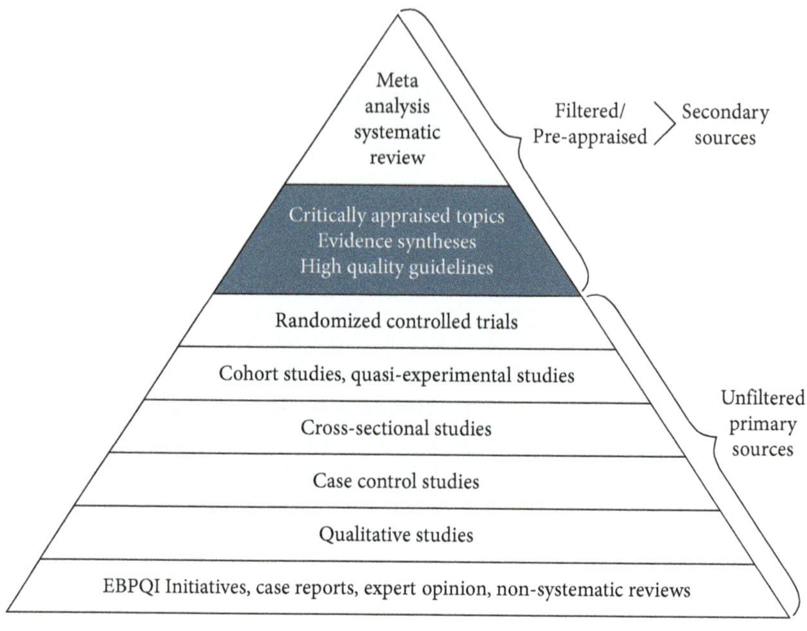

FIGURE 7.1 Hierarchy of evidence pyramid.

Other Types of Evidence

Simply stated, **other evidence** means evidence that is presented or generated without using scientific methods (also known as experimental design). This type of evidence generally fits into one of two broad categories: (a) evidence-based summaries of scientific (research) evidence and (b) evidence gained through practice experience, typically at an organizational level (often referred to as practice-based evidence; Dang et al., 2022; Fineout-Overholt, 2023). At the highest level of other evidence is the evidence generated by systematic synthesis or a summary of existing scientific research (e.g., CPGs). Evidence that is not a synthesis of research can fill gaps in knowledge when there is limited research available and help bridge the transfer of research into patient care. When findings and outcomes across a variety of types of evidence (e.g., EBPQI-generated evidence and research, anecdotal evidence) are in agreement, they provide a more holistic understanding of the body of evidence available to support clinical decision-making and recommendations (Fineout-Overholt, 2023).

Summaries of Evidence

Clinical Practice Guidelines, Consensus Statements, and Position Statements

Clinical practice guidelines, consensus statements, and position statements are sometimes viewed interchangeably, but they are different (see Table 7.1). Although each provides practice recommendations, these recommendations have been developed based on different degrees of evidence and rigor; therefore, they do not provide the same level of evidence.

TABLE 7.1 Universal Terminology for Practice Recommendation Types

Term	Definition
Clinical Practice Guideline	Systematically developed documents created with a validated methodology that includes identifying the literature on specific clinical question(s), using explicit methods of searching and selecting literature, and grading the available evidence. Following this process, recommendations are developed, and the strength of each recommendation is graded.
Consensus Statement	Recommendations developed based on the collective opinion or consensus of an expert panel—often presented when available evidence is limited or conflicting or the intervention's risk versus benefit is not obvious.
Position Statement	Comprehensive document that explains, justifies, and recommends a particular approach to a clinical problem.

Source: Adapted from Joshi et al. (2019).

Quality **clinical practice guidelines** provide the highest level of evidence and are the most trustworthy among clinical practice recommendations because (a) they are systematically developed with transparent methods, and (b) the strength of their recommendations is graded. **Position statements** may provide a high level of evidence if their development is based on a systematic review of research evidence. You must appraise these statements as carefully as you would research evidence so that you can understand how the positions taken were determined. **Consensus statements** reflect the collective opinion of an expert panel; thus, they may be based on limited, new, or conflicting evidence. As they have the most risk for bias, consensus statements provide a lower level of evidence.

Reviews of the Literature Other Than Systematic Reviews

As you learned in Chapter 5, systematic reviews of research involve a rigorous search, appraisal, and synthesis of scientific evidence. Because they use a systematic methodology and are typically based on numerous research studies, systematic reviews inherently have a lower risk for bias and, therefore, are considered a higher level of evidence. However, there are other approaches to exploring the literature on a particular topic, problem, or question, as well as many types of reviews, including literature reviews, scoping reviews, and integrative reviews. You may have noticed that even review types with very similar methodologies have different names (Carter-Templeton et al., 2023).

Literature review is a generic term that describes the examination and summary of available evidence on a topic, sometimes including both research and other types of evidence. There is no standard methodology for conducting literature reviews, so various approaches may be taken (Bowden & Purper, 2022). High-quality unbiased reviews provide strong support for evidence-based practice and are needed to identify what is known (and currently unknown) about a phenomenon to provide a framework for research. The number and type of literature reviews have grown exponentially since the first one appeared in the nursing literature in 1969 (Gruendemann, 1969). Systematic reviews and meta-analyses are considered a high level of research; however, the terms used to identify other types of reviews can be inconsistent. It is critical that methodology be evaluated when appraising a review. Just as with research methods, the methods of any review should be transparent, accurate, complete, and, therefore, replicable. If it is not present, incomplete or unclear, the findings may not be reliable, and the risk for bias is high (Carter-Templeton et al., 2022). Twelve standard review types other than systematic reviews (quantitative or qualitative) and meta-analyses have been identified in the nursing literature (Carter-Templeton et al., 2022; see Table 7.2), but you will likely come across other labels for reviews in your evidence searches.

TABLE 7.2 Other Types of Reviews

Type of Review	Purpose	Methodology
Critical	To critically assess and interpret the literature, usually with a focus on identifying biases, limitations, or assumptions in existing research	Exceeds summarizing studies by offering a critical evaluation of the methods, findings, and theoretical approaches of each included study
Descriptive	To summarize and categorize existing literature without engaging in critical analysis or synthesis	Organizes literature based on themes, methods, or chronological order to provide an overview of the topic's existing landscape
Integrative	To synthesize literature from both theoretical and empirical sources to provide a comprehensive understanding of a research topic or question	Incorporates a wide range of research (quantitative, qualitative) to explore complex phenomena or synthesize theories and evidence
Mapping	To identify the scope, range, and nature of research within a specific field or topic to map the existing literature	Systematically categorizes and describes the literature, often identifying gaps, trends, and patterns
Mixed studies/ mixed methods	To integrate findings from both quantitative and qualitative studies to offer a more comprehensive analysis of a research area	Uses rigorous methods to synthesize findings from diverse methodologies to address complex research questions
Narrative	To provide a narrative synthesis of the literature on a topic with a focus on theories, methodologies, and findings	Uses an often thematic or chronological organization and is qualitative and subjective in nature

Type of Review	Purpose	Methodology
Rapid	To swiftly gather and summarize evidence to inform decision-making or policy	Streamlines the systematic review process, often by narrowing the research question or limiting the search scope
Realist	To provide understanding of how and why a particular intervention does or doesn't work by examining its underlying mechanisms and contexts	Focuses on the theory-driven explanation of the interaction among context, mechanism, and outcome
Scoping	To map the literature on a broad topic, identifying key concepts, evidence, and gaps in research	Involves a systematic search and selection process but is broader and less detailed than a systematic review
State of the art/ science	To present the most current research and developments in a particular field, thereby establishing the research's cutting-edge status	Focuses on the latest and most innovative studies, technologies, methodologies, and findings
Theoretical	To critically analyze the theory behind a research topic, synthesizing and evaluating theoretical frameworks and constructs	Focuses on the evolution of theories and their relationships to the research question or topic
Umbrella	To synthesize multiple reviews on a topic into one coherent overview that summarizes findings from different types of reviews	Compiles evidence from systematic reviews, meta-analyses, and other high-level reviews

Source: Adapted from Carter-Templeton et al. (2023)

A **scoping review** aims to identify and map the amount and type of evidence available on a particular topic, identify and analyze gaps in knowledge, and clarify key concepts associated with that topic. A scoping review does not include a critical appraisal or seek to answer a clinical question (Munn et al., 2018), but it can be rigorous and should follow a strict methodology such as the PRISMA reporting guide for scoping reviews (Tricco et al., 2018; Westphaln et al., 2021). **Integrative reviews** aim to provide a comprehensive and holistic understanding of a health care problem by considering a variety of evidence and knowledge sources. A high-quality integrative review will follow a specific framework for development, including five stages: problem identification, literature search, data evaluation, data analysis, and presentation of findings (Oermann & Knafl, 2021).

Practice-Based Evidence (Experiential or Organizational)

Evidence-Based Practice and Quality Improvement Projects or Initiatives

Reports of EBP and QI projects or initiatives are increasingly found in the literature. Both EBP and QI projects are conducted at an organizational level. **Evidence-based practice projects or initiatives** aim to (a) search and critically appraise the best available evidence, (b) synthesize it with clinical expertise as well as patient preferences and values, and subsequently (c) recommend and support practice changes that improve health care. **Quality improvement projects or initiatives** aim to improve a process or outcome related to an identified problem using a systematic approach, but they may not include a rigorous search for and appraisal of evidence (HQ Solutions, 2023). Given the recognized value of basing practice change on the best evidence and using a systematic process to apply and sustain change, there has been a movement toward combining these two processes and calling them "evidence-based quality improvement" (Levin et al., 2010; Melnyk et al., 2015) or "evidence-based practice quality improvement" (EBPQI; Waldrop & Dunlap, 2024a). Although it is understood that outcomes related to EBPQI are not generalizable, the information found in reports of such projects are transferable and can contribute to the body of evidence used to answer a clinical question. You learned in Chapter 1 that **transferability** is the degree to which an effective intervention and outcome in one context (a specific population and organization) can be applied and achieved in a different context (a different population and/or organization) (Schloemer & Schröder-Bäck, 2018). Transferability will be discussed further in Chapter 12.

Economic Evaluation

Economic evaluations in health care are used to determine the monetary costs and value of interventions or programs. Efficiency of care (including costs) is one of the seven STEEEEP domains of quality care (Table 2.1, Chapter 2). Economic evaluations use a variety of analyses that may include program cost analysis, cost of illness analysis, cost-effectiveness analysis, cost-utility analysis, and cost-benefit analysis (CDC, 2021; Connor et al., 2023; Turner et al., 2021) (see Table 7.3). The EQUATOR Network (n.d.) has reporting guidelines for some of these types of reports.

TABLE 7.3 Definitions of Economic Evaluation Terms

Term	Definition	Example
Cost analysis	A breakdown of a cost summary by individual factors	Evaluation of all expenses and revenues
Cost of illness	The total cost of resources expended because of a health problem	Patient's decreased/lost productivity (indirect costs) and cost of pain and suffering (intangible costs)
Cost-effectiveness analysis	A comparison of one intervention to another (or the current status quo) by estimating cost to gain a particular health outcome	Death prevented or year of life gained
Cost utility analysis	A form of cost-effectiveness analysis that uses quality-adjusted life years as a health outcome	Improved quality of life

Term	Definition	Example
Cost-benefit analysis	A summation of the potential benefits expected from the practice change followed by the subtraction of the total associated costs, with both expressed in monetary units	The cost of a program to help persons with diabetes learn self-management versus the costs of care provision to these patients if they do not manage their own care
Quality-adjusted life-years (QALYs) analysis	A value of health improvement (in years of life) from an intervention; may be compared to the loss of QALYs if no intervention is implemented	Improved quality or more years of life

In the current cost-conscious health care industry, leaders of EBPQI initiatives in health care must be able to demonstrate the cost-effectiveness or cost benefit of a proposed practice change. In a survey by Johnson et al. (2023), 89% of chief nursing officers reported failure to quantify the financial impact of EBP or QI projects as a shortcoming in health care improvement. Economic evaluations can provide an organization with valuable decision-making insights regarding how best to fund interventions and programs, prioritize expenditures, and allocate its limited resources. EBPQI teams should incorporate known cost information whenever possible to inform decision-making for necessary practice change (Conner et al., 2023) and support sustainability. Valuation using a cost-benefit analysis (CBA) or cost-effectiveness analysis (CEA) can be easily applied to EBPQI initiatives: Both methods compare costs (monetary value); however, CBA measures monetary benefits, and CEA measures nonmonetary values (e.g., quality of life, years of life). See comparison in Table 7.4.

TABLE 7.4 Differences Between CBA and CEA

Cost-Benefit Analysis	Cost-Effectiveness Analysis
Measured in dollars	Measured in life years gained or saved
Benefits = total benefits minus costs	CE ratio = intervention cost divided by intervention effect
Based only on quantitative valuation Represented as a ratio of benefit to cost	Based on both quantitative and qualitative valuation
Can also be represented as a return on investment	Results = cost per unit of effectiveness
Outcomes are known	Typically measures longer term outcomes that are not yet conclusively known
Monetary value is definitive over time (absent inflation)	Assumes the desirability of the outcome, but "value" is harder to capture

A CBA of providing noneconomic benefits to nurses to increase retention (as discussed in Example 2, Chapter 3), might focus on several key areas, including (a) the costs of implementing such benefits versus the savings and benefits accrued from reduced turnover, (b) increased job satisfaction, or (c) improved patient care outcomes. Following is a simplified example that illustrates how an organization might approach this analysis.

BOX 7.1: EXAMPLE OF A CBA

A health care facility is experiencing high turnover rates among its nursing staff, leading to increased recruitment and training costs as well as potential declines in patient-care quality. The facility proposes to implement the following noneconomic benefits aimed at improving nurse satisfaction and retention:

- flexible scheduling to allow for work–life balance
- enhanced professional development opportunities, including paid training and certification courses
- a mentorship program that pairs newly hired nurses with experienced nurses
- recognition programs to celebrate nursing achievements and milestones
- a wellness program

Cost Analysis

1. Flexible scheduling system implementation: Costs include the development of a scheduling software or platform modification, estimated at $5,000.
2. Professional development: An annual allocation of $2,000 per nurse for training and certification programs.
3. Mentorship program: Estimated cost of $1,000 per pair for training and program administration.
4. Recognition programs: Annual budget of $10,000 for awards, celebrations, and communications.
5. Wellness program: Online delivery and availability of ANA Healthy Nurse program, which is free to members.

Benefit Analysis

1. Reduced turnover costs: Assuming that the average cost of replacing a nurse (i.e., recruitment, hiring, training) is $40,000 and that the program reduces turnover by 25%, the annual savings on sustaining a nursing staff of 100 could amount to $1,000,000.
2. Increased job satisfaction: Although difficult to quantify, increased satisfaction often leads to improved morale, which correlates with better patient care, thus potentially having a positive impact on hospital ratings and patient choices.
3. Enhanced patient care: Improved continuity of care due to reduced turnover can lead to better patient outcomes, potentially resulting in higher reimbursement rates from insurance due to quality metrics.
4. Attractiveness to potential employees: Being known for a supportive and development-focused culture can make the facility more attractive to high-quality nursing candidates, thereby reducing costs for future recruitment.

Conclusion

The initial direct and indirect costs of implementing the proposed noneconomic benefits for a staff of 100 nurses could total approximately $250,000; however, the potential savings from reduced turnover alone would significantly outweigh these costs. Additional benefits, such as improved patient care outcomes and enhanced attractiveness to potential employees, provide further justification for the investment.

This simplified analysis demonstrates the potential value of noneconomic benefits for retaining nursing staff. Actual results would depend on precise cost figures, the effectiveness of implementation, and how the benefits are perceived by the nursing staff.

Expert Opinion

An **expert opinion** is a recommendation or stated point of view based on the knowledge and experience of an individual (or group of individuals) with recognized expertise on a particular subject. Common sources of expert opinion are opinion editorials, commentaries, editorials, and personal communications (with or from an expert; Dang et al., 2022). Consensus statements by experts, although not based on scientific evidence, may be considered expert opinion. Because expertise is subjective, expert opinion is subject to bias, yet it can offer information that is particularly useful for bridging the gap between research and the provision of direct care to patients. Evidence from various types of expert opinion can provide valuable contributions to the body of evidence needed to answer clinical questions and guide clinical decision-making.

Searching for Other Types of Evidence

You have learned that EBP relies on various evidence types (combined with clinical expertise and patient preferences) to ground appropriate recommendations for best practice changes. Searching for evidence to answer a clinical question requires a systematic approach as well as knowledge of available resources. In Chapter 4, you learned to use the components of your clinical question (PICOT, PPCO), database-specific language such as MeSH terms, and Boolean connectors to start and refine your search in research databases. Many other types of evidence, some of which we have discussed in this chapter, can be found using these same search strategies and databases. The tools and techniques you learned in Chapter 4 can help you to find all relevant evidence.

Your search of terms associated with the population, intervention, comparison, and outcome of your PICOT question (or the problem, population, change, and outcome of your PPCO question) will yield various types of publications beyond research evidence. As you screen each record in your literature search, you will often find that either the title or the methods section of the abstract provides an indication of the type of study or initiative it is. Initially, your search may focus on higher levels of evidence such as systematic reviews and RCTs; however, the screening process offers a valuable opportunity to capture other evidence by looking for titles, terms, or information in the abstract that include wording such as "evidence-based project/initiative," "quality improvement project/initiative," "literature review," "case report," or "economic evaluation." As you turn your focus to other types of evidence, you can narrow your results by adding this same wording (e.g., "quality improvement," "economic evaluation") to your PICOT-based or PPCO-based search terms.

Searching for Clinical Practice Guidelines

Searching for clinical practice guidelines can be challenging because CPGs, unlike research studies and QI reports, are not centrally located in specified databases and easily revealed by traditional searches. CPGs are more likely to be found in an exhaustive number of professional, governmental, and independent databases, repositories, and websites. Given this multiplicity of evidence-based or practice-focused resources, your search for CPGs will be more efficient and effective if you begin with a specific intention.

APRNs should be aware of another important distinction: Although professional organizations often publish national CPGs (most organization-specific CPGs are based on national CPGs), individual clinical practices can have their own site-specific CPGs that APRNs are expected to follow. As a nurse leader or nurse administrator, your clinical decisions about implementing EBP are informed by available evidence and patient input; however, the implementation of CPGs into clinical practice can be impeded by micro-level (individual behavioral, including clinicians and consumers), meso-level (organizational), or macro-level (context and system) challenges (Pereira et al., 2022). Consequently, and sadly, evidence shows that it takes, on average, 17 years for CPGs to be implemented into clinical practice (Beauchemin et al., 2019). It is imperative that APRNs stay currently informed and that nurse administrators and educators stay steeped in the literature so that timely evidence-based management decisions for health care systems can be maintained!

Literature Databases: Practice Guideline Filters

You can find CPGs in many databases. Remember that some databases provide free complete articles, but others require a subscription. Following are a few suggestions. Begin your search as you would for research evidence:

- In CINAHL, enter your search terms, then scroll down through the search options. From the Publication Type dropdown menu, select Practice Guidelines to search for CPGs.
- In PubMed, enter your search terms, then select the search button, and navigate to the filter menu on the left. Under the Article Type filter, select Practice Guideline.

- In Scopus, search within "article title" and "clinical" AND "practice" AND "guidelines" and your topic of interest.

See Table 7.5 in Chapter 4 for additional databases.

Evidence-Based Clinical Decision-Making Resources

Evidence-based clinical resources intended for use at the point of care to aid in clinical decision-making are another link to accessing clinical practice guidelines (see Table 4.2). These sites provide access to various evidence-based tools, materials, and systematically conducted appraisals/syntheses of topics that address clinical questions, and they are generally similar in their accuracy and use (Bradley-Ridout et al., 2021). The downside to these resources is that they require paid access; however, many universities and health care facilities provide access through their library.

TABLE 7.5 Clinical Decision-Making Resources

Resource	Focus	Guidance
DynaMed www.dynamed.com	Health care providers (nurse practitioners, physicians, and physician assistants)	Enter the general condition or concern related to your clinical question. Select the relevant result. Navigate to the left-side menu and select Guidelines and Resources. There is an option to select Prevention and Screening to search for preventive practice guidelines if this is relevant to your clinical question.
Cochrane Database for Systematic Reviews (CDSR) www.cochranelibrary.com	Any health care providers or clinicians	A collection of high-quality systematic reviews to inform health-care decision making
Clinical Key for Nursing https://beta.elsevier.com/products/clinicalkey/nurses	Nurses and other allied health clinicians	Enter the general condition or concern related to your clinical question. Select the relevant result.
UpToDate www.uptodate.com	Physicians and pharmacists	Enter the general condition or concern related to your clinical question. Select the relevant result. Navigate to the left menu options and select Society Guideline Links to search for CPGs.

Professional Nursing and Medical Organization Websites and Journals

Professional health care organizations are the most common developers of CPGs. Professional organization sites and journals are common places to find consensus or position statements. To get started looking, find the professional organization in the specialty that encompasses your clinical issue and questions. For example, if you are interested in CPGs for managing patients in labor, you could consider searching websites for organizations such as the Association of Women's Health, Obstetric, and Neonatal Nurses (AWHONN); the American College of Nurse-Midwives (ACNM); or the American College of Obstetricians and Gynecologists (ACOG). Some organizations restrict access to members only, but many provide free access to CPGs on their website, and most publish their CPGs in their associated professional journals, thus allowing access through literature database searches through CINAHL or PubMed. Referencing position statements published by your professional organization brings a national body of clinicians' expertise to your practice setting and can provide support and evidence for clinical advice and decision-making.

Evidence-Based Practice and Guideline Databases

Although there is no central repository for CPGs, there are resources for searching and accessing quality CPGs; some are sponsored by governments (e.g., USPSTF), some are dedicated guideline databases, and some are larger organizations or databases with dedicated searchable sections for evidence-based recommendations and guidelines. A significant benefit of CPG databases is that most allow open access or access by creating a free account.

One of the most widely recognized CPG sources is the Emergency Care Research Institute (ECRI) Guidelines Trust, which has a mission to advance effective evidence-based health care globally. The ERCI catalogs high-quality CPGs that are vetted with transparent and rigorous criteria for inclusion in their database (Sender, 2019). Guideline Central is another robust repository option; it provides a multilayer filtered search for CPG summaries, pocket guides, and full-text links and is touted as the largest free-access site for current CPGs. An additional feature of Guideline Central is the availability of a free, easy-to-navigate app version (Guideline Central, 2023). If you want to broaden your search to include international CPGs, the Guidelines International Network (2023) has an extensive database of CPGs offered without cost to promote high-quality standards for CPG development, sharing, and implementation to encourage best practice. Lastly, the U.S. Preventive Services Task Force (USPSTF) website is a critical starting point if your clinical question is focused on preventive care. The USPSTF (n.d.) is a panel of experts in preventive and evidence-based care who use a systematic, rigorous approach to developing practice recommendations based on current evidence. Table 7.6 provides some examples of resources to assist your search for CPGs related to your clinical question. Please keep in mind that other specialty nursing/medical organizations may have additional or updated CPGs available.

TABLE 7.6 Resources for Clinical Practice Guidelines Searches

Type	Name	Location
Government/ Global Agencies	Centers for Disease Control and Prevention (CDC)	https://www.cdc.gov/infectioncontrol/guidelines/index.html
	Healthy People 2030	https://health.gov/healthypeople/tools-action/browse-evidence-based-resources
	U.S. Preventive Services Task Force (USPSTF)	https://www.uspreventiveservicestaskforce.org/uspstf/
	World Health Organization (WHO)	https://www.who.int/publications/who-guidelines
Guideline Repositories	Emergency Care Research Institute (ECRI) Guidelines Trust	https://www.ecri.org/solutions/ecri-guidelines-trust
	Guidelines Central	https://www.guidelinecentral.com/guidelines/
	Guidelines International Network	https://g-i-n.net/international-guidelines-library
	Veterans Affairs/ Department of Defense (VA/DoD) CPG	https://www.healthquality.va.gov/
Medical Reference Sites With Dedicated Guidelines Section	Medscape	https://reference.medscape.com/features/guidelines
Professional Organizations	Registered Nurses' Association of Ontario	https://rnao.ca/bpg/guidelines
	American Academy of Pediatrics (AAP)	https://publications.aap.org/pediatrics/collection/523/Clinical-Practice-Guidelines
	American College of Physicians	https://www.acponline.org/clinical-information/clinical-guidelines-recommendations
	American Diabetes Association (ADA)	https://professional.diabetes.org/content-page/practice-guidelines-resources
	American Heart Association (AHA)	https://professional.heart.org/en/guidelines-and-statements/guidelines-and-statements-search
	National Comprehensive Cancer Network (NCCN)	https://www.nccn.org/guidelines/category_1
	American Cancer Society (ACS)	www.cancer.org
	American Association of Nurse Practitioners (AANP)	www.aanp.org
	American College of Nurse Midwives (ACNM)	www.midwife.org
	American College of Obstretrics and Gynecology (ACOG)	www.acog.org
	American Association of Nurse Anesthesiology (AANA)	www.aana.com
	Association of Psychiatric Mental Health Nurse Practitioners	https://apmhnp.enpnetwork.com
	National Association of Nurse Practitioners in Women's Health	https://npwh.org
	National Association of Neonatal Nurse Practitioners	https://apps.nann.org
	Oncology Nurses Society (ONS)	www.ons.org
	National Association of Pediatric Nurse Practitioners (NAPNAP)	www.napnap.org

As part of your search for information and knowledge, it is vital that you seek other forms of evidence to answer your clinical question and fully synthesize the body of evidence. Professional organizations, especially those for APRNs, may differ in their recommendations (e.g., when to start breast cancer screening in low-risk women). For example, the ACS recommends annual mammography starting at 40 years of age, but the USPSTF recommends it starting at 50 years of age. As a clinician, you must weigh the evidence and provide recommendations to your patients that are both based on research and personalized. At times, research evidence may be limited, and other sources may provide the best available evidence with which to make decisions or recommendations. Finding other evidence is sometimes less straightforward than finding pertinent research evidence; however, use of the resources and practical tips we have discussed will give you a good start at collecting a varied body of evidence to support EBP recommendations.

In conjunction with implementing a CPG based on the best available evidence, APRNs and nurse administrators must consider the practical implications and potential challenges of the implementation (Heen et al., 2021). Shared decision-making with patients about practical issues related to guidelines implementation that affect and interest them is an essential part of the APRN role. As nurse leaders, we pride ourselves on being patient centered and holistic in our approach to health care.

Appraising Other Types of Evidence

When you find additional relevant evidence, you must critically appraise it with your EBPQI team. As you will remember from Chapter 4, all **critical appraisal** involves a series of sequential steps: (1) assigning level and quality ratings to each piece of evidence, and if an abundant amount of evidence exists, discarding evidence of low quality; (2) evaluating and summarizing each piece of evidence; (3) synthesizing the individual summaries into a body of evidence; and (4) making a practice recommendation (Fineout-Overholt, 2023). The use of standardized appraisal checklists or tools will enhance the objectivity and transparency of your appraisal and reduce the potential for individual bias (Buccheri & Sharifi, 2017; Tod et al., 2021); moreover, the appraisal process should be completed in teams to improve its accuracy (Dang et al., 2022).

Step 1: Assessing Level and Quality of Other Types of Evidence

At the beginning of this chapter, we discussed the hierarchy of evidence, which provides an essential guide for ranking levels of different evidence types. We caution you, however, to use it wisely, remembering always that the level of evidence does not necessarily predict its quality (Harris et al., 2014). For example, a poorly designed and executed randomized control trial does not carry the same weight or strength as a well-designed one, although both are RCTs. Similarly, the expert opinion of an unrecognized expert will not carry the same strength as that of a nationally recognized expert. A thorough consideration of both the level and quality of your evidence will ensure its strength as well as your confidence to make practice recommendations (Melnyk, 2016). It is imperative that you use a systematic approach to assess and determine quality as you build a body of evidence to answer your clinical question and make a practice recommendation.

As discussed in Chapters 5 and 6, as you assess the quality of research studies, you must determine whether each study is valid, reliable, and applicable (Fineout-Overholt et al., 2010). Applicability describes how well the evidence supports your proposed solution to the clinical problem or issue within the context of your population and can be universally assessed among different evidence types. Traditional elements used to determine validity and reliability may not apply to other evidence if it is not based on the scientific method; however, traditional concepts can be applied through a nonresearch lens while appraising this evidence. For example, when considering an EBPQI initiative, you could appraise validity by looking for a rigorous and systematic literature search that resulted in appraisal and synthesis of the evidence to support the practice change; you could appraise reliability by ensuring that measured outcomes are clearly defined and clinically meaningful (O'Mathuna, 2023; Waldrop et al., 2024). Nonresearch or other evidence appraisal tools assess validity, reliability, and applicability in a meaningful manner specific to the type of evidence. Most of these tools do not result in scoring quality directly; rather, they serve as a guide to highlight critical components associated with quality, thus allowing appraisers an overview from which to make consensus decisions about quality. Appraisal tools intended for use with nonresearch or other evidence can provide a clear and standardized approach to asking the right questions to determine quality.

Clinical Practice Guidelines

As you now know, clinical practice guidelines are practice recommendations made with the goal of optimizing patient care and formulated based on a systematic review of scientific evidence and an assessment of the benefits and harms of related interventions (IOM et al., 2011). It is important to note that not all CPGs are created with the same level of rigor, which can result in varying quality. For example, a CPG on breastfeeding infants in the pediatric intensive care unit developed by the Academy of Breastfeeding Medicine using a systematic review process would be of higher quality than one developed for a specific hospital system by its quality assurance committee based on expert opinion.

There are several tools available that have been explicitly developed to appraise rigor and adherence to quality standards for CPG development. The AGREE II tool (www.agreetrust.org/agree-ii/) is the most widely used and can serve as a framework for CPG development and reporting. For example, your EBPQI team could use this tool to evaluate a CPG that you are considering as potential evidence to support your practice change. The AGREE II tool comprises six quality-related domains: scope and purpose, stakeholder involvement, the rigor of development, clarity of presentation, applicability, and editorial independence. A group of raters (e.g., your team) score the CPG in each domain. An aggregate score is not used, but domain scores of > 70% typically indicate a high-quality CPG. Additionally, the tool prompts the appraisers to rank the overall quality of the CPG and indicate whether they would recommend using the guideline (AGREE Next Steps Consortium, 2017).

EBP and QI Initiatives

EBPQI initiatives are increasingly published in the literature, so researchers must have the ability to determine the quality of these reports. As EBP and QI findings are not research, they are not generalizable; however, they can inform your clinical question and provide important information transferable to your EBP initiative population, organization, and process. To demonstrate quality in development and reporting, EBPQI reports should (a) show the use of a process or model to guide the project, (b) have a clear purpose or aim, (c) align with the evidence (external and internal), and (d) have outcome measurements that are clearly defined and discussed. As with CPGs, guidance has been developed to promote standardized reporting and appraisal of EBPQI initiatives.

Appraisal and reporting tools specific to EBP projects and initiatives are somewhat limited in availability. The Evidence-Based Practice Process Quality Assessment (EPQA) guideline was developed as an appraisal tool and guide to planning and reporting EBP projects (Lee et al., 2013); it uses a checklist format to identify key markers expected in quality EBP projects and initiatives. The Evidence-Based Practice Dissemination Guide can also be used in the appraisal of EBP projects (Dean et al., 2021).

QI projects and initiatives have historically been used and reported among a wider audience of health care professionals, and there is a widely used standard for reporting these projects called the Standards for Quality Improvement Reporting Excellence, or SQUIRE. SQUIRE (2020) 2.0 is a flexible framework for reporting QI initiatives implemented at a systems level with measurable intervention-related outcomes. Considered the gold standard for reporting QI initiatives, these reporting standards provide clear sections and items to be included in reports for publication.

There are several options for QI appraisal tools, such as the Quality Improvement Minimum Quality Criteria Set (QI-MQCS) tool (https://qualitysafety.bmj.com/content/qhc/24/12/796.full.pdf?with-ds=yes) states the minimum criteria for quality for each of 16 domains (Hempel et al., 2015).

A recently developed tool that encompasses all components of EBPQI initiatives is presented as a checklist that includes criteria, descriptions and examples of the criteria, and columns that specify whether the criteria was met, not met, or partially met. Each criterion is scored, and the totals are reflective of the quality of the report (Waldrop et al., 2024). See Appendix B for an example of using the EBPQI critical appraisal tool.

Additional Types of Evidence

As discussed earlier in this chapter, there are many types of nonresearch evidence besides CPGs and EBPQI projects or initiatives, including position or consensus statements, literature reviews, case reports, and expert opinions. Only some types of nonresearch evidence will have a specific appraisal tool; however, you can begin your appraisal by considering the validity (accuracy), reliability (consistency), and applicability within the context of the type of evidence. For example, there is no specific appraisal tool for case studies. A case study is often a clinical report on an individual patient; as such, although it may be published, it is of no higher level of evidence than an unpublished case you might have had in practice, which would constitute "anecdotal" evidence. A report comprised of many cases, however, might be considered a higher level of evidence.

The Johns Hopkins EBP Non-Research Evidence tool (https://www.hopkinsmedicine.org/evidence-based-practice/model-tools) is an appraisal tool tailored to several types of evidence and can be used for consistency in determining quality. The JHEBP Non-Research Appraisal tool is a short checklist with sections for different types of evidence; criteria for assigning quality are included in the tool (Dang et al., 2022). A summary of select resources for various nonresearch appraisal tools can be found in Table 7.7.

Appraising nonresearch evidence for the level and quality of evidence can sometimes feel daunting due to the numerous types of evidence and tools available. Although it is essential to use an appraisal method or tool that is appropriate for the type of evidence, the specific tool used is less important than a systematic and consistent team approach. As a leader, you can leverage your ability to develop or work with a team of experts and novices whose various strengths and frames of reference will lighten the work of critical appraisal!

TABLE 7.7 Resources for Nonresearch Appraisal Tools

Type	Name	Location
Nonresearch evidence (general, may be used with any type of nonresearch evidence)	Johns Hopkins Evidence-Based Practice (JHEBP) Non-Research Evidence Appraisal tool	https://www.hopkinsmedicine.org/evidence-based-practice/model-tools
Clinical practice guidelines	AGREE II instrument	https://www.agreetrust.org/agree-ii/

(Continued)

TABLE 7.7 *(Continued)*

Type	Name	Location
EBPQI projects and initiatives	Evidence-Based Practice Process Quality Assessment (EPQA)	https://pubmed.ncbi.nlm.nih.gov/23387900/
	Quality Improvement Minimum Quality Criteria Set (QI-MQCS)	https://www.ncbi.nlm.nih.gov/pmc/articles/PMC4680162/ (in supplemental materials)
	EBPQI Critical Appraisal Tool	https://journals.lww.com/jncqjournal/fulltext/9900/evidence_based_practice_quality_improvement.154.aspx
Other nonresearch evidence (case reports, economic evaluations, expert opinion)	Joanna Briggs Institute (JBI)	https://jbi.global/critical-appraisal-tools
	Critical Appraisal Skills Programme (CASP) economic evaluation checklist	https://casp-uk.net/casp-tools-checklists/

*Note. * Requires membership subscription and/or fee.*

After assigning a level and quality grade to each piece of nonresearch or other evidence, you can move on to the next step of the critical appraisal process: evaluation.

Step 2: Evaluating Other Evidence

Evaluation is the process of reviewing each piece of evidence and extracting the information relevant to your clinical question. This step is typically reserved for research evidence and includes research components such as study design, variables, data analysis, and findings. However, some types of evidence that measure outcomes, such as EBP and QI initiatives, may also be appropriate to include in the evaluation and can be included in your evaluation table.

Steps 3 and 4: Synthesizing the Body of Evidence and Making Recommendations for Practice

As you consider the final steps of critical appraisal, you may wonder what the difference is between summarizing and synthesizing. In the context of EBP, summarizing involves evaluating, then briefly stating, or recording in an evaluation or summary table the key information from each *individual piece of evidence*, as discussed in Chapter 6. Synthesis involves *combining*, *contrasting*, and *interpreting the evidence*, using your summaries as individual puzzle

TABLE 7.8 RN Turnover and Noneconomic Impact Levels of Evidence Table

Level of Evidence	Article Identified (Number or Author/ Year)	Article Identified (Number or Author/ Year)	Article Identified (Number or Author/ Year)	Article Identified (Number or Author/ Year)	Article Identified (Number or Author/ Year)	Article Identified (Number or Author/ Year)	Article Identified (Number or Author/ Year)	Article Identified (Number or Author/ Year)
RCT								
Experimental								
Cross-sectional	X	X	X	X	X	X	X	X
Case control								
Qualitative								
Other								

pieces with which to build a complete picture or conclusion about what is known about your clinical question (O'Mathuna et al., 2023). Synthesis represents your consideration of the entire body of evidence, including your assessment of the quality, quantity (strength), and consistency of the research and other evidence you have found. Some helpful tools for making this determination are a levels-of-evidence table and a synthesis table. Your levels of evidence table will use one of the systems for the quality of research studies. You could use the one in Figure 7.1 in this chapter (as presented in the following example; Table 7.8).

Remember the example on RN turnover from Chapter 3? When trying to describe the economic impacts of RN turnover, you found that there were also noneconomic impacts. You developed an evidence summary table for each study you included. You can now complete a level of evidence table from those evidence summary tables. As you can see in Table 7.8., all of the studies were cross-sectional studies that described variables at one point in time (cross-sectional study design) and used correlational analyses.

An evidence synthesis table based on the outcomes of interest can help you visualize the consistency of your evidence, as shown in Table 7.9.

After you complete the synthesis process, you should understand the body of evidence available and be able to answer clinical questions and make recommendations for practice. If there is no clear answer to the clinical question, or if an appropriate body of quality evidence does not exist, a recommendation for practice change should not be made. As demonstrated in the mountain model, after all the available evidence has been critically appraised, you may conclude that you must conduct more research before making a recommendation for practice change.

You might end up determining that the existing evidence is not research based. For example, while I (Jayne) was completing a postdoctoral fellowship in EBP, I noticed that DNP-prepared faculty frequently reported challenges or barriers to achieving success in academic roles when the criteria for promotion

TABLE 7.9 RN Turnover and Noneconomic Impact Synthesis Table

Noneconomic Outcome	Article Identified (Number or Author/Year)	Article Identified (Number or Author/Year)	Article Identified (Number or Author/Year)	Article Identified (Number or Author/Year)	Article Identified (Number or Author/Year)	Article Identified (Number or Author/Year)	Article Identified (Number or Author/Year)	Article Identified (Number or Author/Year)
Workgroup cohesion	↔ (no difference)							
RN mental health		↓ (decrease)			↓ (decrease)	↔ (no difference)	↓ (decrease)	
Patient satisfaction	↔ (no difference)		↓ (decrease)	↓ (decrease)			↓ (decrease)	↓ (decrease)
Medical errors		↑ (increase)		↑ (increase)	↑ (increase)	↑ (increase)		

included scholarship. This concerned me because DNP-prepared nurses continue to fill faculty roles in increased numbers, and thoughtful standards for scholarship are needed to advance the nursing profession as a whole. I wanted to lead a team in exploring scholarship standards for faculty who had earned a Doctor of Nursing Practice (DNP) degree. I assembled a team to search for available evidence that addressed this timely topic. Following the steps of EBP, we identified the problem and developed the following PPCO question: "For nurse faculty prepared with the DNP degree, what practices demonstrate impact and clear criteria for scholarship?" (see Table 7.10; Waldrop & Dunlap, 2024b).

TABLE 7.10 PPCO Development

Element	Description	Example
P: Problem	What is the problem in general (external evidence) and specifically in the local context (internal evidence)?	Unclear scholarship standards
P: Population	Who does the problem impact?	Nurses prepared with a DNP degree
C: Change	What has been recommended or done to address the problem? (practice or process changes)	Criteria for scholarship
O: Outcomes	How are outcomes reported (measured)? (It may be the same as the problem originally noted or its components.)	Demonstrated scholarship impact

Source: Waldrop and Dunlap (2024b).

Despite our extensive and iterative search, we found little research evidence that investigated this problem. In the absence of available research evidence, we reviewed and synthesized other types of evidence. As faculty with substantial experience and expertise gained in diverse institutions, we were aware that universities have varied tracks for DNP-prepared faculty including, but not inclusive of, clinical and tenure lines; therefore, DNP scholarship standards from high-ranking intuitions were critically appraised and placed in an evidence synthesis table (accessible if interested in this open-access article: www.sciencedirect.com/science/article/pii/S8755722324000206?via%3Dihub). Using a new inclusive model of DNP scholarship impact (Dunlap et al., 2024), we translated this other evidence, along with the collective expert opinions of the authors, into recommendations. In Chapter 12, we introduce you to this original model that was inspired and informed by other types of evidence, and which we have adapted broadly (for you!) to encompass the work of nurses in academia, practice, and policy settings.

If an initial practice recommendation can be made, you will lead your team to the next step of EBP, which is to integrate clinician expertise and patient values and preferences into the recommendation formulated. You will be introduced to this step in the next chapter.

WELLNESS IN ACTION: GOOD DEED PARTICIPATION

Acts of kindness or engagement in good deeds have been associated with increased health and boosts in well-being (Hui et al., 2020; Poulin et al., 2013). I (Jayne) recently visited a beach with my family during spring break. When we arrived oceanside, our hearts sank seeing the shore littered with trash. The sight felt overwhelming. While I helped our kids apply sunscreen, my husband grabbed a plastic trash bag that we had packed for our own use and began to pick up the trash, one piece at a time. After a few minutes, I told my son that I was going to help pick up trash, and he said, “I will too!” Before long, my daughter, who had been playing in the sand, began to help as well. Within minutes, a nearby family joined our effort, and then another family joined in. Within about 10 minutes, our section of the beach was completely free of debris and looked pretty again. Beach patrol personnel came by and thanked us all for our efforts.

As I looked around at the group, I noticed that the other adults, who had looked as stressed as I felt when we began, appeared content and fulfilled. When my husband decided to pick up those first beer cans, he had no idea that within a few minutes 18 people would be cleaning up the beach alongside him! My kids expressed that they felt proud of themselves for ensuring that other children wouldn’t cut their feet and that the trash wouldn’t be swept into the ocean by the tide and hurt marine life. This experience exemplified for me how one’s engagement as a leader in an act of importance, if only on a small scale, can quickly be taken up as a common goal that makes a meaningful difference and brings satisfaction and pride to all involved. Consider taking these simple steps and serving a small cause on a routine basis:

- Think about something simple you can do as a leader to make a positive impact.
- Make a plan to participate in this good deed or act of kindness regardless of whether it results in a significant outcome.
- Note how you feel afterward and use this insight to inform future good deed engagement.

WRAPPING UP

You must search for and appraise various types of evidence to fully develop and synthesize a body of evidence that allows you to answer a clinical question and make evidence-based practice recommendations. Common nonresearch and other types of evidence used to inform a body of evidence include CPGs, practice statements, consensus statements, EBP and QI projects/initiatives, economic evaluations, and various types of reviews. Given the diversity of other evidence types, a variety of search techniques and resources may be needed to find the best available evidence. Regardless of evidence type, systematic critical appraisal is vital to determining the level and quality of evidence. Higher levels and quality of evidence will strengthen your confidence that you are making sound EBP recommendations. Although considered a lower level of evidence than research evidence, other types of evidence can provide important contributions, especially when research evidence is limited or more information is needed to provide safe, high-quality patient care.

REFLECTION QUESTIONS

1. Using the resources and tips discussed, start a search for other or nonresearch evidence on a topic of your choice using PubMed (https://pubmed.ncbi.nlm.nih.gov), or Guideline Central (www.guidelinecentral.com/guidelines) or the USPSTF (www.uspreventiveservicestaskforce.org/uspstf/topic_search_results).
2. Remember the clinical question about immunizations? Find a clinical practice guideline, consensus statement, or other recommendation on this topic. Using the AGREE II tool with your group, appraise the document you have found. You can use the online AGREE II tool (www.agreetrust.org/) by creating a free account. Select My AGREE PLUS and then the orange Start New button. Alternatively, you can download the pdf version using this link: www.agreetrust.org/wp-content/uploads/2017/12/AGREE-II-Users-Manual-and-23-item-Instrument-2009-Update-2017.pdf
3. Using this QI report (https://journals.plos.org/plosone/article?id=10.1371/journal.pone.0241706), try one of the EBP/QI critical appraisal tools. If you are working in a group, have group members use different tools and compare and discuss them. Was engagement in this activity helpful? Why or why not?

4. Based on the quality of the evidence presented in Table 7.8 and the consistency of the evidence in the synthesis table (7.9) on RN turnover, what would you say is the consistency of the evidence? How would you weigh it with the quality of the evidence? What statement could you make based on the evidence?

REFERENCES

AGREE Next Steps Consortium. (2017). *Appraisal of guidelines for research and evaluation II: AGREE II instrument.* https://www.agreetrust.org/wp-content/uploads/2017/12/AGREE-II-Users-Manual-and-23-item-Instrument-2009-Update-2017.pdf

Beauchemin, M., Cohn, E., & Shelton, R. C. (2019). Implementation of clinical practice guidelines in the health care setting: A concept analysis. *ANS. Advances in Nursing Science, 42*(4), 307–324. https://doi.org/10.1097/ANS.0000000000000263

Bowden, V. R., & Purper, C. (2022). Types of reviews—part 3: Literature review, integrative review, scoping review. *Pediatric Nursing, 48*(2), 97–100.

Bradley-Ridout, G., Nekolaichuk, E., Jamieson, T., Jones, C., Morson, N., Chuang, R., & Springall, E. (2021). UpToDate versus Dynamed: A cross-sectional study comparing the speed and accuracy of two point-of-care information tools. *Journal of the Medical Library Association, 109*(3). https://doi.org/10.5195/jmla.2021.1176

Buccheri, R. K., & Sharifi, C. (2017). Critical appraisal tools and reporting guidelines for evidence-based practice. *Worldviews on Evidence-Based Nursing, 14*(6), 463–472. https://doi.org/10.1111/wvn.12258

Carter-Templeton, H., Wrigley, J., Nicoll, L. H., Owens, J. K., Oermann, M. H., & Ledbetter, L. S. (2023). A bibliometric analysis of review types published in the nursing scientific literature. *ANS. Advances in Nursing Science, 46*(1), 28–40. https://doi.org/10.1097/ANS.0000000000000424

Centers for Disease Control and Prevention. (2022). Autism spectrum disorder: Screening and diagnosis. https://www.cdc.gov/autism/diagnosis/

Centers for Disease Control and Prevention, Office of the Associate Director for Policy and Strategy. (2021, March 3). *Economic evaluation overview.* https://www.cdc.gov/polaris/php/economics/

Connor, L., Dean, J., McNett, M., Tydings, D. M., Shrout, A., Gorsuch, P. F., Hole, A., Moore, L., Brown, R., Melnyk, B., & Gallagher-Ford, L. (2023). Evidence-based practice improves patient outcomes and healthcare system return on investment: Findings from a scoping review. *Worldviews on Evidence-Based Nursing, 20*(1), 6–15. https://doi.org/10.1111/wvn.12621

Dang, D., Dearholt, S., Bissett, K., Ascenzi, J., & Whalen, M. (2022). *Johns Hopkins evidence-based practice for nurses and heathcare professionals: Models and guidelines* (4th ed.). Sigma Theta Tau International.

Dunlap, J. J., & Filipek, P. A. (2020). CE: Autism spectrum disorder: The nurse's role. *The American Journal of Nursing, 120*(11), 40–49. https://doi.org/10.1097/01.NAJ.0000721236.69639.e3

Dunlap, J. J., Waldrop, J. B, Mainous, R. O, Zellefrow, C., Beckett, C., Melnyk, B. M., (2024). Consistent scholarship standards for DNP prepared faculty needed: Actionable insights. *Journal of Professional Nursing, 51*, 58–63. https://doi.org/10.1016/j.profnurs.2024.01.009

EQUATOR Network. (n.d.). *Reporting guideline*. https://www.equator-network.org/?post_type=eq_guidelines&eq_guidelines_study_design=economic-evaluations&eq_guidelines_clinical_specialty=0&eq_guidelines_report_section=0&s=+

Fineout-Overholt, E. (2023). Critically appraising knowledge for clinical decision making. In (Ed.), *Evidence-based practice in nursing & healthcare: A guide to best practice* (5th ed., pp. 153–170). Wolters Kluwer.

Fineout-Overholt, E., Melnyk, B., Stillwell, S. B., & Williamson, K. M. (2010). Evidence-based practice, step by step: Critical appraisal of the evidence: Part II. *AJN, 110*(9), 41–48. https://doi.org/10.1097/01.naj.0000388264.49427.f9

Gruendemann, B. J. (1969). A literature review. *Association of Operating Room Nurses Journal, 10*(6), 57–59. https://doi.org/10.1016/s0001-2092(08)70709-9

Guideline Central. (2023). *About*. https://www.guidelinecentral.com/about/

Guidelines International Network. (2023). *About*. https://g-i-n.net/about-gin

Harris, M., Taylor, G., & Jackson, D. (2014). *Clinical evidence made easy: The basics of evidence-based medicine*. Scion.

Hempel, S., Shekelle, P. G., Liu, J. L., Sherwood Danz, M., Foy, R., Lim, Y.-W., Motala, A., & Rubenstein, L. V. (2015). Development of the quality improvement minimum quality criteria set (QI-MQCS): A tool for critical appraisal of quality improvement intervention publications. *BMJ Quality & Safety, 24*(12), 796–804. https://doi.org/10.1136/bmjqs-2014-003151

Hui, B. P. H., Ng, J. C. K, Berzaghi, E. et al. (2020). *Rewards of kindness? A meta-analysis of the link between prosociality and well-being*. American Psychological Association. https://www.apa.org/pubs/journals/releases/bul-bul0000298.pdf

Hyman, S. L., Levy, S. E., Myers, S. M., & Council on Children With Disabilities, Section on Developmental and Behavioral Pediatrics. (2020). Identification, evaluation, and management of children with autism spectrum disorder. *Pediatrics, 145*(1), e20193447. https://doi.org/10.1542/peds.2019-3447

Jackson, Mick. (Director). (2010). *Temple Grandin* [Motion picture]. IMDbPro. United States

Joshi, G. P., Benzon, H. T., Gan, T. J., & Vetter, T. R. (2019). Consistent definitions of clinical practice guidelines, consensus statements, position statements, and practice alerts. *Anesthesia & Analgesia, 129*(6), 1767–1770. https://doi.org/10.1213/ane.0000000000004236

Lee, M., Johnson, K. L., Newhouse, R. P., & Warren, J. I. (2013). Evidence-based practice process quality assessment: EPQA guidelines. *Worldviews on Evidence-Based Nursing, 10*(3), 140–149. https://doi.org/10.1111/j.1741-6787.2012.00264.x

Levin, R. F., Keefer, J. M., Marren, J., Vetter, M., Lauder, B., & Sobolewski, S. (2010). Evidence-based practice improvement: Merging 2 paradigms. *Journal of Nursing Care Quality, 25*(2), 117–126. https://doi.org/10.1097/NCQ.0b013e3181b5f19f

Melnyk, B. (2016). Level of evidence plus critical appraisal of its quality yields confidence to implement evidence-based practice changes. *Worldviews on Evidence-Based Nursing, 13*(5), 337–339. https://doi.org/10.1111/wvn.12181

Melnyk, B., Buck, J., & Gallagher-Ford, L. (2015). Transforming quality improvement into evidence-based quality improvement: A key solution to improve healthcare outcomes. *Worldviews on Evidence-Based Nursing, 12*(5), 251–252. https://doi.org/10.1111/wvn.12112

Munn, Z., Peters, M. J., Stern, C., Tufanaru, C., McArthur, A., & Aromataris, E. (2018). Systematic review or scoping review? Guidance for authors when choosing between a systematic or scoping review approach. *BMC Medical Research Methodology, 18*(1). https://doi.org/10.1186/s12874-018-0611-x

Oermann, M. H., & Knafl, K. A. (2021). Strategies for completing a successful integrative review. *Nurse Author & Editor, 31*(3–4), 65–68. https://doi.org/10.1111/nae2.30

O'Mathuna, D. P., Finest-Overholt, E., Graham, D. B., & Canada, A. (2023). Critically appraising quantitative evidence for clinical decision making. In B. M. Melnyk & E. Fineout-Overholt (Eds.), *Evidence-based practice in nursing and heathcare: A guide to best practice* (5th ed., pp. 189–265). Wolters Kluwer.

Pereira, V. C., Silva, S. N., Carvalho, V. K. S., Zanghelini, F., & Barreto, J. O. M. (2022). Strategies for the implementation of clinical practice guidelines in public health: An overview of systematic reviews. *Health Research Policy and Systems, 20*(1), 13. https://doi.org/10.1186/s12961-022-00815-4

Poulin, M. J., Brown, S. L., Dillard, A. J., & Smith, D. M. (2013). Giving to others and the association between stress and mortality. *American Journal of Public Health, 103*(9), 1649–1655. https://doi.org/10.2105/AJPH.2012.300876

Reece, J., Johnson, J. Dunlap, J.J. (2023). An updated guide to autism screening: A primer for nurse practitioners. *The Journal for Nurse Practitioners, 20*(2). https://www.npjournal.org/article/S1555-4155(23)00398-7/fulltext

Schloemer, T., & Schröder-Bäck, P. (2018). Criteria for evaluating transferability of health interventions: A systematic review and thematic synthesis. *Implementation Science, 13*(1). https://doi.org/10.1186/s13012-018-0751-8

Sender, J. (2019). ECRI Institute Guidelines Trust. *Journal of the Medical Library Association, 107*(3). https://doi.org/10.5195/jmla.2019.693

SQUIRE. (2020). *Revised standards for quality improvement reporting excellence: SQUIRE 2.0.* http://www.squire-statement.org/index.cfm?fuseaction=Page.ViewPage&pageId=471

Tod, D., Booth, A., & Smith, B. (2021). Critical appraisal. *International Review of Sport and Exercise Psychology, 15*(1), 52–72. https://doi.org/10.1080/1750984x.2021.1952471

Tricco, A. C., Lillie, E., Zarin, W., et al. (2018). PRISMA Extension for Scoping Reviews (PRISMA-ScR): Checklist and explanation. *Ann Intern Med, 169*, 467–473. https://doi.org/10.7326/M18-0850

Turner, H. C., Archer, R. A., Downey, L. E., Isaranuwatchai, W., Chalkidou, K., Jit, M., & Teerawattananon, Y. (2021). An introduction to the main types of economic evaluations used for informing priority setting and resource allocation in healthcare: Key features, uses, and limitations. *Frontiers in Public Health, 9*. https://doi.org/10.3389/fpubh.2021.722927

U.S. Preventive Services Task Force. (n.d.). *About the USPSTF.* https://uspreventiveservicestaskforce.org/uspstf/about-uspstf

Waldrop, J., & Dunlap J. J. (2024a). A new question simplifies the search for evidence. *American Journal of Nursing, 124*(3), 34–37. https://doi.org/10.1097/01.NAJ.0001007676.91191.dd |

Waldrop, J., & Dunlap, J. J. (2024af). The mountain model for evidence-based practice quality improvement initiatives. *American Journal of Nursing, 124*(5), 32–37. https://doi.org/10.1097/01.NAJ.0001014540.57079.72

Waldrop, J. Dunlap, J. J. & Reynolds, S., & (2024). Evidence-based practice quality improvement critical appraisal tool. *Journal of Nursing Care Quality.* https://doi.org/10.1097/NCQ.0000000000000789

Westphaln, K. K., Regoeczi, W., Masotya, M., Vazquez-Westphaln, B., Lounsbury, K., McDavid, L., Lee, H., Johnson, J., Ronis, S. D. (2021). From Arskey and O'Malley and beyond: Customizations to enhance a team-based, mixed approach to scoping review methodology. *MethodsX, 8*, 101375.

IMAGE CREDITS

Fig. 7.1: Jayne Jennings Dunlap and Julee Briscoe Waldrop, *Introduction to Evidence-Based Practice and Quality Improvement for Professional Nursing Practice: A Competency Based Approach*, p. 124. Copyright © 2024 by Cognella, Inc. Reprinted with permission.

CHAPTER 8

Incorporating the Patient Perspective in Quality Care

Elizabeth Walters and Julee Briscoe Waldrop

KEY CONCEPTS

Shared decision-making
Clinical expertise
Patient engagement and family engagement
Health literacy
Diversity, equity, and inclusion
Cultural competency

LEARNING OBJECTIVES

1. Discuss the importance of incorporating patient preference with EPB.
2. Identify benefits and barriers to shared decision-making.
3. Understand the benefits and barriers to shared decision-making.

> Let us never consider ourselves finished nurses.
> We must be learning all of our lives.
>
> —Florence Nightingale

Introduction

Imagine you're at a clothing store looking for an outfit for an important event. A sales associate with the best intentions brings you a stylish outfit that is popular among other customers. While the outfit is fashionable and high quality, it doesn't match your style or the specific requirements you had in mind for the event. You appreciate the associate's recommendation based on their experience and other customers' feedback, but you had a particular look and comfort level in mind. If the associate had asked for your preferences, you would have ended up with an outfit you felt confident and comfortable wearing, enhancing your overall experience. This scenario mirrors the patient experience in health care, in that patients want to be involved in their care decisions rather than merely receive a decision made solely by their health care provider (HCP).

For nurses in advanced roles, the importance of incorporating patient preferences into their care cannot be overstated. Just as you had a specific preference for your outfit, patients desire to have a say in their health care decisions. The outcomes are significantly better when patient preferences are integrated into EBPQI. Research demonstrates that patients who are involved in their health care decisions are more likely to initiate and adhere to their treatment plans (Swift et al., 2017, 2018; King et al., 2005).

As health care becomes increasingly patient centered, the role of APRNs and nurse leaders in facilitating shared decision-making becomes more critical. Engaging patients in discussions about their treatment options, understanding their values and preferences, and incorporating these into clinical decision-making are key components of high-quality care. This chapter explores the importance of integrating the patient perspective in quality care, highlighting the impact of patient engagement on health outcomes, the necessity of cultural competence and humility, and the essential role of therapeutic communication. Through examples and evidence-based strategies, this chapter aims to equip nurses in advanced roles with the tools needed to enhance patient-centered care.

Patient Preference and EBP

Personalizing health care interventions is essential to EBP, which integrates the best available research with clinical expertise, patient preferences, and values (Haverfield et al., 2020; Nutbeam et al., 2018). It ensures that health care delivery is scientifically sound and attuned to patients' needs. Research has consistently shown that integrating patient preferences into health care decision-making leads to better management of chronic conditions and patient outcomes. Studies indicate that patients who are actively involved in their care decisions have better adherence to treatment plans, experience less anxiety, and report higher satisfaction with their care (Haverfield et al., 2020; Nutbeam et al., 2018; Swift et al., 2018).

Patient preference is not merely a desirable add-on but an essential element that respects patients' rights and dignity. Patient-centered care involves comprehending patients' values, which include their attitudes and perceptions about their health and health care, and their preferences, which are their choices regarding treatment options based on these values (Gooberman-Hill, 2012; Llewellyn-Thomas & Crump, 2013).

Consider a scenario when a patient diagnosed with anxiety opts not to take their prescribed medication. This decision might initially seem illogical from a health care provider's perspective, particularly if the provider values medication adherence as crucial for managing anxiety. However, the patient's decision could be rooted in past experiences with side effects or a personal preference for non-pharmacological treatments. By engaging with the patient and exploring these underlying reasons, health care providers can better understand and respect their choices, leading to more effective and satisfactory care plans (Swift et al., 2017, 2018).

Engaging patients in this manner is not just about compliance but collaboration. It shifts the dynamic from a one-sided care delivery to a mutual partnership. Patients who feel their preferences are understood and valued are more likely to participate actively in their care, leading to improved health outcomes. This collaborative approach ensures that care plans are tailored to each patient's unique needs and preferences, thereby enhancing overall patient satisfaction and treatment adherence (Higgins et al., 2017).

If you recall from Chapter 2, the *quintuple aim* in health care includes five primary goals: enhancing the patient experience, improving population health, reducing health care costs, improving caregiver well-being, and promoting equity. So, incorporating patient preferences into evidence-based practice is not just a best practice but a necessity for achieving the quintuple aim (Bodenheimer & Sinsky, 2014).

Improving Population Health and Decreasing Health Care Costs

When patient preferences are considered, the resulting health care plans are more likely to be adhered to, leading to better health outcomes (Swift et al., 2018). For example, in Box 8.1, a patient managing diabetes may prefer dietary changes that fit into their cultural preferences over standard recommendations. By incorporating these preferences into the treatment plan, the patient is more likely to adhere to their diet, which will improve their overall health and reduce the prevalence of uncontrolled diabetes within the population (Nutbeam et al., 2018). This also reduces the likelihood of costly emergency interventions. For example, a patient with diabetes who can self-manage their diet will have lower blood glucose levels, thus reducing the need for frequent hospital visits and expensive treatments (Swift et al., 2017).

Promoting Equity

Incorporating patient preferences also promotes equity in health care and ensures that all patients, regardless of their cultural, socioeconomic, or personal circumstances, receive respectful and appropriate care. For instance, a culturally sensitive approach to care for a patient from a minority background might involve understanding and incorporating traditional healing practices into the treatment plan (Agner, 2020; Brown et al., 2016; Nava et al., 2022).

Improving Caregiver Well-Being

Health care providers experience improved job satisfaction and reduced burnout when they engage in patient-centered care (another component of the quintuple aim [Bodenheimer & Sinsky, 2014]). Providers build stronger therapeutic relationships and experience greater professional fulfillment by incorporating patient preferences into the care plan. For example, a nurse practitioner who collaborates with a patient to develop a personalized care plan for managing diabetes may find the process more rewarding and less stressful, leading to better job satisfaction and reduced turnover (Haverfield et al., 2020).

Patient Engagement

Many factors influence patient engagement, but engaging patients in their care can be straightforward compared to involving their families, especially in complex or culturally sensitive situations. Family engagement is crucial in scenarios such as end-of-life care or pediatric treatment. In many cultures, involving the family in health care decisions is a norm and a sign of respect (Brown et al., 2016). Table 8.1 outlines the major factors.

TABLE 8.1 Factors Influencing Patient Engagement

Factor	Components	Example
Patient commitment	The patient's willingness to participate in health care. Providers need to understanding patient motivations (Higgins et al., 2017).	Patients with anxiety might avoid medication due to past side effects.
Trust	Honest, open communication to build trust and strengthen therapeutic alliance. Providers should be transparent about health conditions and treatment options (Agency for Healthcare Research & Quality [AHRQ], 2020). Active listening to patients' concerns and preferences is essential (Nightingale College, 2022).	Acknowledge patient fears, provide detailed information, and discuss alternatives.
Culture	Communicate with cultural sensitivity and respect for the patient's wishes Ask the patient who needs to be involved—the entire family or specific family members. Be sure to obtain the patient's consent before sharing health information with family members to respect their privacy and comply with legal requirements such as HIPAA (Haines et al., 2017).	In many Asian cultures, family decisions are paramount, and discussing health matters with family members is an essential aspect of care (Nava et al., 2022).

Balancing Family Involvement

Health care providers must balance family involvement with the patient's right to privacy and autonomy. For instance, a patient may feel uncomfortable discussing their mental health issues in front of their family. In such cases, the health care provider should respect the patient's wishes and find a way to engage the family that aligns with the patient's comfort level. This might involve having separate discussions with the patient and family or focusing on family.

Cultural Competence and Cultural Humility

Cultural competence involves understanding and addressing the cultural factors that influence patient care. It is a set of congruent behaviors, attitudes, and policies that come together in a system or agency or among professionals to enable effective work in cross-cultural situations. This competence is essential in health care because it ensures that providers can deliver services that are respectful of and responsive to diverse patients' health beliefs, practices, and cultural and linguistic needs (Brown et al., 2016).

Cultural humility extends beyond cultural competence by fostering an ongoing process of self-reflection and personal development regarding one's cultural biases and interactions with patients from diverse backgrounds (Agner, 2020). Unlike cultural competence, which can sometimes imply that there is an endpoint or level of achievement, cultural humility acknowledges that understanding another's culture is a lifelong learning process.

Enhancing Cultural Competence

Training and Education

Continuous learning about different cultures and health care practices is crucial for developing cultural competence. This involves formal education, such as workshops and courses on cultural competence, as well as informal learning opportunities, like reading about different cultures or engaging with diverse communities (Brown et al., 2016). Health care providers should stay informed about the cultural practices and health beliefs of the populations they serve. For instance, understanding traditional healing practices and common dietary restrictions can significantly impact the way care is provided.

BOX 8.1: EXAMPLE OF CULTURALLY APPROPRIATE PATIENT EDUCATION

While there is not one recommended diet for patients with diabetes, the American Diabetes Association (ADA) recommends a low-carbohydrate and low-sugar diet with an emphasis on whole grains and fruits/vegetables (American Diabetes Association Professional Practice Committee, 2024). Diet is often one of the most challenging aspects for patients, as it surrounds all facets of an individual's life and requires daily choices that support a healthier food intake. The patient's culture influences their dietary choices, often deeply rooted in traditions and social norms. Food selection may directly align with cultural and ethical practices, and for patients with a rich cultural heritage, the foods eaten may come from indigenous practices that span decades (Ghosh et al., 2023; Nemec, 2020). Dietary recommendations for diabetes should be tailored around a patient's cultural preferences to increase individualized approaches and adherence to a healthier diet (Osei-Kwasi et al., 2022). Based on a small study, the adherence rate to a diet recommended by the ADA may be as low as 41% (Katsaridis et al., 2020).

Flores-Luevano et al. (2020) implemented a pragmatic, nonrandomized study to evaluate the effectiveness of a self-management diabetes educational program in a real-world setting among Mexican Americans with a high prevalence of type 2 diabetes mellitus (DM) The Diabetes Education and Empowerment Program (DEEP) is a multicultural program designed for the Hispanic and African American population. The DEEP curriculum includes educating the participants on risk factors, complications, physical activity, diet, medication, proper use of the glucometer, and psychosocial consequences of illness and disease processes. Empowerment through partnership with diabetes providers is a crucial attribute of DEEP's goal. After the intervention, HbA1c decreased from 8.92% to 7.82%, and 67% of participants had a lower HbA1c postintervention. The authors reported that culturally tailored diabetes self-management education programs adopted and delivered in primary care could be important in alleviating diabetes disparities among Mexican Americans. Thus, promoting self-care in an integrated and culturally competent program may be the catalyst for improving glycemic control, self-management behaviors, knowledge, and beliefs (Flores-Luevano et al., 2020).

Patient-Centered Approaches

A patient-centered approach involves tailoring care to meet patients' cultural needs and preferences. This can include considering language, beliefs, and values when developing a care plan. For example, providing medical information in the patient's preferred language or being aware of and respecting cultural beliefs about certain treatments or medications can greatly enhance the patient's comfort and trust in their health care provider. It is also important to ask patients about their cultural needs and preferences directly rather than making assumptions based on their appearance or background (Nava et al., 2022).

Practicing Cultural Humility

Health care providers must regularly reflect on their own cultural biases and consider how these biases might affect patient care. This involves examining one's own beliefs and attitudes toward different cultures and being aware of any prejudices or stereotypes that may influence interactions with patients. Reflective practices might include journaling about patient encounters, seeking feedback from colleagues, or participating in peer discussions about cultural competence and humility.

BOX 8.2: EXAMPLE OF AN ACTIVITY TO IMPROVE CULTURAL HUMILITY

An example of an activity that can improve your cultural humility is the "cultural humility journal." This activity involves keeping a dedicated journal in which you regularly reflect on your interactions with patients from diverse cultural backgrounds. Here is how the activity can be structured:

Daily or Weekly Reflection

- Set aside time each day or week to reflect on encounters with patients from different cultural backgrounds.
- Document specific interactions, focusing on moments where cultural differences were evident.

Use guiding questions to structure the reflections:

- What assumptions did I make about the patient's cultural background?
- How did these assumptions affect my behavior and communication?
- Did I encounter any challenges or misunderstandings? How did I address them?
- What did I learn about the patient's cultural values, beliefs, and practices?
- How did I show respect for the patient's cultural background in our interaction?
- What could I have done differently to improve cultural sensitivity and humility?

Action Plan

- After reflecting on each encounter, identify specific actions or changes in behavior to implement in future interactions.
- Set personal goals for learning more about the cultural backgrounds of the patients served.

Here is an Example Entry

Date: [Insert date]

Patient interaction: [Briefly describe the encounter]

Assumptions made: I assumed the patient preferred traditional Western medicine and did not consider their potential preference for holistic treatments.

Challenges faced: The patient seemed hesitant to discuss their health beliefs, leading to a lack of communication.

Learning outcome: I learned the importance of asking open-ended questions about health practices and being open to alternative approaches.

Action plan: In future interactions, I will ask patients about their preferred treatment methods and ensure they feel their cultural practices are respected.

Patient Empowerment

Encouraging patients to share their cultural needs and preferences openly is another essential aspect of practicing cultural humility. This can be achieved by creating a safe and welcoming environment whereby patients feel comfortable discussing their cultural beliefs and practices. Health care providers should actively listen to patients and validate their experiences and perspectives (Haverfield et al., 2020). For example, asking open-ended questions about a patient's cultural background and how it might influence their health care preferences (as in the action item from the journal activity in Box 8.3) can help build trust and facilitate a more personalized approach to care.

BOX 8.3: EXAMPLE OF IMPLEMENTING A CULTURALLY SENSITIVE APPROACH IN PRACTICE

As an APRN, consider a scenario when you are treating a patient from a cultural background that values traditional healing practices. The patient has been using herbal remedies to manage their diabetes and is hesitant to start insulin therapy. Aware of the cultural importance of these practices, you engage the patient in a conversation about their health beliefs and practices. By acknowledging and respecting the patient's use of herbal remedies, you can discuss how these practices might be integrated with conventional medical treatments. You might suggest continuing the use of safe herbal remedies alongside insulin therapy, explaining how both can work together to manage diabetes effectively. This culturally sensitive approach respects the patient's beliefs and encourages adherence to the treatment plan.

Organizational Strategies

Health care organizations can support cultural competence and humility by implementing policies and practices that promote cultural sensitivity. This includes providing regular training for staff, employing a diverse workforce, and offering translation and interpretation services. Organizations can also create advisory councils that include representatives from diverse communities to provide input on health care practices and policies. By fostering an environment that values and respects cultural diversity, health care organizations can improve patient care and outcomes.

Therapeutic Communication for Nurses in Advanced Roles

Therapeutic communication is a foundational skill for APRNs and nurse leaders and is crucial in building trust and fostering collaborative relationships with patients. Effective communication not only helps in understanding patient needs and concerns, but also significantly impacts patient outcomes and satisfaction (Nightingale College, 2022). It is a purposeful form of conversation designed to advance the physical and emotional well-being of a patient. This type of communication involves both verbal and nonverbal methods to ensure that patients feel understood, supported, and empowered in their health care journey (AHRQ, 2020).

Do's and Don'ts of Therapeutic Communication

Do's

- **Active listening**: Fully concentrate, understand, respond, and remember what the patient is saying. Active listening involves paying close attention to the patient's words, tone of voice, and body language. This means making eye contact, nodding in agreement, and occasionally summarizing what the patient has said to ensure understanding.
  - Example: "I hear that managing your treatment options has been particularly challenging for you. Can you tell me more about your concerns and how they impact your daily life?"
- **Empathy**: Show understanding and compassion for the patient's situation. Empathy involves recognizing the patient's feelings and expressing understanding and concern. It helps patients feel seen and heard, which can significantly enhance the therapeutic relationship.
  - Example: "It sounds really tough to make these decisions while managing other aspects of your life. It sounds like this can overwhelming."
- **Clarity**: Communicate clearly and avoid medical jargon. Patients may not understand complex medical terms, so it is important to explain things in a way that is easy to understand. This can prevent misunderstandings and ensure that patients have a clear grasp of their health and treatment options.
  - Example: "Let's go over the different treatment options available for your condition and discuss their benefits and potential side effects."
- **Open-ended questions**: These questions encourage patients to share more detailed information about their health and concerns. Open-ended questions cannot be answered with a simple yes or no, prompting patients to provide more comprehensive responses.
  - Example: "What are some thoughts you have about the treatment options we've discussed?"
- **Reflective statements**: Reflecting back what the patient has said shows that you are listening and helps clarify their feelings and thoughts.
  - Example: "It seems like you're worried about the potential side effects of the medication. Am I understanding that correctly?"
- **Clarification**: Asking for clarification ensures that you understand the patient's concerns correctly and shows the patient that you are engaged and interested in their well-being.
  - Example: "Can you explain what you mean when you say you are hesitant about starting this treatment?"

Don'ts

- **Interrupting**: Avoid cutting off the patient while they are speaking. Interruptions can make patients feel rushed and undervalued, potentially leading to incomplete information and a lack of trust.
- **Judgment**: Refrain from making assumptions or judgments about the patient's experiences. Patients need to feel that they can speak openly without being judged for their choices or experiences.
- **Distractions**: Ensure that the interaction is free from unnecessary distractions. Focus fully on the patient during the interaction to show respect and concern for their issues.

BOX 8.4: DETAILED EXAMPLE OF THERAPEUTIC COMMUNICATION TECHNIQUES

Your patient, Ms. Smith, has been diagnosed with rheumatoid arthritis. She is meeting with you to discuss treatment options. Ms. Smith is hesitant about starting a new medication due to concerns about potential side effects and the impact on her daily life.

- **Active listening**
    - APRN: "Ms. Smith, I understand that you're feeling uncertain about starting the new medication. Can you tell me more about your concerns and what specifically worries you?"
    - Ms. Smith: "Well, I'm worried about the side effects I've read about, especially fatigue. I already struggle to keep up with my daily activities and taking care of my grandchildren."
- **Empathy**
    - APRN: "It sounds like the idea of new side effects is really stressful for you, especially considering how they might affect your daily activities. I can see how that would be a major concern."
- **Open-ended questions**
    - APRN: "What are some specific activities you are worried might be impacted by the medication?"
- **Reflective statements**
    - Ms. Smith: "I'm worried that the medication might make me too tired to take care of my grandchildren or even do my daily chores."
    - APRN: "It seems like your ability to stay active and take care of your grandchildren is very important to you, and you're concerned that the medication might interfere with that."
- **Clarification**
    - APRN: "When you say you're worried about feeling too tired, are there specific past experiences with medications that have made you feel this way?"
- **Empowerment and support**
    - APRN: "Let's look at some options together. There are different types of medications available, and we can discuss their side effects and how they might fit into your lifestyle. What do you think about exploring a medication that has a lower risk of causing fatigue?"

The detailed example in Box 8.4 demonstrates your use of therapeutic communication techniques to understand Ms. Smith's concerns. You provided clear information and worked collaboratively to find a treatment plan that respected her preferences and fit her lifestyle. This approach addressed Ms. Smith's fears and empowered her to make an informed decision about her treatment, ultimately leading to better adherence and satisfaction.

Benefits of Therapeutic Communication

Effective therapeutic communication fosters strong patient relationships characterized by trust, respect, and empathy. This encourages patients to openly share their concerns and actively participate in their care, leading to better health outcomes. Additionally, therapeutic communication enhances patient satisfaction because patients feel valued and understood.

In conclusion, therapeutic communication is vital for all nurses in advanced roles. By adhering to the do's and avoiding the don'ts, you can create a supportive environment that promotes patient engagement and improves health outcomes. Ms. Smith's example demonstrates how using active listening, empathy, open-ended questions, reflective statements, and clarification can help patients feel supported and understood, ultimately leading to better management of their health conditions.

Shared Decision-Making

Shared decision-making (SDM) is a collaborative process that ensures health care decisions align with the patient's preferences and values. It involves both the patient and the health care provider working together to make informed choices. For NPs and nurse leaders, SDM is crucial as it bridges the gap between clinical expertise and patient autonomy, ensuring that care is both evidence based and patient centered. AHRQ (2020) is an excellent resource for more information on SDM, with online training for health care professionals. For APRNs, engaging in SDM means acknowledging the patient as an expert in their own life experiences and preferences, while the APRN contributes their clinical expertise.

For nurse leaders, SDM is crucial in creating protocols and policies that reflect patients' and health care staff's needs and values. It fosters a culture of collaboration and inclusivity, ensuring that all stakeholders are heard and respected. Implementing SDM at an organizational level can lead to more effective and sustainable health care practices.

Factors Influencing SDM

Health Care Provider Factors

- **Communication skills**: The ability to convey information clearly and empathetically is crucial for effective SDM. APRNs must ensure that patients understand their options, the potential benefits, and the risks associated with each choice (Deniz et al., 2021). Effective communication involves both verbal and nonverbal skills. APRNs should use simple, clear language, avoid medical jargon, and employ techniques like active listening and empathy to make patients feel heard and understood.
    - Example: An NP discussing treatment options for hypertension might say, "Let's go over the different medications available. Each has its benefits and potential side effects, and I want to ensure we choose the best option for your lifestyle and health goals."
- **Attitude and beliefs**: APRNs must be open to incorporating patient preferences into care plans. This requires a mind-set that values patient autonomy and respects their values and beliefs. APRNs should be aware of their own biases and ensure they do not overshadow the patient's preferences.
    - Example: If a patient expresses a preference for a holistic approach to managing their chronic pain, the NP should explore integrative therapies alongside conventional treatments rather than dismissing the patient's choice.
- **Clinical knowledge and experience**: APRNs must stay updated with the latest EBPs to provide patients with accurate and relevant information. Their clinical experience also plays a role in understanding the nuances of different treatment options and potential outcomes.
    - Example: An NP advising a patient on managing diabetes might share insights from recent studies and personal clinical experiences to help the patient make an informed decision.

Patient Factors

1. **Health literacy**: Understanding of health information and services is crucial for SDM. Patients with higher health literacy are better equipped to engage in discussions about their care. APRNs should assess the patient's level of health literacy and tailor their communication accordingly (Nutbeam et al., 2018).
    - Example: An NP might use visual aids, simplified language, and teach-back methods to ensure a patient understands the instructions for a new medication regimen.
2. **Experience and preferences**: Patients bring their prior experiences with health care and their individual values to the decision-making process. These experiences can influence their preferences and choices. APRNs need to explore these aspects to understand the patient's perspective fully.
    - Example: A patient with a history of adverse side effects from medications may prefer nonpharmacological treatments. The NP should discuss these experiences and provide alternatives that align with the patient's values.

Steps in SDM

To effectively engage in SDM, NPs and nurse leaders can follow a structured approach presented with an example in Table 8.2.

TABLE 8.2 NP Example of SDM

Step	Description	NP Example Patient: Mr. Johnson Diagnosis: Anxiety
1	First, seek your patient's participation.*	NP: Mr. Johnson, would it be alright with you if we discussed your symptoms and possible treatment options?
2	Define and explaining the problem.	NP: Mr. Johnson, your symptoms are consistent with anxiety, which is a condition that causes your natural fight-or-flight response to turn on in situations when it isn't needed, such as when you're in elevators, new social situations, or getting a blood draw.
3	Evaluate available options.	NP: Let's look at the best available evidence for managing anxiety. There are clinical practice guidelines, evidence-based tool kits, and research studies that can help us decide on the most effective treatment for you.
4	Discuss pros and cons of the options.*	NP: We can use medication, therapy, or a combination of both to manage anxiety. Medications can help reduce symptoms quickly but might have side effects. Therapy can provide long-term coping strategies but might take longer to see results. Let's review these options in more detail.
5	Clarify patient values and preferences.*	NP: What are your preferences for managing your anxiety?
6	Discuss patient's self-efficacy and abilities.	NP: Let's make sure the decisions we make can be implemented effectively. Do you have the time and resources to attend regular therapy sessions? Mr. Johnson: I usually have Wednesdays off from my job, and my health insurance covers in-network providers, so as long as I can go to an in-network provider on Wednesdays, it should be okay. NP: We will work to find a therapist in your network with openings on Wednesdays.
7	Describe health care provider's professional knowledge and recommendations.	NP: The research shows us that therapy is a great option to help manage anxiety. I have had many patients who have been successful in managing their anxiety symptoms with the tools they learned in therapy. That is an excellent treatment option based on your preference to avoid medications.
8	Clarify the patient's understanding.	NP: Please review your plan for anxiety management with me.

(Continued)

TABLE 8.2 *(Continued)*

Step	Description	NP Example Patient: Mr. Johnson Diagnosis: Anxiety
9	Make or defer decision.*	NP: Based on our discussion, we will start with therapy. I'll make an appointment for you with a therapist who has openings on Wednesdays. If therapy alone isn't enough, we can consider adding medication later.
10	Keep the conversation going.*	NP: Let's schedule a follow-up appointment in 6 weeks to review your progress. We'll check how therapy works for you and make any necessary adjustments.

**Components of SHARE (AHRQ, 2020)*

Through this detailed example, the NP uses therapeutic communication techniques to understand Mr. Johnson's concerns, provide clear information, and work collaboratively to find a treatment plan that respects his preferences and fits his lifestyle. This approach addresses Mr. Johnson's fears and empowers him to make an informed decision about his treatment, ultimately leading to better adherence and satisfaction.

Nurse Leader Example

Consider a scenario when a nurse leader, Sarah, implements a new patient care protocol in her department. The protocol involves changing the approach to managing chronic pain, and she wants to ensure that her team and the patients are on board with the new changes. The shared decision-making framework is still an applicable communication framework (see Table 8.3).

TABLE 8.3 Nurse Leader Example

Step	Description	Nurse Leader Conversation
1	Define and explaining the problem.	NL: Team, we are considering a new protocol for managing chronic pain. Our current approach may not be addressing all patient needs effectively. Chronic pain is a complex issue that requires a comprehensive strategy.
2	Evaluate available options.	NL: We can take several approaches, including nonpharmacological interventions like physical therapy, cognitive behavioral therapy, and changes to our medication management practices. Let's review the best available evidence and guidelines for these options.

Step	Description	Nurse Leader Conversation
3	Discuss pros and cons of the options.*	Nurse leader: Nonpharmacological interventions can reduce dependency on medications and provide long-term benefits, but they may require more resources and time. Medication changes might provide quick relief but come with potential side effects. We need to balance these factors.
4	Clarify patient values and preferences.*	Nurse leader: I'd like your thoughts on these options. What have you found to be effective in your practice? What feedback have you received from patients? Team member: Many of our patients have expressed interest in alternative therapies and are concerned about long-term medication use.
5.	Discuss patient's self-efficacy and abilities.	Nurse leader: Do we have the resources and capabilities to implement these nonpharmacological interventions effectively? Are there training or logistical challenges we need to address? Team member: We might need additional training in cognitive behavioral therapy and resources for physical therapy sessions.
6.	Describe health care provider's professional knowledge and recommendations.	Nurse leader: Research supports the integration of nonpharmacological interventions for chronic pain management. Many health care providers have successfully implemented similar protocols with positive outcomes.
7.	Clarify the patient's understanding.	Nurse leader: Let's ensure we are all on the same page. Can someone summarize our plan for implementing the new protocol?
8.	Make or defer decision.*	Nurse leader: Based on our discussion, we will pilot a program that includes more nonpharmacological interventions. I'll arrange for the necessary training and gather the required resources. We will start with a small group of patients and evaluate the outcomes.
9.	Keep the conversation going.*	Let's schedule regular check-ins to review the progress of the new protocol and gather feedback from staff and patients. Our first meeting will be in a month.

In this example, the nurse leader engages her team in SDM, ensuring that the new protocol aligns with staff capabilities and patient preferences. By fostering a collaborative environment, the nurse leader ensures that the changes are more likely to be accepted and successfully implemented, ultimately improving patient care and satisfaction.

WELLNESS IN ACTION: EMBRACING THE BEGINNER'S MIND

I (Julee) made a mistake last week doing something relatively new to me. I had been feeling competent, and with this mistake, I was taking a step backward. I perseverated until a young acquaintance reminded me of the concept of the *beginner's mind*, or "shoshin." It is a foundational element in Zen Buddhism and mindfulness practices. It encourages approaching life with openness, eagerness, and a lack of preconceptions, much like a beginner would. This mind-set allows for greater curiosity and a deeper appreciation of everyday experiences, reminding me that I am a beginner and without discomfort, there is no growth. Benefits of the beginner's mind are (a) enhanced creativity to approach problems with a fresh perspective, which can lead to innovative solutions and creative thinking; (b) letting go of expectations and judgments, which can reduce stress and anxiety; and (c) everyday activities becoming more enjoyable as you learn to appreciate them anew (Suzuki, 2020).

Try one of these options to cultivate a beginner's mind:

- Mindful observation: Take a moment each day to observe something familiar as if you are seeing it for the first time. This could be a flower, a tree, or even your own breath.
- Journaling: Write about your experiences from a beginner's perspective. What new details do you notice? How does this change your perception?
- Learning new skills: Engage in an activity that you are unfamiliar with. Allow yourself to make mistakes and learn without the pressure of expertise.

Incorporating the beginner's mind into your daily routine can transform mundane tasks into opportunities for growth and enjoyment. Embrace the curiosity and openness of a beginner to enrich your life experiences. By fostering a beginner's mind, you can cultivate a sense of wonder and joy in your everyday life, leading to greater overall well-being.

WRAPPING UP

Incorporating the patient perspective in quality care is essential for delivering effective, empathetic, and patient-centered health care. For NPs and nurse leaders, this approach not only enhances the therapeutic relationship but also significantly improves patient outcomes and satisfaction. By prioritizing patient preferences, engaging families, practicing cultural competence and humility, employing therapeutic communication, and facilitating shared decision-making, health care providers can create a more inclusive and responsive health care environment.

Understanding and respecting patient values and preferences are fundamental to patient-centered care. Patient engagement relies on health care providers' ability to listen actively, communicate empathetically, and involve patients in their care decisions. This approach ensures that care plans are tailored to meet each patient's unique needs and expectations, leading to higher satisfaction and better health outcomes. Additionally, involving families in care decisions, when appropriate, can enhance support systems and adherence to treatment plans, especially in culturally sensitive contexts.

Cultural competence and humility are critical in addressing patients' diverse needs. By continuously educating themselves and reflecting on their biases, health care providers can deliver care that respects and integrates cultural differences. This builds trust and promotes equity in health care, ensuring that all patients receive high-quality, respectful care. Therapeutic communication further strengthens this relationship by fostering an environment where patients feel valued and understood, encouraging them to participate actively in their care.

SDM is a cornerstone of patient-centered care, emphasizing collaboration between health care providers and patients. By following a structured approach to SDM, NPs and nurse leaders can ensure that treatment plans are both evidence based and aligned with patient preferences. This collaborative process enhances patient autonomy, improves treatment adherence, and ultimately leads to better health outcomes.

In summary, incorporating the patient perspective in quality care is not just beneficial but necessary for achieving optimal health care outcomes. By embracing these principles, APRNs and nurse leaders can create a health care environment that is effective, efficient, compassionate, and responsive to the needs of all patients. This holistic approach to care fosters a partnership between patients and providers, ensuring that health care delivery is scientifically robust and deeply humane.

REFLECTION QUESTIONS

1. Do you know your cultural IQ or CQ? Go to this website to take a quick assessment: https://commonpurpose.org/resources/free-tools/cq-test. Reflect on the results, and based on what you have learned in this chapter ask yourself if there are opportunities for self-improvement.
2. A 55-year-old patient, John, has been diagnosed with early-stage prostate cancer. There are multiple treatment options available, including active surveillance, surgery, radiation therapy, and hormone therapy. Each option has its own risks, benefits, and potential impact on John's quality of life. John is understandably anxious and uncertain about which treatment to choose. His health care team recommends a shared decision-making approach to help him make an informed choice that aligns with his values and preferences.

    a. What strategies can be employed to elicit and respect John's values, preferences, and concerns regarding his treatment options?
    b. How can the health care team effectively communicate complex medical information to John to help him make an informed decision?

c. What role can a decision aid (e.g., brochures, videos, decision support tools) play in facilitating John's understanding and decision-making process?
d. How can the team balance providing expert recommendations with supporting John's autonomy in choosing his treatment plan?

REFERENCES

Agency for Healthcare Research and Quality. (2020). *The SHARE approach—health literacy and shared decisionmaking: A reference guide for health care providers.* https://www.ahrq.gov/health-literacy/professional-training/shared-decision/tool/resource-4.html

Agner, J. (2020). Moving from cultural competence to cultural humility in occupational therapy: A paradigm shift. *The American Journal of Occupational Therapy, 74*(4). https://doi.org/10.5014/ajot.2020.038067

American Diabetes Association Professional Practice Committee. (2024). 1. Improving care and promoting health in populations: *Standards of care in diabetes—2024. Diabetes Care, 47*(1), S11–S19. https://doi.org/10.2337/dc24-s001

Bodenheimer, T., & Sinsky, C. (2014). From triple to quadruple aim: Care of the patient requires care of the provider. *Annals of Family Medicine, 12*(6), 573–576. https://doi.org/10.1370/afm.1713

Brown, E. A., Bekker, H. L., Davison, S. N., Koffman, J., & Schell, J. O. (2016). Supportive care: communication strategies to improve cultural competence in shared decision making. *Clinical Journal of the American Society of Nephrology, 11*(10), 1902–1908. https://doi.org/10.2215/CJN.13661215

Deniz, S., Akbolat, M., Çimen, M., & Ünal, Ö. (2021). The mediating role of shared decision-making in the effect of the patient-physician relationship on compliance with treatment. *Journal of Patient Experience*, 8. https://doi.org/10.1177/23743735211018066

Flores-Luevano, S., Pacheco, M., Shokar, G. S., Dwivedi, A., & Shokar, N. K. (2020). Impact of a culturally tailored diabetes education and empowerment program in a Mexican American population along the US/Mexico border: A pragmatic study. *Journal of Clinical Medicine Research, 12*(8), 517-529. https://doi.org/10.14740/jocmr4273

Gooberman-Hill, R. (2012). Qualitative approaches to understanding patient preferences. *The Patient: Patient-Centered Outcomes Research*, 5(4), 215–223. https://doi.org/10.2165/11633720-000000000-00000

Haines, K. J., Kelly, P., Fitzgerald, P., Skinner, E. H., & Iwashyna, T. J. (2017). The untapped potential of patient and family engagement in the organization of critical care. *Critical Care Medicine, 45*(5), 899–906. https://doi.org/10.1097/CCM.0000000000002282

Haverfield, M. C., Tierney, A., Schwartz, R., Bass, M. B., Brown-Johnson, C., Zionts, D. L., Safaeinili, N., Fischer, M., Shaw, J. G., Thadaney, S., Piccininni, G., Lorenz, K. A., Asch, S. M., Verghese, A., & Zulman, D. M. (2020). Can patient-provider interpersonal interventions achieve the quadruple aim of healthcare? A systematic review. *Journal of General Internal Medicine, 35*(7), 2107–2117. https://doi.org/10.1007/s11606-019-05525-2

Higgins, T., Larson, E., & Schnall, R. (2017). Unraveling the meaning of patient engagement: A concept analysis. *Patient Education and Counseling, 100*(1), 30–36. https://doi.org/10.1016/j.pec.2016.09.002

Katsaridis, S., Grammatikopoulou, M. G., Gkiouras, K., Tzimos, C., Papageorgiou, S. T., Markaki, A. G., Exiara, T., Goulis, D. G., & Papamitsou, T. (2020). Low reported adherence to the 2019 American Diabetes Association nutrition recommendations among patients with type 2 diabetes mellitus, indicating the need for improved nutrition education and diet care. *Nutrients*, *12*(11), 3516. https://doi.org/10.3390/nu12113516

King, M., Nazareth, I., Lampe, F., Bower, P., Chandler, M., Morou, M., Sibbald, B., & Lai, R. (2005). Impact of participant and physician intervention preferences on randomized trials: a systematic review. *The Journal of the American Medical Association*, *293*(9), 1089–1099. https://doi.org/10.1001/jama.293.9.1089

Llewellyn-Thomas, H. A., & Crump, R. T. (2013). Decision support for patients: values clarification and preference elicitation. *Medical Care Research and Review*, 70(1 Suppl), 50S-79S. https://doi.org/10.1177/1077558712461182

Nava, A., Estrada, L., Gerchow, L., Scott, J., Thompson, R., & Squires, A. (2022). Grouping people by language exacerbates health inequities—The case of Latinx/Hispanic populations in the US. *Research in Nursing & Health*, *45*(2), 142–147. https://doi.org/10.1002/nur.22221

Nemec, K. (2020). Cultural awareness of eating patterns in the health care setting. *Clinical Liver Disease*, *16*(5), 204–207. https://doi.org/10.1002/cld.1019

Nightingale College. (2022). *Are you ready to employ therapeutic communication techniques in your nursing practice?* https://nightingale.edu/blog/therapeutic-communication/

Nutbeam, D., McGill, B., & Premkumar, P. (2018). Improving health literacy in community populations: A review of progress. *Health Promotion International*, *33*(5), 901–911. https://doi.org/10.1093/heapro/dax015

Osei-Kwasi, H., Akparibo, R., Ojwang, A., Asamane, E., Olayanju, A., & Ellahi, B. (2022). Design and implementation of a culturally tailored diet and lifestyle intervention for African and Caribbean people residing in Manchester: Insights from a process evaluation. *Proceedings of the Nutrition Society*, *81*(OCE5). https://doi.org/10.1017/s0029665122002592

Swift, J. K., Callahan, J. L., Cooper, M., & Parkin, S. R. (2018). The impact of accommodating client preference in psychotherapy: A meta-analysis. *Journal of Clinical Psychology*, *74*(11), 1924–1937. https://doi.org/10.1002/jclp.22680

Swift, J. K., Greenberg, R. P., Tompkins, K. A., & Parkin, S. R. (2017). Treatment refusal and premature termination in psychotherapy, pharmacotherapy, and their combination: A meta-analysis of head-to-head comparisons. *Psychotherapy*, *54*(1), 47–57. https://doi.org/10.1037/pst0000104

Suzuki, S. (2020). *Zen mind, beginner's mind* (50th anniv. ed.). Shambhala.

CHAPTER 9

Advanced Quality Improvement Competencies

Staci S. Reynolds

KEY CONCEPTS

QI leadership
SMART goals
Plan-do-study-act
Run charts
Statistical process control charts
Capacity

LEARNING OBJECTIVES

1. Explore the background and definition of QI.
2. Identify the nurse's role as a QI team leader.
3. Discuss how to measure improvements in QI.

Coming together is a beginning, staying together is progress, and working together is success.

—Henry Ford

Introduction

The philosophy that undergirds this chapter is summarized in its corresponding quote by Dr. Donald Berwick, one of the founders of the Institute for Healthcare Improvement (IHI, 2018). Dr. Berwick's words emphasize that QI, or more precisely, the process of improving the quality of care, is the responsibility of everyone on the health care team, from novice to expert. Advanced nurses who understand the importance of QI are committed not only to performing their job (e.g., caring for patients during a shift) but to improving their job through QI initiatives. QI, also known as process improvement (PI), is a framework used to systematically improve care at the local level (National Academies of Sciences, Engineering, and Medicine et al., 2018).

In Chapters 1–3, you were introduced to the concepts of quality and safety and the steps of the EBP process. In this chapter, we provide you with an introduction to QI that covers its background as well as various models, frameworks to guide initiatives, and strategies to successfully measure improvements found during EBPQI initiatives. As a nurse, you may have been members of QI teams or impacted by changes implemented during a QI project. Now, in advanced nursing practice, you will play a larger role; with expertise in a specialty area, you will be able to provide additional knowledge and may be responsible for leading QI initiatives. We hope that as a future nurse leader, you will find the tools and practical information in this chapter useful as you commit to improving and sustaining the quality of patient care.

Defining QI

Within the nursing profession, there are three levels of clinician inquiry: research, EBP, and QI, as we explained in Chapter 1 (Carter et al., 2021; Roe-Prior, 2022; Dunlap et al., 2024). Each of these levels seeks to improve the quality of care provided to patients, but they approach that aim in different ways. Nursing research is inquiry driven and seeks to generate new knowledge using a systematic problem-solving approach and a formal research design (Polit & Beck, 2021); EBP is a systematic problem-solving approach driven by *evidence* (hence the term *evidence*-based practice) which seeks to translate research findings into clinical practice (Melnyk & Fineout-Overholt, 2022); and QI is a data-driven problem-solving approach that seeks to improve workflow processes that are specific to the local area (Provost & Murray, 2022). Additionally, a primary goal of QI is to reduce variation in a process and achieve predictable results so that care is equitable, consistent, and reliable across patients. For example, suppose that you or your nurse practitioner (NP) colleagues write orders for different antibiotics based on your personal preferences. The variations in prescriptions could lead to inconsistent care and result in some patients not receiving optimal, evidence-based care. An antimicrobial stewardship QI initiative could provide structure and guidance for knowing which antibiotic(s) to prescribe based on evidence, thus reducing the variation between NP practice and improving the overall quality of care provided.

Although the three levels of clinical inquiry in nursing are distinct, they can overlap. For example, projects can integrate best evidence from research with EBP to improve local workflow processes (QI). Throughout this textbook, we have referred to this synergy between levels as EBPQI, depicted by the mountain model (Waldrop & Dunlap, 2024). Combining EBP and QI can significantly enhance a project's impact on the quality of patient care (Reynolds & Granger, 2023). Let's consider again the example from the previous paragraph about variation in prescribing antibiotics. Suppose you are an NP who seeks to explore this issue. You might begin by looking in the literature and the Center for Disease Control and Prevention (CDC) website (best *research* evidence), as well as collaborating with your infectious disease colleagues (clinician expertise), while also considering your patient population, and their preferences, to identify best practices for prescribing antibiotics (EBP). Next, you could review the current processes used by NPs in your work setting in prescribing antibiotics (QI). Let's further suppose that you find that the variation in NPs' practices is the result of not having data and information readily available within the electronic health record's (EHR) order panel for antibiotics (e.g., culture results) that provides guidance on what antibiotics would be most effective. As a leader in patient care, you could form a multidisciplinary team, including other nurses in advanced roles, such as a nurse informaticist and clinical nurse specialist (CNS), to develop a clinical decision support tool embedded into the EHR to guide all clinicians in choosing the best antibiotic for individual patients. This project would improve the quality domains of safety, effectiveness, as well as patient centeredness (see Chapter 2). You have now used both EBP and QI (EBPQI) to provide a more effective strategy and improve patient care!

Background of QI

Providing quality care to patients has been an essential principle of care practice since the time of Hippocrates. As we discussed in Chapter 1, clinicians have been working for hundreds of years to improve quality of care. During the Crimean War, Florence Nightingale (1863) notably highlighted improvements in basic sanitation measures that nurses could implement to reduce mortality. Nightingale began with meticulous data collection to identify variation in the processes of care provided to soldiers. When variability in handwashing was reduced and overall compliance with this practice improved, the health outcomes for soldiers improved significantly.

As mentioned in Chapter 2, professional organizations have developed resources to provide clinicians with the knowledge and skills needed to improve the delivery in quality of care. In addition, numerous accreditation and regulatory organizations have enacted guidelines and laws to hold clinicians accountable for implementing knowledge and have authorized penalties for failing to provide evidence-based care.

One international organization that has been a leader in QI is IHI, founded by Berwick. Although IHI (2022) was officially established in 1991, its work began in the late 1980s as part of the National Demonstration Project on Quality Improvement in Health Care. The goal of IHI is to redesign health care in a way that decreases errors, waste, delays, and unnecessary health care costs through use of practical QI methods. IHI has many resources that provide clinicians with the knowledge and skills needed to conduct QI initiatives. (See Chapter 13 for continuing education opportunities through IHI.)

Identifying QI Opportunities

Now that we have reviewed how QI began and why it is important, we can discuss how to conduct QI initiatives in health care settings. As a nursing leader, you will find there is no shortage of opportunities to improve the quality of care; the issue will not be *what* needs improving, but how you *prioritize* the many potential EBPQI initiatives you are faced with. Ideas for identifying a problem were presented in Chapter 2.

Once you have chosen a problem on which you want to focus, you should begin by describing the current status. For this initial phase in the process, strategies and tools such as benchmarking and balanced scorecards are useful. Balanced scorecards are tools that help you and your team visualize how your unit or organization is performing compared to other units or organizations; they are used to identify areas for improvement, communicate strategies for improvement, and track progress toward specific improvement goals. These tools provide data that can serve as a baseline: a quick snapshot of the level of quality being generated by current care processes and the areas in which improvement is needed. Benchmarking involves comparing characteristics of hospitals or units to see how your setting compares with similar settings on quality metrics. Benchmark data routinely comes from external agencies, such as the (a) National Healthcare Safety Network (NHSN; reports health care-associated infections), (b) National Database for Nursing Quality Indicators (NDNQI; measures nurse-sensitive indicators), and (c) The Joint Commission (TJC; provides voluntary evaluation and accreditation for hospitals and health care organizations). See Chapter 2 for further information on these external agencies.

Balanced scorecards are often used to examine internal data and perhaps to benchmark units against their previous performance. For example, a medical/surgical unit's fall rate may be benchmarked against performance in the prior calendar year. Balanced scorecards, or a similar type of unit-based "report card," should be viewed regularly because they typically contain important quality metrics that can help nurse leaders easily determine areas in need of QI.

Most often, your desire to engage in QI will be fueled by data. You may look at benchmarked data or the data on your clinic/unit's balanced scorecard and realize that processes are not as effective or efficient as they could be. You may have a clinical experience of a process that is inefficient or ineffective and resolve to improve it.

BOX 9.1: BALANCED SCORECARD EXAMPLE FOR THE MEDICAL INTENSIVE CARE UNIT (MICU) AT NATIONAL HOSPITAL

This example of a balanced scorecard for an outpatient NP-led heart failure clinic reveals several areas of opportunity for QI. Based on the provided metrics, average patient wait times and overall patient satisfaction are underperforming. As such, you should focus your nursing QI efforts on these areas.

Quality Metric	Target	Current
Influenza immunization	90%	85%
Falls with injury per 1,000 visits	0.07	0.5
Average patient wait time to see a provider in clinic (in minutes)	10 min	38 min
Average days to next available appointment	14	35
Patient satisfaction with access (% top box)	50%	12%
Patient satisfaction with the clinic (% top box)	50%	51%
Percent of clinic no-shows	10%	13%

KEY:

Blue:	Exceeds expectations
Green:	Fully achieves/meets targets
Yellow:	Between prior year's average performance (or similar) and fully achieves
Red:	Below prior year's average performance

Prioritizing QI Projects

Your examination of data from balanced scorecards and benchmarks as well as your clinical practice experiences will likely provide several potential QI initiative ideas. As shown in Box 9.1, our hypothetical clinic has more than one metric that is underperforming. On which metric(s) will you focus? As you decide, you must think through these key questions:

- Is this topic a recurring or chronic issue?
- Is it specific and measurable?
- Does it have an operational or financial impact?
- Does the topic align with the organization's goals?

There are several tools available to help you narrow down your topic list and focus on specific QI initiatives. The first option is a **PICK chart**, which is a Lean Six Sigma tool used to prioritize improvement ideas. It has four quadrants, measured in terms of "payoff" (low or high) and "difficulty" (easy to hard). These quadrants represent four categories into which ideas are sorted: possible idea (low payoff and easy), implement idea (high payoff and easy), challenge idea (high payoff and hard), and kill idea (low payoff and hard). To identify priority topics, team members sort ideas into the most suitable

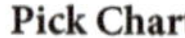
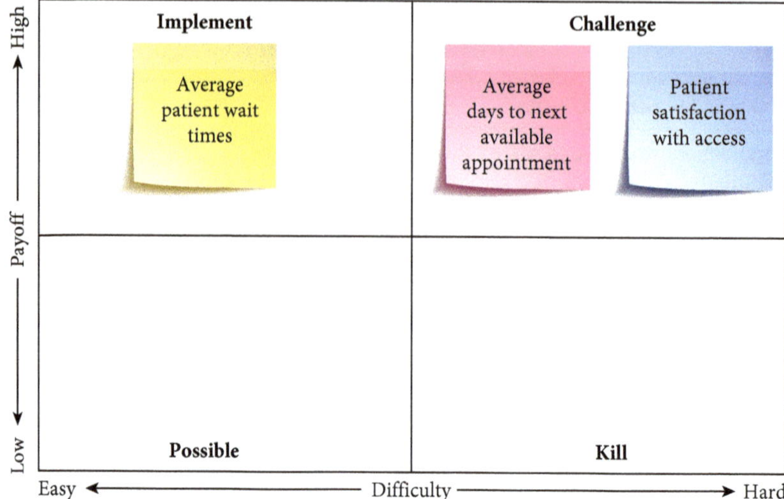

FIGURE 9.1 PICK chart example.

quadrants. The ideas in the kill quadrant should generally not be considered. The ideas in the possible quadrant are not a priority to pursue. The team may consider whether some of the ideas in the challenge quadrant might be worth pursuing in the future, given the high payoff, if the effort can be made easier. The ideas in the implement quadrant, however, are easy to implement and yield a high payoff, so they are likely your best choices. See Figure 9.1 for an example of a PICK chart.

Another option for prioritizing your ideas is the aptly named **prioritization matrix** (Granger, 2008; IHI, 2016). There are numerous templates available online, but you can make your own matrix with criteria that are important to your organization. Solving a problem or achieving an improvement goal can require time, effort, and perhaps funding. A prioritization matrix can help you to calculate which competitive projects are most urgently needed, will be most beneficial or impactful, can be addressed with available resources, and are of greatest interest to your team members. The criteria (ideally developed by your team) could result from your consideration of the key questions we mentioned earlier or from your answers to other questions, such as the following:

- Resources (Are needed resources readily available?)
- Feasibility (Is the opportunity actionable/feasible?)
- Urgency (How soon does this issue need to be addressed?)

You will want to consider and discuss questions such as these with your team to determine your criteria. After you have determined the criteria, devise a useful rating scale (e.g., 1–5, 1–10) and rate each item as a team in terms of its importance to address. Total the scores and make your final selection(s) after a full discussion to ensure consensus within your team. The selections do not necessarily need to be the items with the highest rating, although higher scores often indicate higher priority.

BOX 9.2: PRIORITIZATION MATRIX FOR THE MEDICAL INTENSIVE CARE UNIT AT NATIONAL HOSPITAL

A prioritization matrix can help health care institutions identify priority areas. In the NP-led heart failure clinic at National Hospital, three areas of opportunity were identified. Figure 9.1 provides an example of the prioritization matrix. Each of the criteria was rated by the multidisciplinary team on a scale (1 = *not at all a priority* to 5 = *extremely high priority*). When the scores were added, average patient wait times received the highest score. As such, the leadership team may consider focusing their EBPQI efforts on improving this metric.

	Average Patient Wait Times	Average Days to Next Available Appointment	Patient Satisfaction With Access
Does the topic align with the organization's goals?	5	5	5
Is there a large financial impact?	4	3	2
Is the opportunity actionable? (e.g., areas of opportunity are available)	5	4	3
Are needed resources readily available?	5	1	2
Total:	19	13	12

Writing an Aims Statement

After a QI initiative topic has been identified, your team should develop a SMART aim statement (as discussed in Chapter 4). Clinicians are often excited and want to begin implementing changes and improvements immediately; however, before beginning an EBPQI initiative, it is important to clarify a solid aim that you and the team are attempting to accomplish. A well-written aim statement can be (although it need not be) a formal document, sometimes referred to as a charter (IHI provides a clear template for this to guide you). A clear aim is an effective and valuable way of letting the team, as well as other leaders, know the goals of your project and of defining the timeframe of the initiative. It can aid your selection of team members and help the team avoid unwanted variations from the original purpose, which can waste time and resources. A SMART aim statement is the generally accepted standard for writing aims or goals that are effective, measurable, and useful for focusing team efforts (Bjerke & Renger, 2017).

Let's return to the heart failure clinic example from National Hospital. In Box 9.2, the team prioritized working on average patient wait times as their QI project. Their aim statement may look something like this: "Reduce average patient wait times by 20% in the NP-led heart failure clinic at National Hospital within 6 months." As you develop your aim, take time to consider your wording carefully, work as a team, and be prepared to refocus the aim if necessary. Create a solid aim statement that will contribute to a successful project. Remember that a problem well stated is a problem half solved!

An aim statement is different from a PICO or PPCO question, which is used for discovery of evidence, as described in Chapter 3. An aim statement guides the EBPQI initiative, but PICO or PPCO questions provide a framework to guide the *literature search*. As you will recall, not all elements of the PICO format need be used. A PICO question for the clinic project might look something like this: "Within an outpatient heart failure clinic (P), what evidence-based practices (I) could reduce patient wait times (O)?" A PPCO question might be a better choice in this instance; the first (P) could refer to the general problem of clinic wait times, and the PPCO question might look something like this: "Within an outpatient heart failure clinic (P), what evidence-based practices (C) address patient wait times (O)?" Using these questions, the team would identify search strategies and terms (e.g., outpatient clinic, ambulatory clinic, evidence-based practices, wait times) to guide the literature review. PICO questions do not contain measurable aims and outcomes. An aim statement, on the other hand, should follow the SMART format and include the overall outcome of interest to the team that is measurable (e.g., reducing patient wait times by 20% within 6 months).

Models of Quality Improvement

Once a priority topic has been identified, your QI initiative can begin. There are many different models for improvement in health care. Although they all have the same goal (improve quality of care), each model works to accomplish this goal in a slightly different way. In this chapter, we discuss several QI models commonly used in health systems. You will want to find out what model your health care organization uses so that you can align your project with it. See Table 9.1 for an overview of different QI models.

TABLE 9.1 Overview of Different QI Models

Model	Overview
LEAN	Focuses on efficiency and waste reduction (see Table 9.2 for eight types of waste); LEAN methodology is based on five principles: (a) Define value. (b) Map value stream. (c) Create flow. (d) Establish pull. (e) Pursue perfection. See Box 9.3 for an example of a value stream map (Lawal et al., 2014).

Model	Overview
DMAIC	Define: Define/identify the problem. Measure: Measure a baseline state. Analyze: Analyze the data received in the baseline state. Improve: Implement and evaluate improvements. Control: Put in place sustainability measures (Shankar, 2009).
PDSA	One of the most common QI models available; incorporates iterative plan-do-study-act (PDSA) cycles: Plan: Identify what the team aims to accomplish (this step is similar to the define phase in DMAIC). Do: Implement test(s) of change. Study: Analyze the data to see if the test(s) of change have improved practice. Act: Decide if test(s) of change should be continued, modified, or stopped (IHI, 2018).

TABLE 9.2 Eight Types of Waste Described in the Lean QI Model

Type of Waste	Examples
Defects	Hospital-acquired conditions (falls, infections, pressure injuries); avoidable readmissions
Overproduction	Duplication of laboratory tests, unnecessarily lengthened hospital stays
Waiting	Patients spending time in waiting rooms between provider consultations and blood collection in the lab
Transportation	Transport of patients between various departments; nurses gathering supplies and moving between rooms for one procedure
Inventory	Surplus supplies and medications; stockpiling outdated forms
Motion	Increased walking by hospital staff due to poor building design
Overprocessing	Patients entering repetitive information on multiple forms; nurses inputting repetitive data into multiple areas of the electronic health record
Untapped human potential	Health care personnel not working at the top of their license/scope of practice

Based on the value stream map, the team identifies several areas of opportunity for improvement in the check in process. For example, to *create flow*, the team may decide to have the nurses in the clinic draw the patients' labs or hire a phlebotomist for the heart failure clinic, so patients do not have to go to another clinic.

BOX 9.3: LEAN PROCESS FOR THE CLINIC PROJECT

For the heart failure clinic project to reduce patient wait times, the value (or aim) has been identified. The team can now map the value stream. Let us suppose that they want to map the process from when patients register at the clinic until they are assessed by the NP. Figure 9.2 identifies value added and nonvalue-added steps.

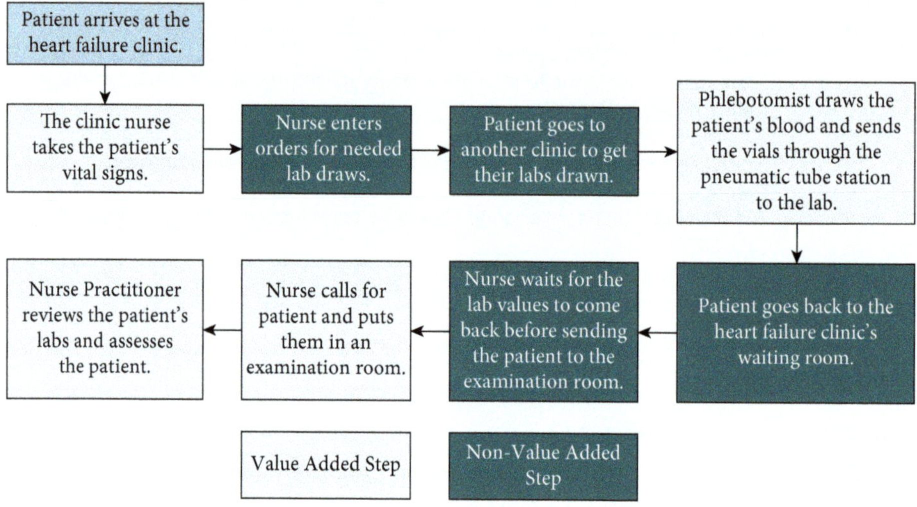

FIGURE 9.2 Value stream map.

Let's suppose that the heart failure clinic project uses the PDSA model for improvement (see Table 9.1). The team's first step (plan) is to identify a goal.

That's easy because the answer to "What are we trying to accomplish?" is the same as the aim statement: "Reduce patient wait times by 20% in the NP-led heart failure clinic at National Hospital within 6 months." The next step is to figure out how the team will know whether a change is an improvement. To do this, the team must identify measures to obtain feedback on whether changes are having a desired impact. Using the rates provided by the hospital's balanced

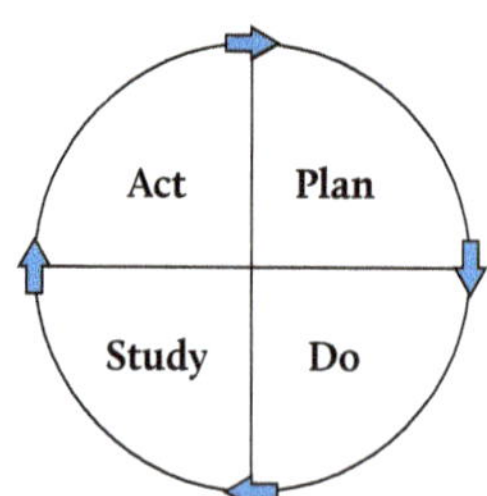

What are you hoping to achieve?
How will you know that what you changed worked?
What practice change can you make that will lead to improvement?

FIGURE 9.3 IHI's model for improvement.

scorecard (Box 9.1), the outcome measure that will determine whether a change has made an improvement will be "average patient wait time to see a provider in clinic (in minutes)." To help the team visualize whether improvements are being made, measures should be displayed on run charts or statistical process control charts to facilitate learning. Unlike simple pre- and postimplementation data, run and statistical process control charts provide feedback on measures throughout the initiative.

The next question in the model for improvement process is "What change can we make that will result in improvement?" Sometimes the answer is obvious, and the team easily identifies interventions that can address the issue successfully. Unfortunately, potential interventions or changes are not always apparent. In such cases, it is not uncommon for teams to resort to ineffective ways of developing change, such as using "more of the same" (e.g., more training, more people) or trying to develop "one perfect fix." Teams can get stuck as they search for an idea or try to understand the problem(s) in the current process. This is why we suggest using known tools and strategies rather than brainstorming.

There are many tools to assist with identifying changes; for example, you could use a fishbone diagram, flowchart, histogram, Pareto chart, or driver diagram. A fishbone diagram, also known as a cause-and-effect diagram, displays possible causes and effects of a problem on a graph, along with the potential factors responsible (e.g., people, the environment, materials, methods, equipment). Figure 9.4 is an example of a fishbone diagram for the example in Box 2.5 of a heparin dosing error in a neonate.

A flowchart, also known as a process map, visually represents the sequences of steps of a process. Laying out a process as it currently operates can help the team identify points at which inefficiencies regularly occur.

Histograms and Pareto charts both allow teams to recognize and analyze patterns that may be hiding in tables. A Pareto chart, which is a type of bar chart,

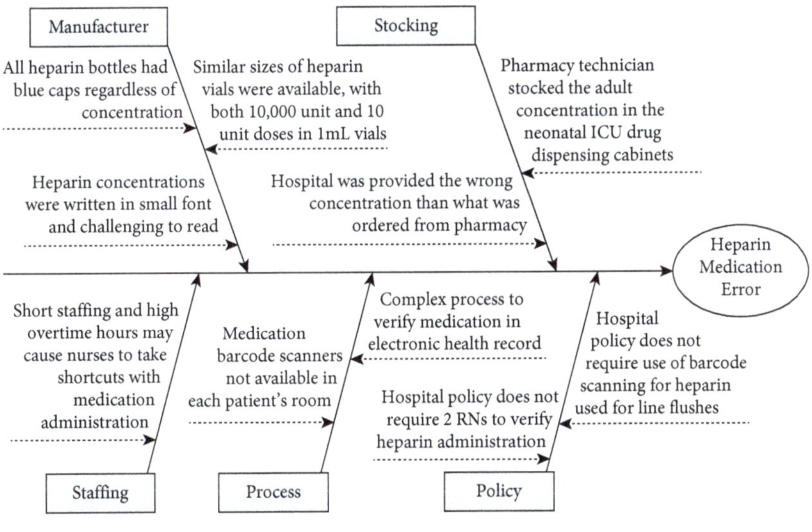

FIGURE 9.4 Fishbone diagram.

displays contributing factors in order (from the largest to the smallest effect), thus allowing viewers to easily identify factors that have the largest effect and warrant the most attention. A Pareto chart is an effective tool that can help your team target their improvement efforts to have the greatest impact (Provost & Murray, 2022). For example, let's say that nurses in the heart failure clinic regularly track patient complaints related to wait times. This data, put into a Pareto chart, can show the clinic leaders the process areas with the most opportunity for improvement (Box 9.4). Additional information on these tools, including examples, can be found in the IHI's QI essentials toolkit (www.ihi.org/resources/tools/quality-improvement-essentials-toolkit).

BOX 9.4: PARETO CHART EXAMPLE FOR THE NP-LED HEART FAILURE PROJECT

A Pareto chart provides a visual display of areas of opportunity. Various data categories are plotted on the *x*-axis, and frequency is plotted on the *y*-axis. The bars are ordered from left to right according to frequency (from highest to lowest). According to the Pareto principle (also known as the 80/20 rule), in any group of factors that contribute to an overall effect, roughly 80% of the effect is attributable to 20% of the causes. The Pareto chart in Table 9.5 provides patient complaints related to wait times. Patients being required to go to another clinic for lab draws have the highest percentage of complaints, which indicates areas of opportunity accounting for about 30% of the issues (orange line, which represents the cumulative percentage). As such, the team may consider focusing their efforts on reducing wait times around lab draws. This also aligns with opportunities noted within the value stream map, showing nonvalue-added activities in the process between patient registration and getting lab draws completed.

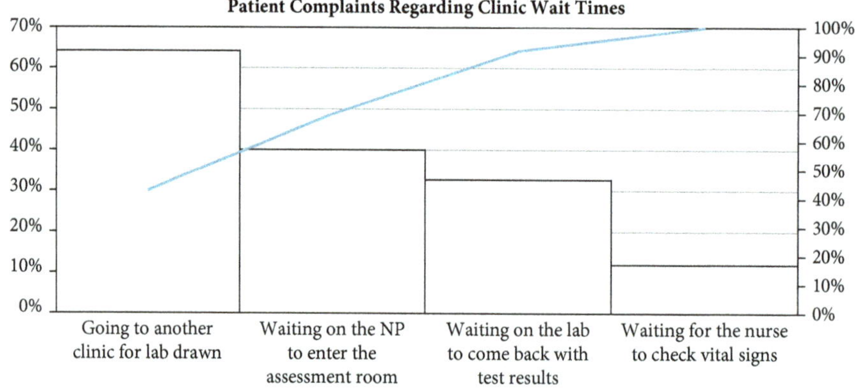

FIGURE 9.5 Patient complaints regarding clinic wait times.

When the first three questions of the model for improvement have been answered, the team can move on to conduct PDSA cycles, which begin with **planning** the changes that will be implemented and tested. During the planning phase, the team ensures that the problem is well defined and that metrics are in place to measure the outcome; these metrics should be directly related to the aim statement.

In the **do** phase, which follows the planning phase, the team implements the test of the change that was identified from question 3. For the heart failure clinic, they decided to first implement a process whereby the NP puts in orders for lab draws the day prior to the patient coming to the clinic. Patients are sent a message via their portal to first go to get their labs drawn prior to registering at the clinic; tweaks to this process can be made by the staff at the clinic on a week-to-week basis. Another test to implement, although one that will take additional time, is to hire a phlebotomist who is dedicated to the heart failure clinic. The lead NP will need to use their advanced nursing competencies to work with the administration to develop a business case for the extra staff member. During this phase, data should be collected, and initial analysis should occur. Beginning data collection and analysis at the start of the change allows the team to see whether the change is making an improvement or if modifications need to be made (in the act phase).

Next, in the **study** phase, the team reviews the impact and outcomes of their test of change. Data are analyzed in more detail to see whether a change or improvement has occurred and, if so, to determine its magnitude. The use of run charts or statistical process control charts can help the team to monitor trends in performance and detect changes in outcomes quickly. In the **act** phase, the final phase, the team determines whether the changes can be implemented as they are or if further modifications are needed to refine the approach. If the change has been successful, the team must develop a long-term monitoring and evaluation plan to sustain the gains. Ongoing monitoring can alert the team if performance begins to deteriorate (which is common after an initial QI project wraps up). If the change has not been successful (i.e., data show no improvements), another approach or test of change should be implemented and another PDSA cycle begun.

Measuring Data for QI

A common QI saying is "What gets measured gets done." Data are used ubiquitously in health care, which is fortunate for nurses because QI in health care requires feedback to show us where to focus our efforts and whether our implemented changes have improved a process. Regular measurement and reporting of data keeps teams focused, as they use this information to make decisions and improve results. Data used for improvement are typically collected by those working within the health care system to observe process performance, obtain ideas for improvement, and test changes to see whether an improvement has been made and is being maintained.

To ensure that data are measured accurately and consistently by members of the health care team, your team should develop operational definitions for each of their metrics. An operational definition is an agreement that a metric will be measured in the same way each time. There should be a definition, agreed on by your team at the beginning of the project, for the following:

- What data will be collected?
- When will this data be collected (e.g., daily, weekly, monthly)?
- How will the data be collected (e.g., from the EHR, through patient surveys)?
- Who will collect this data?
- Where will this data be collected?

Often an operational definition is converted into a checklist or form that delineates what is meant by "appropriate" or "complete" and helps multiple data collectors remain consistent in their use of the operational definition. To ensure consistency, it is helpful to create a checklist form for data collection.

Family of Measures

Now that you have determined how your team will measure data, you must think about developing a family of measures including outcome, process, and balancing measures. Because health care systems are extremely complex, a single measure is inadequate to determine improvement. Multiple measures are necessary to best evaluate the impact of changes to improve a practice or process. Creating a family of measures will help you to answer question 2 of the PDSA model for improvement: "How will we know whether a change is an improvement?" An overall project aim, as described previously, usually includes the main *outcome* measure or what the aim is for the overall project. All improvement activities should include one or more outcome measures.

Continuing with our heart failure clinic example, the outcome measure of interest would be the average patient wait time to see a provider in the clinic (in minutes). However, the project should also include some process and balancing measures. *Process* measures are useful because they are connected to the process of achieving the outcome measure(s) and typically show improvement before the outcome measure does. They provide early indicators of whether the changes being made are improvements. In the Pareto chart in Figure 9.5 the biggest area of opportunity was related to patients needing to go to another clinic for lab draws. Measuring the time between patients being checked in at the heart failure clinic and having their labs drawn may be a good process metric. Completing this process (lab draws) in a timely manner will help improve the outcome (average patient wait times to see a provider in the clinic). *Balancing* measures aid in detecting unintended consequences (e.g., reduction in patient satisfaction). In a QI initiative, you want to ensure that while focusing on improving one aspect, the team does not inadvertently negatively impact another area of care.

Typically, a set of 3-8 measures are recommended for improvement initiatives. Do not include too many measures, especially process measures, because collecting data for too many measures can reduce the time your team has to test changes and make the project's data collection process overwhelming. For each measure, your team should include what they are measuring, the operational definition

TABLE 9.3 Family of Measures for the MICU QI Project

Type of Measure	Measure	Operational Definition	Data Source
Outcome	Average patient wait time to see a provider in clinic (in minutes)	The average number of minutes between when a patient registers at the clinic to the time the NP comes into the examination room	Hospital's balanced scorecard
Process	Time between patients being registered at the heart failure clinic and having their labs draw	The average number of minutes between when a patient registers at the clinic to the time they begin to have their blood drawn by the phlebotomist	Audits conducted by QI team members using a standard audit form
Balancing	Patient satisfaction	The percent of top box overall patient satisfaction	Hospital's balanced scorecard

of the measure, and the data source for the measure. If helpful, the team can consider putting this information in a table to keep it organized, as in Table 9.3.

Run Charts

Once your team has identified a family of measures and operational definitions for each measure, it is time to plot the data on a run chart or control chart. Charts provide a visual display of data that are usually hidden within tables or text. A run chart, also known as a trend chart, is easy to construct and simple to interpret and provides a visual tool that allows the team to learn about the change process. Additionally, run charts can help the team determine whether a change has resulted in improvement and if gains are sustained. Although run charts can be developed on paper, it is most common to use a spreadsheet software program, such as Microsoft Excel (using the line graph feature). Time should be displayed on the *x*-axis (e.g., in weeks, in months); the *y*-axis will display the unit of measurement (e.g., wait time in minutes). The following data points should be plotted on the chart: the metric's data, median, and target. It is helpful to give the graph a title and label the *x*- and *y*-axis appropriately. Plotting data on run charts should begin as soon as you have your first data point; if available, you can plot prior baseline data (Provost & Murray, 2022).

Once PDSA cycles begin, the median should be frozen and extended into the future, which will allow the team to identify improvements. Sometimes improvement is visually obvious; however, when this is not the case, probability-based "rules" for interpreting a run chart can be used to determine "signals" of improvement, or nonrandom evidence of change. Whereas a run chart can be developed from the beginning of the initiative, to use probability-based rules, at least 10 data points should be used to create the median. If one or more rules are identified, this indicates a signal of improvement. The two most common rules are the following:

- **Shift:** Six or more consecutive points, either all above or all below the median; values that fall on the median do not add to or break a shift.
- **Trend:** Five or more consecutive points, all going up or down.

It is important to review the run chart critically to determine whether a signal is an improvement (rather than a variation) and to avoid misinterpretation. For example, an improvement for the heart failure clinic would be if there were five data points all going down, indicating that the average wait times were decreasing. If all five data points were going up, this would indicate that the average wait times were increasing, opposite of the desired direction.

BOX 9.5: RUN CHARTS OF THE FAMILY OF MEASURES FOR THE HEART FAILURE CLINIC PROJECT AFTER PDSA CYCLES BEGAN

After the PDSA cycles began in week 10, the median was frozen and extended into the future (noted with a dashed median line). It is visually obvious that there have been improvements in both average clinic wait times and the time between patients being checked in at the heart failure clinic and having their labs drawn. Signals of improvement were also noted using probability-based rules. After PDSA cycles began, there were six data points below the median for the outcome measure, with eight data points below the median for the process measure, indicating a shift. Additionally, both measures saw a trend, with five or more data points all going down. For the balancing measure, there were relatively no changes, indicating that the tests of change have not impacted the patient's satisfaction with the clinic.

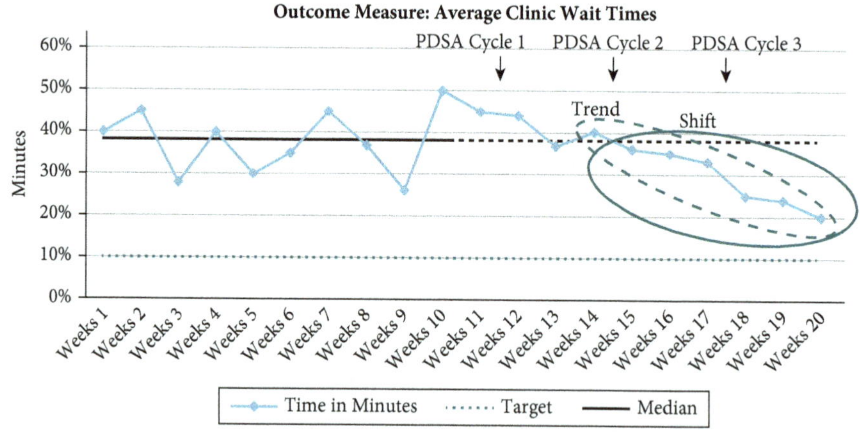

FIGURE 9.6 Outcome measure: Average clinic wait times.

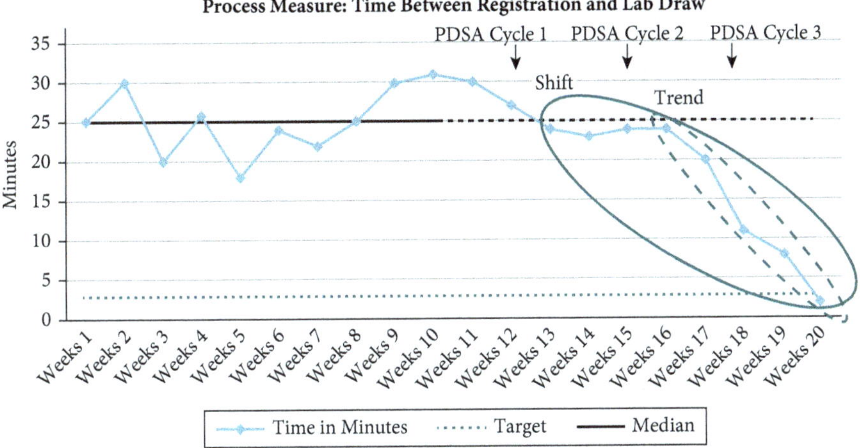

FIGURE 9.7 Process measure: Time between registration and lab draw.

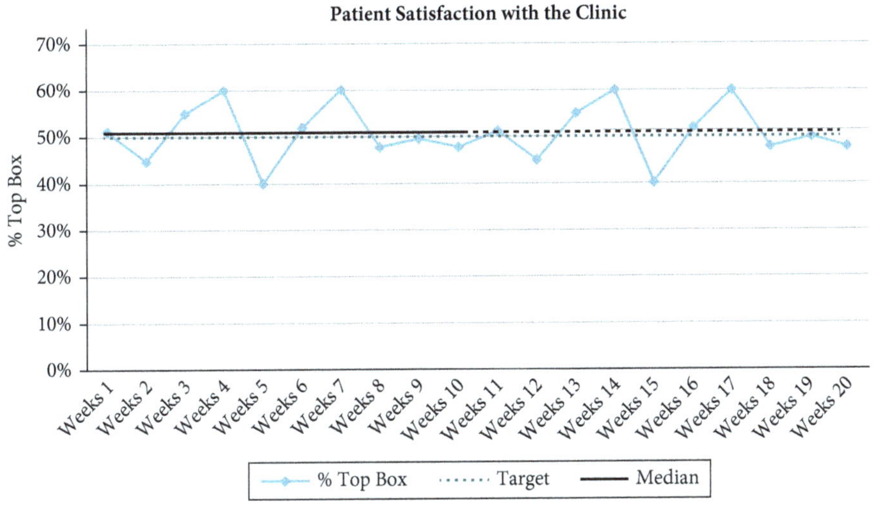

FIGURE 9.8 Balancing measure: Patient satisfaction.

When tests of change result in improvements, it may be useful to create a new, second median for the new data representing improved performance. Some judgment is required to decide whether the improvement has been sustained long enough to warrant a new median. For example, in the process measure run chart, improvement began immediately following the start of the PDSA cycles and was sustained; as such, the team may consider calculating a new median with data from weeks 13 to 20.

Data collection should continue until the gains are sustained; once sustained, the frequency of data collection can be reduced (e.g., from once a week to every other week or every month). It is important to continue data collection long-term and plot the data on the run chart; if the data gets worse, the team will see this and can act quickly to remedy the situation.

Statistical Process Control Charts

A statistical process control chart (also known as a SPC chart, control chart, or Shewhart chart) is another tool that can help teams visualize improvements in their data related to process characteristics. There are common variations present in any process; a control chart is useful because it can identify the source of process variation and process changes over time. In addition to the data line and target, a control chart contains three additional lines: mean, upper control limit (UCL), and lower control limit (LCL). The UCL is calculated by taking the mean *plus* three times the standard deviation; the LCL is calculated by taking the mean *minus* three times the standard deviation (also known as three sigma deviations from the mean). The UCL and LCL help determine whether variation in the data is in "control" (within the two lines) or out of control (outside the two lines), thus allowing the team to monitor the stability and variation within a process and alerting them to problems that might need to be corrected. Similar to "signals of improvement" identified in run charts, a control chart can detect "special causes of variation" (e.g., causes that are uncommon or unpredictable) in the data due to the addition of the UCL and LCL.

Both run charts and control charts are useful and provide valuable data for a QI project, but they have some important differences. Control charts are more rigorous but require more data. A run chart requires at least 10 baseline data points to calculate the median to use probability-based rules, but a control chart requires at least 20 baseline data points to calculate the mean, UCL, and LCL. Teams that do not have 20 baseline data points can use a run chart, but if enough baseline data is available, the team should consider using a control chart. If 20 baseline data points are available and the UCL and LCL have been calculated, the team should lock these limits and extend them into the future; this will help the team judge the process moving forward and identify indicators of special cause variation (Provost & Murray, 2022).

Similar to the rules for interpreting a run chart, there are also rules for appropriately interpreting a control chart. The occurrence of any one rule is an indication of special cause variation. Rules can provide evidence of an improvement to a process or show "losing" gains made previously. These are the most common rules:

- **Shift:** Eight or more data points, all above or below the mean
- **Trend:** Five or more consecutive data points, all increasing or decreasing
- **Out of UCL or LCL:** A single data point is outside of the control limits

BOX 9.6: STATISTICAL PROCESS CONTROL CHARTS FOR THE HEART FAILURE CLINIC PROJECT AFTER PDSA CYCLES BEGAN

Box 9.4 uses control charts rather than run charts to present data similar to that presented in Figure 9.3.

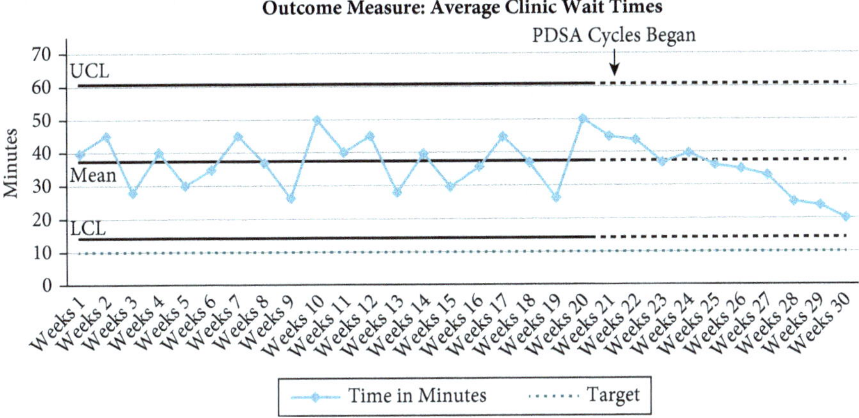

FIGURE 9.9 Outcome measure: Average clinic wait times.

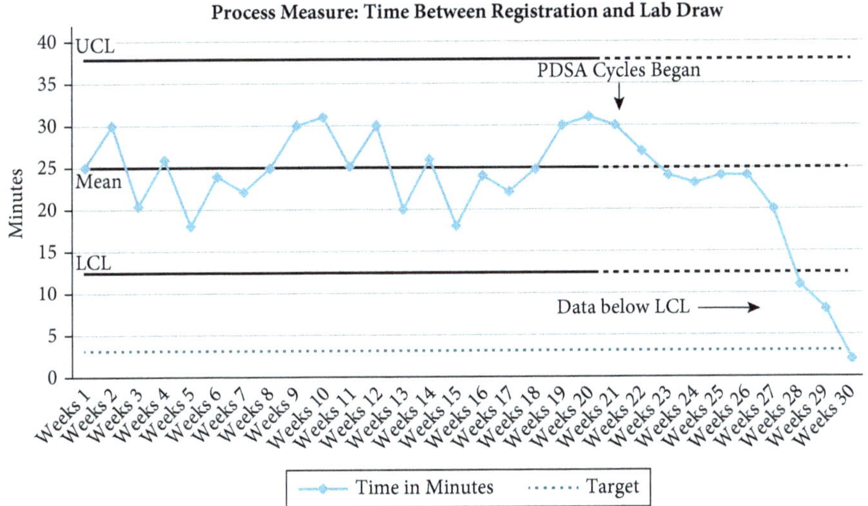

FIGURE 9.10 Process measure: Time between registration and lab draw.

To monitor progress in EBPQI initiatives, it is essential to display the data visually so you can identify when improvements are being made. Whether your team chooses run charts or statistical process control charts, data visualization tools should be used. Once charts are made, information should be continuously fed back to your frontline team (those who are making the change in practice) so that they can view their progress and either celebrate successes or discuss future tests of change.

Capacity and Capability in QI

Capability and capacity are used interchangeably in the literature and mean the same thing. Capability is a prediction of the future performance of a process. Future performance is dependent on the stability of the system and factors associated with that: (a) The measure of interest must be well defined and specified; (b) the process measure must be stable; and (c) any special cause variation should be eliminated before trying to calculate a projection for the future capability of the system. Because of these three reasons, a control chart is important to use prior to doing the capability analysis. However, there are some instances when you may see a run chart used instead, such as if the team decides that the information from control charts is too complex for frontline staff to understand. This is an important consideration as we talk about how leaders perform in systems; if the tools you're using to convey information are above the level of your learners or staff, the message will not be conveyed. Another reason run charts may be used instead of control charts is because of a software restriction; organizations may not have the software or the ability to use software to calculate the control limits on the control chart. Lastly, a run chart may be used if the team decides they need to show a rapid visual example of the improvement as run charts are simple to construct and interpret. If you need to convey a simple message in a short amount of time, a run chart can be used. However, control charts do add benefits with the additional granularity of using control limits. With control charts, you can better view the baseline and much more clearly understand the stability of the system.

To assess capacity, you first need a comprehensive, granular historical market data set. Many organizations rely on trends within their own internal data to extrapolate a forward-looking view of their expected utilization and capacity needs. However, such forecasts are limited in their ability to predict how external market trends and events will impact the organization. As such, a good capacity-planning tool is powered by the following foundational data sets:

- A detailed forecast of the population within the market
- A market-wide data set that provides visibility into utilization and share among all payers and providers at the local market level that can then be augmented with internal data
- A comprehensive inventory of internal and competitive services capacity in the market, both in terms of the number of clinical full-time employees and the number of hospitals and clinics

The second core element of calculating process capability is knowing the definitions and the targets you are striving for. Often we have poor alignment of our target definitions or goals with what our actual future goal state would be. When the goals and definitions are standardized, everyone can clearly communicate across settings what the goals and targets are and align the definitions with these goals.

The third core element is the granularity of the data needed to really assess whether the goals have been achieved. Examples of granular data may include patient demographics (e.g., race, sex, age), disease state, payer/provider, service line/care setting, and ZIP code. Collecting data at this level of granularity across every unit or hospital or clinic is a large investment (both financial and personnel to train your staff to collect and enter data appropriately). When assessing capability, leaders need to weigh the pros and cons with collecting this level of granular data and understand how much detail you need to have to be able to achieve your target.

The next step is to define the measurement target, which is a central aspect to QI. It's important to identify a target, define your operational definitions, and assess a family of measures that all work together to influence the target. Some examples of process capability targets may be customer satisfaction or wait times, provider availability, or cost of delivery. For example, more and more, clinic visits are being scheduled virtually through telehealth; some examples or capability targets for telehealth are these:

- satisfaction with the new process for patients (including using new technology, not having to drive to the hospital, pay to park, etc.)
- satisfaction of the providers and staff
- wait times for a clinic appointment
- increased provider availability and an increased number of encounters
- decreased time for a consultation
- how this would impact the cost of care delivery (or the efficiency)

For our telehealth example, let's say Figure 9.11 shows the baseline data; you can see that the capacity is not meeting the demand; there is much more demand for telehealth visits than there is capacity. If we did a QI project to improve capacity, we may look at all of these measures (in our family of measures) to see how they are affected.

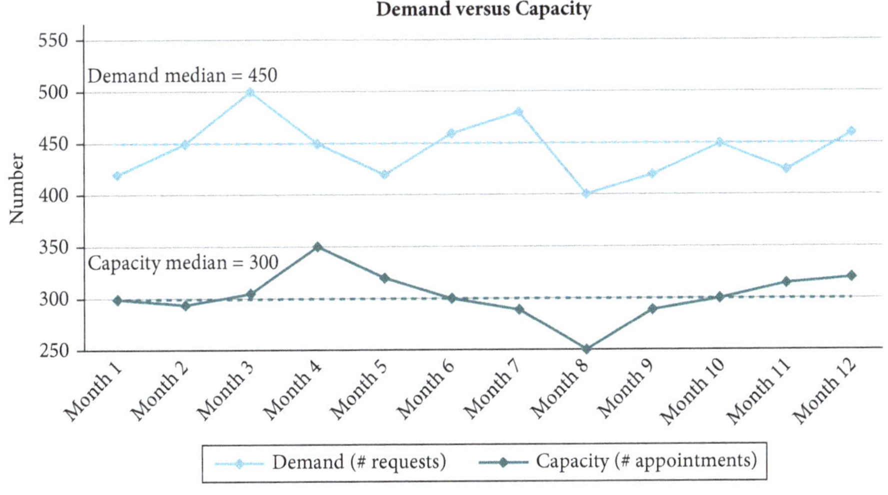

FIGURE 9.11 Run chart of demand versus capacity.

As you are assessing capability, you need to think through contributing factors, including distribution, variation, and stability. These are precursors to being able to predict or determine the predictability of future variation. These are important things to consider as you assess your baseline data before you do a quality improvement project. Next, you could identify barriers to achieving your target using tools previously mentioned in this chapter. For the telehealth example, you may reach out to your colleagues to see what barriers or concerns they have related to using this technology; these barriers can also help shape your family of measures, including outcome, process, and balancing measures. In addition to making sure the capacity of the telehealth visits was optimized (which is your outcome), there are many other metrics to consider as we have discussed, such as patient/provider satisfaction, cost, and time.

Sustainability in QI

During the beginning phases and throughout a QI initiative, there is generally enthusiasm when gains are made; however, once the initial initiative drive is over, it can be easy for staff to fall back into previous patterns of behavior. As such, it is important for QI teams to think about future sustainability measures, even when first beginning to construct a QI initiative.

After PDSA cycles have been instituted and your team has obtained data on outcomes, the team should review whether the initial aim was met. If the aim was not achieved, you and your team should consider continuing your PDSA journey. If gains were made, your team needs to ensure that the improvements will "stick."

There are several key points that QI teams need to consider when they are thinking about sustainability. First, they must stabilize systems that are in place, or, in other words, hardwire them into the culture and workflow. Second, they must avoid the pitfall of person-dependent systems, so if one person leaves the health care system, the sustained gains can be maintained. Whereas it is helpful to have a "project leader," the team needs to ensure that this person is not responsible for all aspects of the project. Lastly, the team should consider long-term monitoring of the process and outcome measures. For our heart failure clinic initiative, this would entail continuously monitoring wait times long-term and plotting the data on either a run chart or statistical process control chart. Plotting the data on a chart will help the team readily identify times when gains are not being sustained (Granger, 2020).

Using additional tools can also help with your sustainability plan; one such tool is the National Health Service (NHS) sustainability model from the United Kingdom (see https://www.england.nhs.uk/improvement-hub/wp-content/uploads/sites/44/2017/11/NHS-Sustainability-Model-2010.pdf) This model delineates 10 factors associated with the likelihood of sustainability after a successful change in clinical practice. The factors are grouped into the domains of process, staff, and organization-related factors. This tool can help identify which factors serve as the strongest levers in the change and could provide the best potential for effective sustainability. Factors within each domain are scored and added, providing an overall sustainability score. Preliminary evidence suggests a score of 55 or higher offers reason for optimism; scores lower than 35 would require significant effort

BOX 9.7: NHS SUSTAINABILITY MODEL EXAMPLE

Using the heart failure clinic example, the QI team, led by an NP, scores each of the factors associated with sustainability. The total score was 65.4, indicating a high likelihood of sustainability.

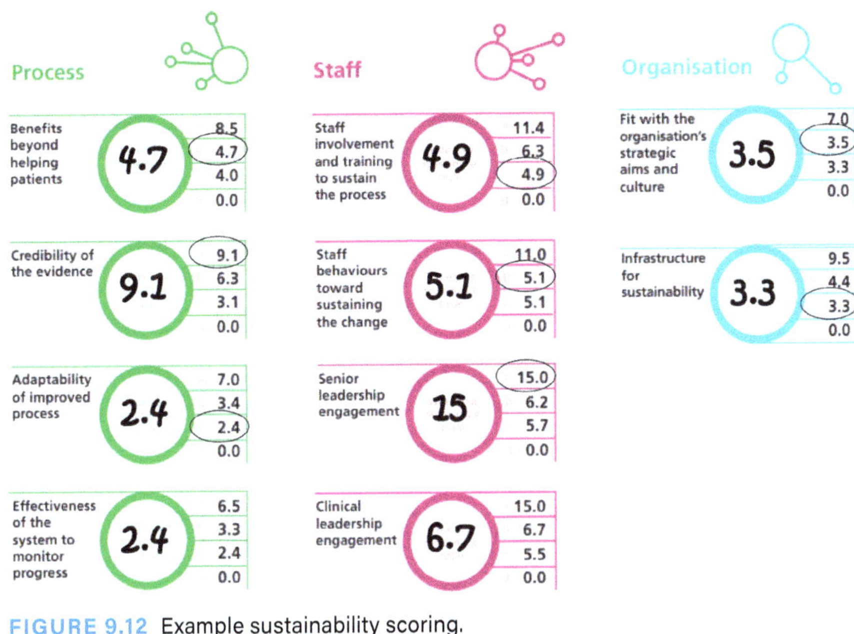

FIGURE 9.12 Example sustainability scoring.

and suggests that you need to take some action to increase the likelihood that your project will be sustainable. Taking these actions early in the improvement process will help ensure success is sustainable in the long-term. See Box 9.7 for an example.

Scale and Spread Change

After a QI initiative, the team must review the results to determine if the change could (or should) be spread to other clinics/units within the health care system. There are three main scenarios that can occur after you review aims from a QI project. First, you may recognize that success has been achieved and your aim has been met. Another option is that the initiative has been unsuccessful. This may be due to a lack of resources or a lack of focus on the QI project (often following an initiative, it's easy to have your focus pulled to another topic). Sometimes, the aim was not achieved due to unanticipated challenges or a creep of the scope. There may be unanticipated challenges in the way that the aim was conceived or the way the plan was put in place or may include losing financial resources, losing personnel, or changes in the patient's scenario. Remember, when looking to spread an initiative, only successful projects should be spread, not those that were unsuccessful or are still a work in progress.

Next, we will discuss leadership and financial aspects that can help to maintain the scope, progress, and spread of successful improvement. First, it's important for the leadership team to understand the changes and the benefits that have been gained. QI is an ongoing valuable tool, but if it's invisible to the leadership team, the value of the tool can be lost. So, it's important that the team continually puts sustained improvements before the leadership team so that the gains are appreciated and the value continues. Another aspect of the leadership and finance team is to ensure that those leaders are committed in an ongoing way to sustaining the change. Reiterating the costs and value of the improvements to these teams may open doors for the business case.

With a supportive leadership team, the next step is to focus on how to spread the improvement to another area; this can involve sharing improvements with other staff, units, or teams at the same hospital site or with teams at other sites. It also means translating the process or approach to other conditions. Teams with experience on the topic and the process of quality improvement are useful in educating and training other teams. Using a similar approach for other conditions usually makes it simpler the second time around, and learnings from the first example can be applied in the second case, and the process may go smoother.

When preparing for spread, teams that are successful are excited and ready to share the work they've done. If the change was relatively easy, the teams may be more willing to adopt and spread the change immediately. Also, the process of spread is highly social; spreading a change across different units and different team members is dependent on a social dynamic. This dynamic can be positively affected by communicating clearly, providing the steps involved, the challenges experienced, and how those challenges were overcome. One group of individuals can be effectively used to convince the other to change. For the spread to be effective, teams must be ready, willing, and able to change; let's discuss each of these further.

First, *readiness* to accept a change is necessary; spread teams must agree that the redesigned system is an improvement. It's helpful for a member of the improvement team to explain the rationale for changes. The team should describe the process of testing and the success that was gained through the improvement project; describing a few failures is often helpful to humanize the process and reassure those who are trying to spread the redesign. Spread teams will be more ready to change if they see a pathway that is reasonable.

Willingness is the second component to change. Once the spread team hears the rationale for the change, they need to assimilate that information within their own context. It cannot be assumed that changes that worked for one team will work for another without modification; sometimes, tweaks should be made to fit particular circumstances or clinical areas. The third component of spreading improvement is *ability.* Once a spread team embraces the change as valuable and worthwhile, they will need time, support from leadership, and resources to make the change. Leadership is instrumental in ensuring the spread team has what it needs to redesign a system and sustain the benefits.

How does spread happen? As with any change process, it is important to have a plan. The spread plan will outline what will happen, who will be involved, as well as the timeframe over which the change will occur. Most often, the spread is monitored with the same metrics that were used with the improvement team. A plan is reassuring to the staff and facilitates the transition effectively; the spread plan contains four main components; see Table 9.4.

TABLE 9.4 Components of an Effective Spread Plan

Step	Component
1	List the changes that are needed for the spread to occur.
2	Evaluate the new system through process mapping and identify key differences in the new clinic/unit as compared to the original clinic/unit where the improvement was made; these will be the areas the spread team will focus on to make changes, much like the original improvement team did with the gap analysis.
3	Make an action plan, including how you will capture information to monitor and what those measures will be.
4	Consider using PDSA cycles when there are associated impacts due to differences between the original improvement clinic/unit and the spread clinic/unit.

Once the spread team is satisfied that the redesign has been adopted, with or without modifications, follow the sustainability steps; this will ensure that the sustained, redesigned system will stick at the new site. How quickly spread can happen depends a lot on the change. Anticipated impacts of the change on the spread team and the culture of the organization all matter when spreading improvement to a new clinical location.

When spreading improvements, teams need to have the necessary materials and the complete documentation of job descriptions (including the key personnel that are involved in the change). It's important throughout the process not to rush the team in either their organization or the startup phase. Also, the team should have the desire to improve systems in this new clinical setting; the change from the previous clinic/unit cannot simply be pasted into a new unit without the real desire and motivation of the team to adopt the change. Lastly, spread teams perpetuate the cycle of continuous quality improvement; however, they cannot do this if they don't own the adoption of the improvement as a need for their own patient population.

Leadership Support

One key ingredient to successful QI initiatives is leadership support. In advanced nursing practice, you will be looked at to provide this needed support, but what does this mean, exactly? To effectively guide quality, patient-centered care, nurse leaders require leadership skills that often take the form of "nonclinical" or "soft" skills, such as effective communication, enthusiasm, emotional intelligence, and interpersonal skills. Using Dale Carnegie's classic book *How to Win Friends and Influence People*, Reynolds (2021) provides practical concepts that nurse leaders can use to provide needed leadership support:

- Begin in a friendly way: Build personal relationships with your staff and colleagues.
- Ask questions instead of giving direct orders: Instead of *telling* staff what they should do to improve practice, seek ways to *ask* and engage them in the process.
- People inherently like ideas they come to on their own better than those that are handed to them: Again, engage others in developing tests of change for a QI initiative rather than using a top-down approach without their input.
- Show respect for their opinions: Even if some solutions identified by staff are not feasible, keep an open dialogue and respect their ideas; these ideas may morph into other feasible tests of change!
- Begin with praise and honest appreciation: Show small tokens of appreciation to team members; this can serve to boost their morale.
- Praise every improvement: This is especially true when beginning a QI initiative! Not every PDSA cycle will result in clinically meaningful changes. Instead of getting frustrated and discouraged, praise even small improvements by staff.
- Give the other person a fine reputation to live up to: People will work with vigor and confidence if they believe they can improve. As a leader, make sure to spread praise among team members rather than take all the credit for yourself.
- Use encouragement to make the fault seem easy to correct: The whole point of PDSA cycles is to continuously improve processes; if one test of change implemented during a PDSA cycle doesn't work, implement a new one! If a fault seems easy to correct, staff will jump at the opportunity to improve. If you allow the flexibility needed in your PDSA cycles, staff will be more flexible and open to trying something new.
- Dramatize your ideas: Staff nurses are inundated with things they "need to do better" based on scorecard results. Simply telling the clinic nurses that wait times need to be reduced because that is a metric underperforming on the balanced scorecard won't cut it. Providing patient stories about the detriments of long wait times and how this influences their day may make the change more important to staff members.
- Finally, throw down a challenge: Often, if we give someone a challenge, they will rise to meet it. This could include some friendly competition with the staff to reduce their wait times with some celebration if they meet the goal.

This is not an exhaustive list of how to provide leadership support. Reflect on previous leaders you have worked with that showed support for various initiatives. What actions did they take? Or, just as important, what actions did they *not* take? As a leader, people will follow your lead. If you don't take the initiative seriously, neither will your colleagues and/or staff. Be sure to positively support initiatives that seek to improve the quality of patient care.

WELLNESS IN ACTION: DANCE

As a leader, have you considered dancing with your team? Dance can be used solo or in groups to celebrate, shake off some stress, or both. Some EBP immersions involve dancing as a way to move and have fun after extended periods of sitting and learning intense content. Dancing has several documented health benefits. It can boost memory and support cognition (Predovan et al., 2019; Verghese et al., 2003); increase mindfulness and enhance life quality (Laird et al. 2021); and improve heart, muscle, and bone health through physical movement such as twisting and turning (CDC, 2023). The next time you feel stress or desire a change in energy level after a mentally taxing experience (maybe that moment is right now and you are ready to celebrate getting to the end of this chapter), consider dancing out your stress/energy. Just find a comfortable place, crank up your favorite song (or playlist), and start moving, solo or with others!

If you enjoy your dance experience, you might schedule a regular dance session into your life plan or just continue to use this wellness activity spontaneously (or maybe both). Dance can be a solo or group activity, so you get to pick your desired place and the people who will join you. The goal is to make you feel better during dancing, after dancing, and as you improve your health. No matter the dancing style you choose, try to make dance a part of your overall wellness routine, and have fun doing it!

WRAPPING UP

This chapter provided an overview of (a) the fundamentals of quality improvement, including a brief history; (b) methods of identifying and prioritizing QI projects; and (c) various QI models and tools used to guide initiatives. Additionally, we discussed how to measure and monitor tests of change that are made to improve care processes and provided tips on how to sustain these gains. As a nurse leader, you will go beyond participating in QI initiatives to being the ones who lead, develop, implement, and evaluate QI initiatives. Don't forget that improving the quality of patient care is the job of everyone on the health care team!

REFLECTION QUESTIONS

1. As a nurse in an advanced role interested in leading an EBPQI initiative, how will you prioritize a topic on which to focus when numerous areas of improvement are needed?
2. Your team is interested in improving efficiency and reducing waste. Which quality improvement models should you discuss using and why?
3. Why is a blending of EBP and QI an optimal approach for your team's improvement initiatives?

REFERENCES

Bjerke, M. B., & Renger, R. (2017). Being smart about writing SMART objectives. *Evaluation and Program Planning, 61*, 125–127. https://doi.org/10.1016/j.evalprogplan.2016.12.009

Carter, E. J., Usseglio, J., Pahlevan-Ibrekic, C., Vose, C., Rivera, R. R., & Larson, E. L. (2021). Differentiating research and quality improvement activities: A scoping review and implications for clinical scholarship. *Journal of Clinical Nursing, 30*(17–18), 2480–2488. https://doi.org/10.1111/jocn.15668

Centers for Disease Control and Prevention. (2021, April 1). *National Healthcare Safety Network*. https://www.cdc.gov/nhsn/index.html

Granger, B. B. (2008). Practical steps for evidence-based practice: Putting one foot in front of the other. *AACN Advanced Critical Care, 19*(3), 314–324.

Granger, B. B. (2020). Six simple steps to sustainability: A checklist for ongoing monitoring of clinical practice improvements. *AACN Advanced Critical Care, 31*(2), 203–209. https://doi.org/10.4037/aacnacc2020667

Institute for Healthcare Improvement. (2016). *Priority matrix: An overlooked gardening tool*. https://www.ihi.org/education/IHIOpenSchool/resources/Pages/AudioandVideo/Priority-Matrix-An-Overlooked-Gardening-Tool.aspx

Institute for Healthcare Improvement. (2018). *How to improve with the model for improvement*. https://www.ihi.org:443/education/IHIOpenSchool/resources/Pages/QI-102-How-to-Improve-with-the-Model-for-Improvement.aspx

Institute for Healthcare Improvement. (2022). *History*. https://www.ihi.org:443/about/Pages/History.aspx

Lawal, A. K., Rotter, T., Kinsman, L., Sari, N., Harrison, L., Jeffery, C., Kutz, M., Khan, M. F., & Flynn, R. (2014). Lean management in health care: Definition, concepts, methodology and effects reported (systematic review protocol). *Systematic Reviews, 3*, 103. https://doi.org/10.1186/2046-4053-3-103

Melnyk, B. M., & Fineout-Overholt, E. (2022). *Evidence-based practice in nursing & healthcare: A guide to best practice*. Lippincott Williams & Wilkins.

Montalvo, I. (2007). The National Database of Nursing Quality Indicators (NDNQI). *OJIN: The Online Journal of Issues in Nursing, 12*(3). https://doi.org/10.3912/OJIN.Vol12No03Man02

National Academies of Sciences, Engineering, and Medicine, Health and Medicine Division, Board on Health Care Services, Board on Global Health, & Committee on Improving the Quality of Health Care Globally. (2018). *Crossing the global quality chasm: Improving health care worldwide*. National Academies Press.

Nightingale, F. (1863). *Notes on hospitals* (3rd ed.). R. a. G. Longman editors.

Provost, L. P., & Murray, S. K. (2011). *The health care data guide: Learning from data for improvement*. Jossey-Bass.

Provost, L. P., & Murray, S. K. (2022). *The health care data guide: Learning from data for improvement* (2nd ed.). Jossey-Bass.

Reynolds, S. S. (2021). How to win friends and influence people—as a nursing leader. *Nurse Leader, 19*(1), 87–89. https://doi.org/10.1016/j.mnl.2020.07.013

Reynolds, S. S., & Granger, B. B. (2023). Implementation science toolkit for clinicians: Improving adoption of evidence in practice. *Dimensions of Critical Care Nursing, 42*(1), 33–41. https://doi.org/10.1097/DCC.0000000000000556

Roe-Prior, P. (2022). Questioning the answers, answering the questions: Evidence-based practice, quality improvement, and research. *Journal for Nurses in Professional Development, 38*(2), 114. https://doi.org/10.1097/NND.0000000000000861

Shankar, R. (2009). *Process improvement using Six Sigma: A DMAIC guide*. Quality Press.
Waldrop, J., & Dunlap, J. J. (2024). The Mountain Model for Evidence-Based Practice Quality Improvement Initiatives. *The American journal of nursing, 124*(5), 32–37. https://doi.org/10.1097/01.NAJ.0001014540.57079.72

IMAGE CREDITS

Fig. 9.1a: Copyright © 2014 Depositphotos/tatus.
Fig. 9.3: Adapted from Gerald J. Langley, et al., *The Improvement Guide: A Practical Approach to Enhancing Organizational Performance*. Copyright © 2009 by Institute for Healthcare Improvement.
Fig. 9.12: Adapted from NHS Institute for Innovation and Improvement, "Sustainability Model," https://www.england.nhs.uk/improvement-hub/wp-content/uploads/sites/44/2017/11/NHS-Sustainability-Model-2010.pdf, p. 22. Copyright © 2010 by NHS Institute for Innovation and Improvement.

CHAPTER 10

Leading EBPQI Initiative Implementation

Julee Briscoe Waldrop and Jayne Jennings Dunlap

KEY CONCEPTS

Implementation
Stakeholders
Adoption
Human subjects protection
Buy-in
Barriers
Facilitators

LEARNING OBJECTIVES

1. Select implementation process for EBPQI initiatives.
2. Review the importance of human subjects protection.
3. Explore purpose statements and multidisciplinary team formation.
4. Discuss integration and sustainability of practice changes.

> Leadership is the capacity to translate a vision into reality.
>
> —Warren Bennis

Introduction

If you have read this far, you likely have identified a health care problem to be addressed by your team. In fact, anyone who has experienced or provided health care has probably noted a problem or issue that merits attention, so it is important that, as a leader, you listen to all who are directly involved with patient care, including interdisciplinary team members, and prioritize improvements that can be accomplished with available resources through translation of the best available evidence in your local setting. Identifying a problem is only the first step toward improvement, however; as a leader, you must be prepared to implement improvement through practice change. Health care is not perfect, so nurse leadership is needed to address problematic issues and improve the system to optimize patient care quality and safety.

It is time to focus on the implementation of your team's EBPQI initiative—that is, the specifics of actually *doing* the initiative for which you have been preparing. As you know, the mountain model framework provides guidance for all EBPQI initiatives and can be used in conjunction with other detailed EBP or QI models during the implementation of practice changes.

The Iowa model revised: evidence-based practice to promote excellence in healthcare (Cullen et al., 2022) is the most frequently used EBP process tool in Magnet facilities (Speroni et al., 2020) and provides a roadmap for addressing all types of health care issues. In this chapter, we will use the Iowa model as a guide within the EBPQI process.

The Trigger

Before we take the next step of your leadership journey, let's quickly review what you've done so far: In Chapter 2, you identified a trigger upon which to act—a key part of your leadership role. You will recall that *trigger* refers to a practice problem or issue that you have identified and want to address.

State the Question or Purpose

In Chapter 4, you learned to use your leadership focus to write various types of questions to guide your team's search for evidence, and you used one of those options (e.g., PPCO) to get your team started. You also learned how to write a purpose statement and SMART aims. As your team begins the implementation process, you must specify the desired outcome of your EBPQI initiative; this will help you communicate successfully, particularly with stakeholders (e.g., those with budgetary oversight in your organization), about the benefits of supporting your initiative.

Determine Organizational Support (and Whether It Is a Priority)

If your organization does not support your initiative or has valid reasons (e.g., insufficient resources, anticipated personnel changes) to delay implementation of your team's recommended practice change, don't give up! Consider asking your

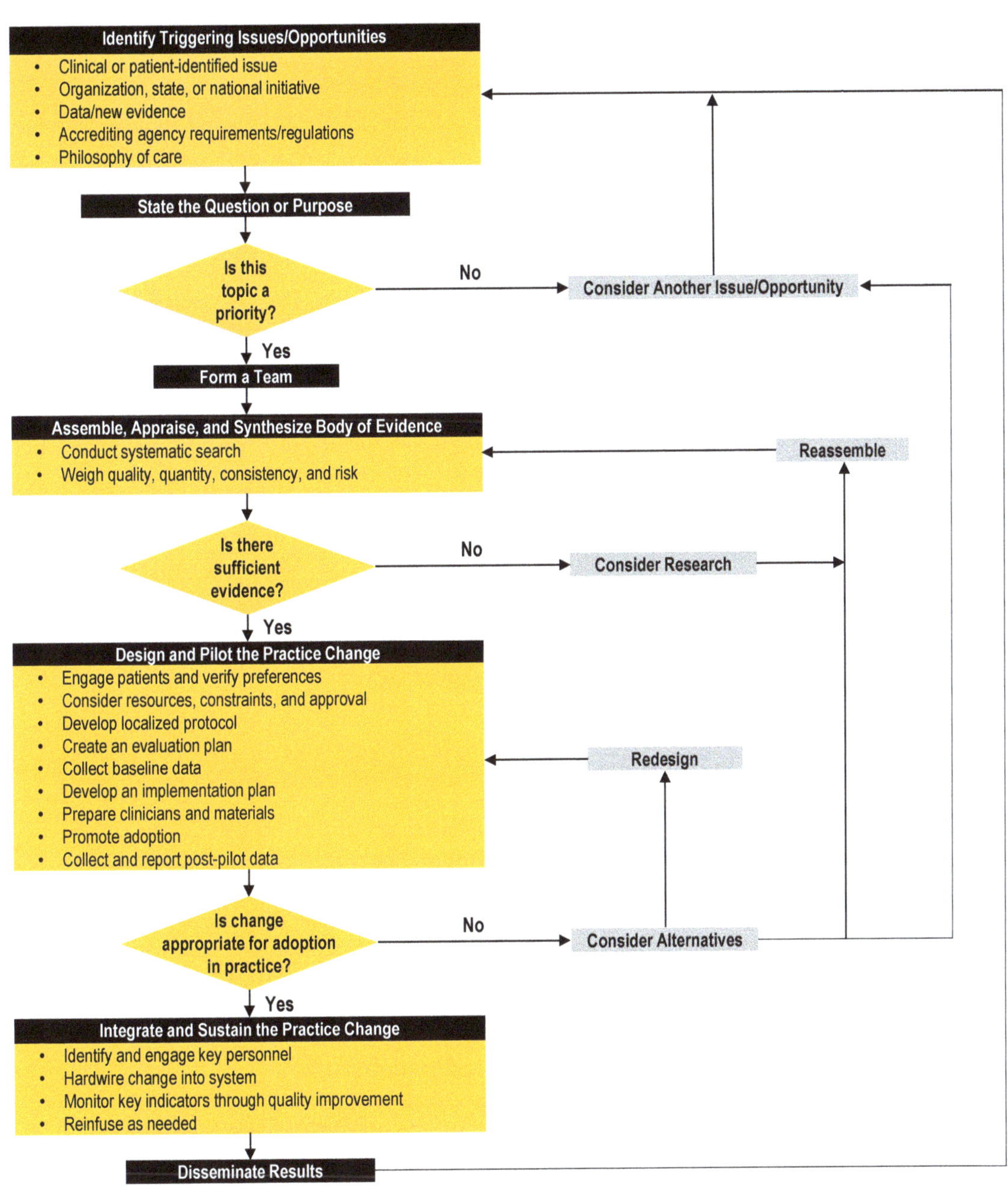

FIGURE 10.1 Updated Iowa model.

leaders to share their concerns or outline issues that they would like addressed before approving implementation. If you agree with their points, consider whether your team can produce acceptable solutions. If organizational solutions are already in the planning stage, you can seek an opportunity to join the team as a leader. Of course, if your organization agrees with your recommended process change, you can pat yourself on the back and move ahead to form a team (if you have not already done so). Otherwise, consider what you have learned from this experience and be on the lookout for the next problem to solve as a nurse leader. Every experience in your nursing leadership career will make you wiser and more prepared as a problem solver and patient advocate.

Form Your Team

Before you form or finalize your team, you must thoughtfully identify any people, environments, processes, or products likely to be affected by the proposed practice change. Determine whether and how behaviors, situations, or settings will be impacted when the innovation is implemented. As you determine who might make the strongest team members, remember that a successful solution considers multiple viewpoints; try not to overlook any persons or roles involved in your solution. Your first official undertaking as a team will be to gather evidence on the problem in general and in your local context; this effort will benefit from your team members' diverse experiences and input.

Conduct a Systematic Search of the Evidence (the Literature)

A systematic search of the evidence is the hallmark of EBP (and thus a primary focus of this book). It forms the foundation of the mountain model (Waldrop & Dunlap, 2024) because research or practice change will be unfounded, and potentially dangerous, without it. However, as you learned in Chapters 5–7, to answer the essential question of whether sufficient evidence exists to change practice, your team must use an evidence-searching question to search the literature, followed by critical appraisal skills to judge the literature. If you determine that the answer to your critical question is no, your team will undoubtedly feel disappointed, but occasional disappointment is expected when working with evidence. Moreover, you will find that identifying a lack of (or gap in) available evidence on a topic often offers a purposeful opportunity to engage in research (at the mountain base) to fill that gap and thus produce a more solid foundation of new knowledge to support problem solving in the future.

Consider Research

You have become familiar with the common characteristics of research studies (e.g., design, sample, measurement tools, statistical analysis of results), and because you care about people's health, most of the research studies you have read likely have included human beings. The most important part of a research study is its participants (sometimes called subjects). Always value them. Ask yourself, "What are their rights?" and "What are the responsibilities of the organizations who fund the research or employ the researchers?" Most importantly, you and your team must determine and commit to doing whatever is needed to ensure your subjects' safety, privacy, and dignity.

As an example, let's suppose that in an RCT, participants with cancer will be randomly assigned to receive either an experimental new drug to treat cancer or the standard treatment. You might find yourself wondering, "What if this new drug works better, yet only some receive it?" or "What if it provides no benefit to participants who could have taken a more beneficial drug instead?" You may even worry, "What if the experimental drug causes harm?" All researchers must consider the potential risks and benefits of the research process and ensure human subject protection, so you may wonder how it is possible to do this and still answer such research questions. Rest assured that you have explicit guidance to follow in this respect! Fortunately, national governing bodies exist that regulate research conducted with humans with the primary purpose of protecting them from harm. Historically, this has not always been the case.

History of Human Subjects Protection

One of the first research disasters occurred in 1929–1930 when a researcher trying to prevent tuberculosis gave newborns the oral bacillus Calmette-Guerin vaccine. Of the infants in the study, 72 died within their first year of life, 135 became ill but recovered, and 44 stayed well and became resistant to further tuberculosis infection. The parents were never informed of the risks of the vaccine. This tragedy led to official guidelines in 1931 on human experimentation, which addressed such issues as therapeutic intent, informed consent, and nonmaleficence; however, these guidelines did not prevent World War II atrocities committed by the Nazi and Japanese regimes on prisoners in concentration camps in the name of research. As a result of the trials for physicians who had participated in unethical and harmful research, the Nuremberg Code (1947) was written with the expectation that it would apply to human experimentation whenever and wherever conducted (Katz, 1996). As the code did not address the needs of children or other special populations, these moral, ethical, and legal concepts informed the World Medical Association's (n.d.) Declaration of Helsinki in 1964, which still guides research practice today. Unfortunately, the declaration's development did not prevent some research ethics violations from occurring (White, 2020).

You may have heard of the 40-year-long "Tuskegee Study of Untreated Syphilis in the Negro Male." Begun in 1932, this infamous study's purpose was to observe the natural course of the infection, if left untreated, over many years. Researchers enrolled Black men (299 with syphilis and 201 without) who were poor and living in rural Alabama. The participants were promised free medical care in return for participation but were given placebos, and when an effective cure (penicillin) became available, they were left uninformed and untreated so that the study could continue. When researchers' conduct was discovered and reported in 1969, their shocking experiment triggered Congress to pass the National Research Service Award Act of 1974 (Pub L No. 93-348), of which Title II created the National Commission for the Protection of Human Subjects of Biomedical and Behavioral Research (CDC, 2022).

Although the commission issued several reports, the Belmont Report (1976) had the largest influence on the conduct of human subjects research (Office of Human Research Protections [OHRP], 2010). This report established what is known as the "common rule" that any activity comprising an element of medical research (i.e., research that tests a theory, as opposed to medical practice, which has a known and expected result) should undergo review for the protection of human subjects). Currently, research with human subjects in the United States is clarified, guided, regulated, and overseen by the OHRP as part of the U.S. Department of Health and Human Services (DHHS). Four ethical principles guide the protection of human subjects in research: respect for persons, beneficence, justice, and nonmaleficence.

The principle of **respect for persons** is grounded in the ethical conviction that (a) individuals should be treated as autonomous agents able to choose to participate (i.e., volunteer) or decline to participate in research, and (b) persons with diminished autonomy (e.g., individuals who are incarcerated or living with developmental disabilities) are entitled to protection (OHRP, 2010).

The principle of **beneficence** refers to the moral obligation to treat participants in an ethical manner, respect their decisions, protect them from harm, and make efforts to secure and maximize possible benefits for them. The benefits and risks of a research study must always be fully explained to potential participants as part of the process of obtaining their "informed consent."

Justice refers to fairness, equity, and appropriateness in distributing the benefits and possible burdens of research. Each eligible participant in research should have an equal opportunity for selection. No person should feel undue coercion or influence to participate in research. Additionally, no person involved should be harmed, either through your actions or inaction; this ethical concept constitutes the principle of **nonmaleficence**.

In 1978, the National Commission for the Protection of Human Subjects completed a companion report stating that institutional review boards (IRBs) were the primary mechanism for ensuring that the rights of human subjects are protected. There are many federal requirements regarding the composition and function of individual IRBs. The DHHS has regularly updated the regulations for the protection of human subjects (45 CFR 46 and 21 CFR 50), most recently in 2019 (OHRP). Many health care institutions conducting research have an IRB charged with protecting humans involved in research at their institution. These boards are composed of local members of the organization and representatives of the public. If your research involves human subjects, you must seek the appropriate IRB approval to determine whether and how you can proceed.

Human Participation in EBPQI Initiatives

EBPQI initiatives often do not meet the criteria of **human subjects research** (HSR). For example, suppose you have strong evidence that can be translated into a practice change, and you decide to use this existing research as an impetus to make a change that could benefit patients, providers, or the organization. The change to your customary practice with patients (or humans in other roles) will generate internal data that determine whether the change resulted in the improvement you intended. However, whether the change in practice might be considered HSR will depend not only on what you measured but on how you measured it; for example, did your actions or their consequences affect or change human behavior?

The Federal Policy for the Protection of Human Subjects, known as the Common Rule (OHRP, 2017), governs the use of human subjects for research by any institution that receives federal funding, and almost all university-associated IRBs abide by its regulations as well. IRBs apply different levels of review and oversight based on the following two critical questions to evaluate (a) whether EBPQI initiatives and other types of research might be HSR and (b) the amount of oversight needed to ensure that humans are protected:

> Question 1: Is the activity a systematic investigation designed to develop or contribute to generalizable knowledge?

If the answer to this question is no (and it generally will be), it will likely be the only question you will need to answer to obtain an IRB determination of NHSR (i.e., not HSR) for your EBPQI initiative. EBPQI initiatives are performed in a systematic way, but their purpose is to solve a problem for your local unit or organization only. The outcomes may be transferable but not generalizable (see Chapter 1 for a review of this concept).

> Question 2: Will you collect any identifiable information from living people?

Identifiable information refers to personal details, such as name, birth date, address, and age. There is generally no reason for you to collect this type of information from the people involved in your EBPQI initiative; if you are not collecting this information, you can answer no to this question. Please note that, historically, there has often been an overemphasis on demographic information in EBPQI, which may not be meaningful to the initiative and could detract from its purpose and aims. Your EBPQI team should exercise thoughtfulness prior to seeking this information and have a rationale ready to justify a decision to collect identifiable information. As outlined in Figure 10.2, the level of oversight for protecting human subjects increases according to the potential for risks to humans or participants.

- NHSR: Does not meet the criteria for HSR
- Exempt or expedited: HSR with no more than minimal risk (beyond that of daily living)

Full Board	- Studies are more than "minimal risk." - Studies are reviewed once a month. - Example: Interventions that involve physical or emotional discomfort & studies with deception of participants.
Expedited Review	- Studies are not greater than "minimal risk." - Studies fit under one of nine categories defined by the federal regulations (45CFR-46). - Example: Studies that collect identifiable information through surveys, interviews, and so on.
Exempt Review	- Studies not greater than "minimal risk." - Studies fit under one of six categories defined by the federal regulations (45CFR-46). - Example: Research with de-identified records & anonymous surveys.
Not Human Subjects Research	- Research that is not generalizable. - Research that does not collect identifiable information or biospecimens from living individuals. - Example: Program reviews & oral histories.

FIGURE 10.2 Levels of human subjects protection.

- Exempt: Exempt from specific regulations and requirements
- Expedited: Must follow specific regulations and requirements (e.g., informed consent)
- Full board review: HSR that involves greater than minimal risk or vulnerable subjects; requires full board review by the IRB

As an ANP leader, you are well trained and positioned to engage in health-related research using your many skills: You have learned how to communicate responsibly and accurately with patients; you can administer protocols for treatments and drugs; and you know how to document your interactions and interventions with patients/participants as well as their responses. In the foreword of this textbook, the contributors each provided a brief story about their decision to enter ANP. Suzy Lockwood's story describes her early interactions with a researcher and how these inspired her to pursue a research-focused doctorate. Can you see yourself in this role?

Let's return to our earlier essential question, "Is there sufficient evidence to change practice?" This time, suppose that the answer is yes. You are now ready to initiate a change in your practice, unit, or organization with your team based on your review of the evidence. Your team will accomplish this by using evidence from the field of implementation science.

Implementation science is the scientific study of methods to promote the systematic uptake of research findings and other evidence-based practices to improve health services and care (Eccles & Mittman, 2006). In other words, by making something easier to do than not do, you make doing it relatively advantageous!

Implementation science is the study of the practices used in implementing practice changes. Results from implementation science research studies describe best practices that you can use to *encourage people/systems to accept or make a change*, and QI describes how you can *support them by facilitating their effort to make a change* (Granger, 2018). This field developed when it became evident that simple linear EBP and QI models were not as effective as had been hoped in improving health and health care.

The study of implementation has demonstrated that implementing change is not usually as linear a process as following a step-by-step model (e.g., IHI PDSA cycles). Systems are dynamic, people are diverse, and cultures may be deeply entrenched and resistant to change. You should be ready for unpredictable factors and adaptable to continued change in your plans (Braithwaite et al., 2018). Adaptability and iterative changes are the hallmarks of effective improvement, and implementation science offers strategies you can use to increase the success of your endeavors because multiple strategies are generally required (Leeman et al., 2021). The Expert Recommendations for Implementing Change project aimed to develop common nomenclature for discrete implementation strategies. This project identified nonthematic clusters and 73 discrete implementation strategies (Kirchner et al., 2020; see Table 10.1).

TABLE 10.1 Implementing Change

Theme	Example Strategies
Use evaluative and iterative strategies	Assess for readiness Identify barriers and facilitators Audit and provide feedback
Provide interactive assistance	Provide clinical supervision Facilitate
Adapt and tailor to content	Promote adaptability Tailor strategies
Develop stakeholder interrelationships	Identify and prepare champions Identify early adopters Recruit, designate, and train for leadership
Train and educate stakeholders	Conduct educational meetings Create a learning collaborative
Support clinicians	Create new clinical teams Revise professional roles
Engage consumers	Prepare patients/consumers to be active participants Intervene with patients/consumers to enhance uptake and adherence
Utilize financial strategies	Fund and contract for the clinical innovation Develop disincentives
Change infrastructure	Change record systems Mandate change

Source: Adapted from Kirchner et al. (2020)

Engage Stakeholders

Once you have articulated your initiative aims (Chapters 3 and 9), you can design and pilot your team's proposed practice change. The first step in this process involves engaging **stakeholders** (persons with related interests or concerns). Stakeholder input should be incorporated early in the design and piloting phases of EBP (Laures & Fowler, 2020), with key involvement from health care end users. Ideally, you will have asked key stakeholders to be on your EBPQI team, perhaps as health care codesigners; this will involve forming equal partnerships among (a) people who work within the system, (b) consumers within the system, and (c) health care change designers (Ward et al., 2018). Incorporating the perspectives of patients, families, and clinicians is vital to achieving effective practice change design (Kildea et al., 2019). Stakeholder engagement is ranked as the most significant facilitator of implementing change in health care; similarly, a lack of stakeholder engagement is the most significant barrier to the successful implementation of change (Alatawi et al., 2020).

You will recall the importance of appraising evidence (covered in Chapters 5, 6, and 7). Now is the time to use your appraisal skills on data specific to your proposed change to identify stakeholders your team should contact regarding your initiative. Special interest groups and advisory boards can provide stakeholder connections. Representation from the impacted population is important because failure to consider patient perspectives reduces the likelihood that practice change will be adopted (Mathieson et al., 2019). There are many ways to engage target individuals, including conversation, focus groups, individual interviews, and patient surveys (Cullen et al., 2022). You can use the stakeholder input you gather to verify local practice change preferences.

Organizational Assessment and Identifying Facilitators and Barriers

You must now engage in real-time critical reflection on the resources you will need, personally and professionally, to ensure that your practice change can be well executed. You should think deeply about potential resources, anticipated barriers to change, and needed approval pathways. Some ANP leaders may abandon the initiative at this point due to multiple constraints or failure to see a clear path forward for change. Throughout this textbook, however, we have exposed you to leadership-focused evidence-in-action strategies for personal application. Lean on those supports as you prepare to fully appraise what your team will need to obtain from your workplace to implement positive change for the patients you serve.

Here are some examples of items and materials specific to your proposed change that you might consider:

- Time: How much time is needed, and over what span? How can you make a solid case for your organization to provide the time needed for the initiative? (Remember that behavior change may take substantial time to realize.)

- Assistance: Who is needed? Remember that no EBPQI effort is completed solo. Does your organization have an EBP or QI department with access to supportive resources? Are training and technical assistance available? Would the research department render aid to an EBPQI initiative? If not, could neighboring organizations provide support? Consider both materials and statistical expertise as supportive resources. Specialized help from a statistician can reduce your workload tremendously.
- Leadership: Regular communication with local (and possibly system) leadership with budgetary oversight facilitates essential resource negotiation. These leaders can help jumpstart and maintain change momentum.
- Approval: Where does initiative approval begin and end within your organization? Follow the organizational policy approval path closely and, as previously warned, do not begin the practice change until the IRB determines that the project designation and permission has been granted.

One way to identify facilitators and barriers is to complete an environmental assessment or scan of factors within and outside of your organization that may impact the practice change. This can be accomplished in several ways. A SWOT (strength, weakness, opportunities, threats) analysis provides a visual map of the existing organizational context to increase awareness of factors that will play into the proposed practice change (see Table 10.2).

TABLE 10.2 Example: EBPQI Initiative to Improve Vaccination Rates

Internal	Strengths ▪ Clinic administration is supportive as they desire to improve this preventative benchmark. ▪ You have a good team dedicated to the initiative. ▪ You can serve as a strong EBP mentor.	Weaknesses ▪ There are some providers who are resistant to any new idea. ▪ The regional manager is worried about the possibility of additional time per patient.
External	Opportunities ▪ If your initiative is successful in the pilot clinic, it might be considered as a practice change across the entire organization. ▪ Once completed, you can work with your team to present the results at a conference or as a publication.	Threats ▪ Staffing shortages have impacted your clinics. ▪ There are several new hires who recently onboarded into the clinics.

A SOAR analysis (strengths, opportunities, aspirations, results) is another method of identifying barriers and facilitators. SWOT describes the organization's current status, but SOAR's advantage is that it focuses more on the future—on what you want to make happen and the results that will, ideally, be achieved. We recommend listing each barrier you identify and creating a proactive path to address it (Table 10.3).

TABLE 10.3 Example: EBPQI Initiative to Improve Vaccination Rates

Current	Strengths • Clinic administration is supportive of the initiative and desires to improve this preventative benchmark. • You have a good team dedicated to the initiative. • You have a strong EBP mentor.	Aspirations • You reach or exceed the national vaccination benchmark. • The team continues to work together to improve other problems. • Your team may become EBP mentors one day.
Future	Opportunities • If your initiative is successful in the pilot clinic, it might be considered as a practice change across the entire organization. • Once completed, you can work with your team to present the results at a conference or as a publication.	Results • A successful EBPQI initiative can increase public health outcomes to meet or exceed the national average for vaccination rates. • Professional development opportunities also increase satisfaction in the workplace. • Both results will help the organization retain employees.

Initiatives have an increased likelihood of failure when implementation is not integrated by all stakeholders (Sibbald et al., 2021), so be sure to create awareness and interest among those who will be involved in your team's EBPQI change. To successfully adopt an EBPQI change, you must identify and engage key personnel in practical ways and build on sustained engagement early and often. Change agents can help your team leverage comparisons between the local practice and EBP to develop meaningful motivation to depart from the status quo. For example, in a clinic-based EBPQI initiative, you will want to continually involve influential health care workers with topical expertise across organizational levels, as well as patients and community leaders to keep the change momentum going. Positive peers with intimate EBPQI involvement can improve learning and provide the team with messages to reduce cultural barriers and make practice change stick.

What is meant by a specific change in practice? A majority of clinical practice recommendations are broadly written and may not fit some specific patient populations or practice settings; this is why EBP change must be adapted to specific patient populations in the local environment as part of the QI process. Develop an organization protocol that addresses practice change; this may include EBPQI procedures and practice statements (see the mountain model). You will use the identified EBPQI recommendations (i.e., the "what" or innovations/interventions/changes) to create a new localized protocol with your stakeholders. As you use evidence to codesign the local practice change protocol, consider the complexities of the recommended change and try to simplify recommendations as appropriate and if feasible to reduce cognitive load (Cullen et al., 2022).

As your team's initiative will incorporate QI principles along with the EBP change, it is important that you use QI tools to further assess change within your environment (many of these tools were presented in Chapter 9). You will need to compile EBP information and package change recommendations within the local practice context.

In Chapter 3, you were provided with two examples for EBPQI initiatives—one on vaccine hesitancy and one on nurse turnover rates. In the example on vaccine hesitancy, you knew that the vaccination rate for primary immunization series completed by 36 months was 60% and well below the national average of 76%. You developed a PPCO question and identified evidence to support a practice change that had been demonstrated to reduce vaccine hesitancy and improve vaccination rates in research and other EBPQI initiatives. You found strong evidence that provider conversations that used motivational interviewing techniques and provided evidence-based information and strong recommendations would be the cornerstone of your practice change (O'Leary et al. 2024). You now decide to use a process map (Figure 10.3), and you identify three separate parts to improving vaccination rates: (a) knowing which patients are not up-to-date (or are behind schedule), (b) the provider conversation, and (c) subsequent vaccination determination and vaccine administration. From this external evidence and the internal evidence on your clinic's vaccinations, your team decided to implement some evidence-based practice changes in your clinic.

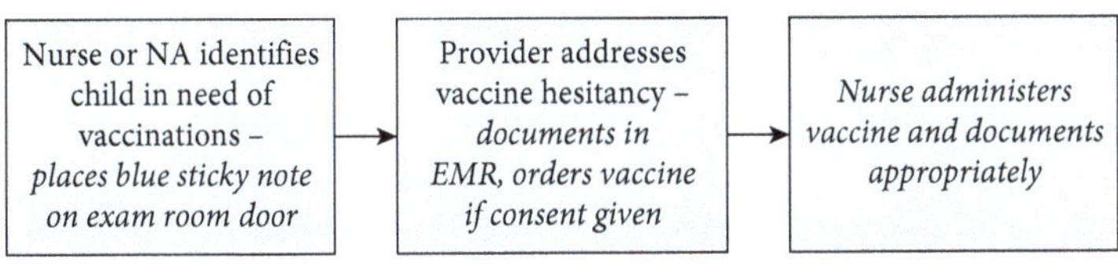

FIGURE 10.3 Vaccination process map.

Vaccination Hesitancy Practice Changes

The primary intervention based on the evidence was for providers to discuss vaccinations and document this in the EMR. For providers to easily know which parents/caregivers to have the conversation with, these patients had to be identified and flagged before the provider entered the exam room. Once a conversation had occurred, the nurse had to follow through with administering the vaccine(s) and documenting this in the EMR and as a charge (O'Leary et al., 2024).

Your team developed the process measure first because, in almost every case, processes must change before outcomes change, and you can usually monitor process change immediately after implementation without waiting to see its impact on outcomes. The SMART process measure you first developed was as follows: In 90% of vaccine-eligible patients, documentation of a discussion will be present at 3 months postpractice change implementation. However, because you had used a process map, you saw that a crucial step had to occur before the provider could have and document the conversation—they needed to easily know who to have that conversation with! You asked your team, therefore, to develop another process measure related to the identification and notification of the provider. Process measure 2 was as follows: 95% of children < 3 years old will be identified, and the notification system will be used (blue sticky note on the door). Your outcome measure (i.e., vaccination rates for children 3 and under will increase by 10% 6 months after implementing the practice change[s]) would show whether your actions had made a difference. To ensure that you were not causing unanticipated issues, your team developed a balancing aim: 90% of providers will report the practice change as feasible to implement. See Table 10.4.

Nurse Turnover

In the nurse turnover clinical example from Chapter 3, you will recall that your hospital's turnover rate was 35%, and the national average was 22%. Your hospital had set a goal of reducing the rate to 25% without increasing salaries. In this example, you focused on adding noneconomic value to employment at your hospital, as this had been shown to be an important factor in nurse retention (Bae, 2023). Your team developed a PPCO question to guide your evidence search. Your evidence synthesis included research and other evidence demonstrating that nurse well-being is associated with lower turnover intent (Bae, 2023; Woodward & Willergorodt, 2022) and that nurses who report feeling valued and supported in maintaining work–life balance have higher job satisfaction (Woodward & Willergorodt, 2022).

System Changes to Decrease Nurse Turnover

Based on the evidence, your team proposes that the hospital partner with the American Nurses Association's (ANA) Health Nurse Healthy Nation (HNHN) initiative, whose goal is to "improve the health of the Nation's 5.2M nurses—one nurse at a time." The HNHN initiative challenges nurses and partner organizations to take action in six areas: physical activity, rest, nutrition, quality of life, safety, and mental health by providing a web-based platform of content and resources. This partnership comes at no cost to the organization and allows all nurses, whether or not they are members of ANA, to participate. Because you know that setting metrics or benchmarks can be motivating, you encourage the organization to join at the champion level. This is the highest engagement level and requires the organization to submit quarterly reports on nurses' progress. But how will your team know whether nurses are engaging in the HNHN program?

Measurable Aims

In order for the HNHN program to be effective, nurses first need to know about it. A member of your team is from human resources, and they propose a kick-off week preceded by disseminating information about the HNHN program. A process aim might be that 50% of all nurses will participate in one of the HNHN opportunities within 6 months of availability. The organization also wants to maintain the workplace climate, so a balancing measure to this effect can also be included. Because you know that making healthy behavior changes is not easy, you also know that this first round of changes will need to be monitored. If there is not much change, data and feedback can lead to continued change until there is a solid move toward improvement.

Do you see how the aims you wrote are relevant to the practice changes your team has included in your bundle? Now is a good time to get specific about "who, what, when, where, and how" each aspect of this bundle will be conducted. See Table 10.5.

TABLE 10.4 Specifics of Practice Change Bundle: Vaccination Hesitancy

What (Practice Change)	Who	When	Where	Why (Evidence Should Provide the Answers)	How (Implementation Strategy)
Providers will be notified of parents/caregivers with whom to have conversations.	Nurse/NA	On work-up admission	In exam room	Although all well visits should include vaccination recommendations, children who are not up-to-date with recommended vaccinations require additional discussion time to address concerns. An individualized plan increases vaccination rate.	Nurse/NA will identify children who are not up-to-date on vaccinations and notify provider by placing a blue sticky note on the exam room door.
Provider will initiate and document a conversation on vaccine hesitancy. Education of staff/family	Provider, nurse	During well-child visit	In exam room (or via phone or video call if telehealth visit)	Evidence has demonstrated that provider concern, willingness to listen to and discuss parent concerns about vaccines, and recommendations to vaccinate lead to increased vaccination.	Provider has discussion, documents in EMR, and orders vaccines (if parent or caregiver consents). Engage consumers, patients, and family as active participants.
Vaccines are administered.	Nurse	Following provider vaccination order	In exam room	Vaccines administered per ACIP/CDC recommendations and organizational policies	No change
Evaluation of compliance with practice changes, outcomes interventions, and outcome.	EBPQI team members	Daily for observation of sticky note compliance Weekly for conversation, documentation, and provider feedback Monthly for vaccination rates, falls rate	Clinic walkthrough Sample of charts Verbal question during huddle Random sample of charts Review of data from billing or other documentation systems for immunizations Quality department	All those involved in the EBPQI initiative want to feel that what they are doing is making a difference. Frequent and regular feedback improves individual and team motivation and willingness to continue with the change.	Evaluative and iterative strategies Audit and feedback

TABLE 10.5 Specifics of Practice Change Bundle: Nurse Turnover

What (Practice Change)	Who	When	Where	Why (Evidence Should Provide the Answers)	How (Implementation Strategy)
Awareness campaign	Human resources will lead but other EBPQI team members will support	Nurses Week	Everywhere nurses work in the organization	A healthier nurse workforce is safer and doesn't change employment.	Multiple communication strategies (posters, email, text, in-person visits to units)
Participation in HNHN	All nurses on EBPQI team All nurses in organization	First week available Continued enrollment	Online	Nurses know what is required to be healthy.	Motivation and accountability
Turnover rates	HR	Monthly	Employment data	Part of routine HR process and main outcome of EBPQI	This data is already routinely collected by HR.
Nurses' answers on organizational climate	HR Other team members encourage completion	Surveys conducted bi-annually	Online	Part of routine HR processes	This data is already routinely collected by HR.

You can begin your team's initiative with a broad timeline and develop a more specific one when you are ready to implement change. Timelines in EBPQI are not written in stone and may need to be adapted depending on how smoothly the initiative implementation progresses.

Clinicians and materials should be thoroughly prepared prior to initiation of the practice change; you can accomplish this preparation through team training and educating stakeholders according to local needs using strategies such as simulations, formal presentations, unit or clinic in-services, required continuing education modules, or lunch-and-learn sessions. We recommend additional preparation including but not limited to the following activities:

- Use evidence-based active learning to engage stakeholders when possible.
- Link the practice change to organizational goals and values.
- Share reliable evidence with practice recommendations early and often.
- Select change champions to lead locally.
- Ensure that any needed supplies are accessible where locally needed.
- Make supportive resource materials available, including pocket guides, checklists, algorithms.
- De-implement materials that are unneeded or no longer in use (Cullen et al., 2022).

De-implementation describes the "stopping" of practices that are no longer "best" or representative of the "standard of care." There are frameworks and models to guide you in the de-implementation process (Walsh-Bailey et al., 2021). De-implementing old practices in order to implement new best practices and gold standards is essential but not always easy, particularly when nurses and other health care personnel have been engaging in practices that need to be stopped for a long time. Your evidence search might even lead your team to de-implement a practice as your practice improvement! (Leeman et al., 2021). As a leader, remember to let the evidence guide your team's determination of practices, or elements of practice, that should be de-implemented and unlearned in order to update practice policy, procedures, and workflow. When electronic resources are available at the bedside, chairside, or tableside, we recommend digitally embedding reminders to increase frontline adoption with end users. You should complete these steps prior to your scheduled pilot start date.

The Iowa model and the model of change emphasize the importance of pilot testing before implementing practice change and encourage nurses to consider organizational context prior to the pilot (Cullen et al., 2022; Langley et al., 2009). For example, in the practice change to improve immunization rates, you might start with one provider-nurse team, to determine if your process for identifying patients, notifying the provider and conducting the conversation is feasible or needs adjusting before rolling it out with the whole clinic. After this weeklong pilot, let's suppose that the feedback reveals the provider is forgetting to have the conversation once they enter the room even though they noticed the sticky note on the door. Your team brainstorms ways to improve this part of the process. One of the nurses suggests that the provider remove the sticky note from the door as they enter the room, and restick it on the computer as a continued reminder. Your team changes the "how" component of this part of the process, the change is communicated to all involved, and the pilot proceeds accordingly.

Despite detailed planning, unexpected issues are likely to arise because that is simply the nature of working with people and organizations! We are confident that, by this point, you understand that your team's localized EBPQI change must be tailored appropriately to the needs of your local setting and patient population. As the practice change implementation progresses, engage the team in troubleshooting problems as they appear and develop responses/modifications/adaptations as indicated (Cullen et al., 2022).

Once the pilot is stable, it is time to include the rest of the clinic/unit in the practice change bundle. How you evaluate the clinic/unit-wide implementation will be based on your team's aims. The EBPQI team members will be responsible for collecting data on compliance with the bundle as well as on the vaccination rate and communicating it with all who need or want to know (as per Table 10.4.). We will move on to the evaluation component of EBPQI in the next chapter.

WRAPPING UP

You have now been introduced to the basics of leading the implementation of an EBPQI initiative: Let the evidence guide your team's best-practice decision, proceed through your organizational process, and obtain approval from leadership.

Be sure to lead implementation of your practice change thoughtfully by providing team members with timely, evidence-based guidance throughout the duration of your EBPQI initiative. Remember that implementing an EBPQI initiative is a team-based activity for which your skills as an ANP leader are critical.

Persistence and curiosity are key features of successful leader and team engagement in the practice change process. Should you encounter barriers to implementing your team's change, discuss and address them with your team and upper level leadership in a timely manner. Implementation and sustainability require continuous monitoring, so you will learn how to evaluate and set up regular monitoring of your team's practice change in the next chapter.

You've come a long way on your nurse leadership journey! Let's pause here to relax and think about one of our favorite ways to reduce stress—inhaling a pleasant aroma.

WELLNESS IN ACTION: INHALED AROMATHERAPY

Exposure to some fragrances can increase endorphin levels in the body and promote relaxation and feelings of happiness (Sánchez-Vidaña et al., 2017). Positive olfactory engagement may also increase comfort and productivity. We (Julee and Jayne) often gift one another candles, as we have found that soft light and pleasant fragrances positively impact us both. Pictured to the right is the first scented candle we chose for each other to use while writing our prelicensure EBPQI textbook in our home workspaces. Watching our candles burn down, enjoying a pleasant aroma in a relaxing atmosphere, served as a reminder of the time we were spending as we shared important work. If you prefer to avoid a flame, consider trying a battery-powered candle or a nonburning scent-generating device. We encourage you to explore candles or other aromatherapy devices. Choose a scent that invokes pleasant feelings, gift yourself a little aromatherapy, then note how you feel. If you find it soothing or helpful, consider incorporating aromatherapy into your routine.

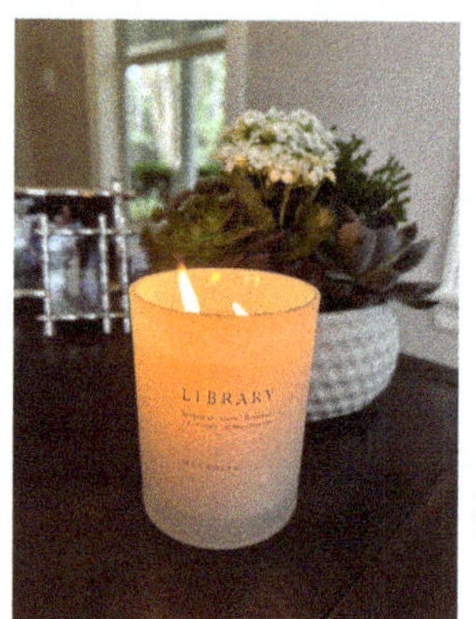

Image 10.1

REFLECTION QUESTIONS

1. What areas of strength and vulnerability related to a future EBPQI initiative of interest did you identify?
2. What strategies could you use to overcome a potential barrier to your best practice change?
3. What leadership steps would you need to take as your team designs a potential practice change for pilot purposes?

REFERENCES

Alatawi, M., Aljuhani, E., Alsufiany, F., Aleid, K., Rawah, R., Aljanabi, S., & Banakhar, M. (2020). Barriers of Implementing Evidence-Based Practice in Nursing Profession: A Literature review. *American Journal of Nursing Science, 9*(1), 35. https://doi.org/10.11648/j.ajns.20200901.16

Bae, S-H. (2023). Comprehensive assessment of factors contributing to the actual turnover of newly licensed registered nurses working in acute care hospitals: A systematic review. *BMC Nursing, 22*, 31. https://doi.org/10.1186/s12912-023-01190-3

Braithwaite, J., Churruca, K., Long, J. C., Ellis, L. A., & Herkes, J. (2018). When complexity science meets implementation science: A theoretical and empirical analysis of systems change. *BMC Medicine, 16*(1), 63. https://doi.org/10.1186/s12916-018-1057-z

Centers for Disease Control (2022, December) *Tuskegee Study—timeline.* https://www.cdc.gov/tuskegee/about/timeline.html

Cullen, L., Hanrahan, K., Farrington, M., Tucker, S., & Edmonds, S. (2022). *Evidence-based practice in action*. Sigma Theta Tau International.

Dunlap, J., Waldrop, J. Brewer, T. & Mainous, R. (2024). Differentiation and Integration of research, evidence-based practice, and quality improvement. *Journal of Nursing Education.* Published ahead of Print. https://doi.org/10.3928/01484834-20240514-01

Eccles, M. P., & Mittman, B. S. (2006). Welcome to *Implementation Science. Implementation Science, 1*(1), 1. https://doi.org/10.1186/1748-5908-1-1

Granger B. B. (2018). Science of improvement versus science of implementation: Integrating both into clinical inquiry. *AACN Adv Crit Care, 29*(2), 208–212. https://doi.org/10.4037/aacnacc2018757

Institute for Healthcare Improvement. (n.d.). *Quality improvement essentials toolkit*. https://www.ihi.org/resources/Pages/Tools/Quality-Improvement-Essentials-Toolkit.aspx

Journal, Y., & McCall, T. (2007). *Yoga as medicine: The yogic prescription for health and healing* (no-value ed.). Bantam.

Katz, J. (1996). The Nuremberg Code and the Nuremberg Trial: A reappraisal. *JAMA, 276*(20), 1662–1666. https://doi.org/10.1001/jama.1996.03540200048030

Kildea, J., Battista, J., Cabral, B., Hendren, L., Herrera, D., Hijal, T., & Joseph, A. (2019). Design and development of a person-centered patient portal using participatory stakeholder co-design. *Journal of Medical Internet Research, 21*(2), e11371. https://doi.org/10.2196/11371

Kirchner, J. E., Smith, J. L., Powell, B. J., Waltz, T. J., & Proctor, E. K. (2020). Getting a clinical innovation into practice: An introduction to implementation strategies. *Psychiatry Research, 283*, 112467. https://doi.org/10.1016/j.psychres.2019.06.042

Langley, G. J., Moen, R. D., Nolan, K. M., Nolan, T. W., Norman, C. L., & Provost, L. P. (2009). *The improvement guide: A practical approach to enhancing organizational performance* (2nd ed.). Jossey-Bass.

Laures, E., & Fowler, C. (2020). The power of the pilot. *Journal of PeriAnesthesia Nursing, 35*(5), 543–547. https://doi.org/10.1016/j.jopan.2020.02.009

Leeman, J., Rohweder, C., Lee, M., Brenner, A., Dwyer, A., Ko, L. K., O'Leary, M. C., Ryan, G., Vu, T., & Ramanadhan, S. (2021). Aligning implementation science with improvement practice: A call to action. *Implementation Science Communications, 2*(1), 99. https://doi.org/10.1186/s43058-021-00201-1

Mathieson, A., Grande, G., & Luker, K. (2019). Strategies, facilitators and barriers to implementation of evidence-based practice in community nursing: A systematic mixed-studies review and qualitative synthesis. *Primary Health Care Research & Development, 20*, e6. https://doi.org/10.1017/S1463423618000488

Office of Human Research Protections. (2010, January 28). *The Belmont report*. https://www.hhs.gov/ohrp/regulations-and-policy/belmont-report/index.html

Office of Human Research Protections. (2016, February 16). *45 CFR 46*. https://www.hhs.gov/ohrp/regulations-and-policy/regulations/45-cfr-46/index.html

Office of Human Research Protections. (2017, October 11). *What regulations protect research participants?* https://www.hhs.gov/ohrp/education-and-outreach/about-research-participation/protecting-research-volunteers/principal-regulations/index.html

O'Leary, S. T., Opel, D. J., Cataldi, J. R., & Hackell, J. M. Committee on Infectious Diseases, Committee on Practice and Ambulatory Medicine, Committee on Bioethics. (2024). Strategies for improving vaccine communication and uptake. *Pediatrics, 153*(3), e2023065483. https://doi.org/10.1542/peds.2023-065483

Sánchez-Vidaña, D. I., Ngai, S. P., He, W., Chow, J. K., Lau, B. W., & Tsang, H. W. (2017). The effectiveness of aromatherapy for depressive symptoms: A systematic review. *Evidence-Based Complementary and Alternative Medicine, 2017*, 5869315. https://doi.org/10.1155/2017/5869315

Satchidananda, S. S. (2012). *The yoga sutras of Patanjali* (revised ed.). Integral Yoga Publications.

Sibbald, S. L., Van Asseldonk, R., Cao, P. L., & Law, B. (2021). Lessons learned from inadequate implementation planning of team-based chronic disease management: Implementation evaluation. *BMC Health Services Research, 21*(1), 134. https://doi.org/10.1186/s12913-021-06100-4

Waldrop, J., & Dunlap, J. J. (2024). The mountain model for evidence-based practice quality improvement initiatives. *Am J Nurs., 124*(5), 32–37. https://doi.org/10.1097/01.NAJ.0001014540.57079.72

Walsh-Bailey, C., Tsai, E., Tabak, R. G., Morshed, A. B., Norton, W. E., McKay, V. R., Brownson, R. C., & Gifford, S. (2021). A scoping review of de-implementation frameworks and models. *Implementation Science, 16*(1), 100. https://doi.org/10.1186/s13012-021-01173-5

Ward, M. E., De Brún, A., Beirne, D., Conway, C., Cunningham, U., English, A., Fitzsimons, J., Furlong, E., Kane, Y., Kelly, A., McDonnell, S., McGinley, S., Monaghan, B., Myler, A., Nolan, E., O'Donovan, R., O'Shea, M., Shuhaiber, A., & McAuliffe, E. (2018). Using co-design to develop a collective leadership intervention for healthcare teams to improve safety culture. *International Journal of Environmental Research and Public Health, 15*(6), 1182. https://doi.org/10.3390/ijerph15061182

White, M. G. (2020). Why human subjects research protection is important. *The Ochsner Journal, 20*(1), 16–33. https://doi.org/10.31486/toj.20.5012

Woodward, K. F., & Willgerodt, M. (2022, July/August). A systematic review of registered nurse turnover and retention in the United States. *Nurs Outlook, 70*(4). https://doi.org/10.1016/j.outlook.2022.04.005

World Medical Association. (n.d.). *WMA Declaration of Helsinki—Ethical principles for medical research involving human subjects*. https://www.wma.net/policies-post/wma-declaration-of-helsinki-ethical-principles-for-medical-research-involving-human-subjects/

IMAGE CREDITS

Fig. 10.1: Jayne Jennings Dunlap and Julee Briscoe Waldrop, *Introduction to Evidence-Based Practice and Quality Improvement for Professional Nursing Practice: A Competency Based Approach*, p. 180. Copyright © 2024 by Cognella, Inc. Reprinted with permission.

Fig. 10.2: University of Iowa Hospitals & Clinics, "Updated Iowa Model," https://uiowa.qualtrics.com/CP/File.php?F=F_3lxS6fsUbWlBfKK. Copyright © 2015 by University of Iowa Hospitals & Clinics. Reprinted with permission.

Fig. 10.3: Jayne Jennings Dunlap and Julee Briscoe Waldrop, *Introduction to Evidence-Based Practice and Quality Improvement for Professional Nursing Practice: A Competency Based Approach*, p. 186. Copyright © 2024 by Cognella, Inc. Reprinted with permission.

CHAPTER 11

Leading Evaluation of EBPQI Initiatives

Julee Briscoe Waldrop and Elizabeth Walters

KEY CONCEPTS

Selecting measures
Outcomes measures
Data trending
Statistics interpretation

LEARNING OBJECTIVES

1. Identify the steps of the evaluation process.
2. Compare and contrast evaluation types.
3. Determine appropriate statistical measures.
4. Develop strategies for evaluation based on initiative and context.

> Take responsibility for your own happiness, never put it in other people's hands.
>
> —Roy T. Bennett

Introduction

To use resources to change practice and not evaluate whether the change led to the desired outcome is irresponsible. Nurse leaders are charged with the responsibility to manage valuable health care resources, and part of the stewardship of these resources includes evaluation. This chapter will provide you with the knowledge and tools you need to lead the fulfillment of this crucial obligation.

The Evaluation Process

Evaluation is a systematic and objective assessment of your EBPQI initiative to determine its efficacy (success in producing the intended result) and potentially areas for improvement. This usually involves data collection and analysis. The outcomes of the data analysis will inform the decision to adopt the practice change, continue to work on improvement, or sometimes let it go. Evaluation can be performed at different stages of the process, including before (i.e., baseline data), during (formative; process; i.e., is the change you intended happening), and after (summative; i.e., final results) implementation. Review the typical steps involved in the evaluation process in Table 11.1.

TABLE 11.1 Steps in the Evaluation Process

1	Purpose	Evaluation should have a purpose. In EBPQI, the purpose is usually to determine whether the practice changes that were implemented resulted in improvements. Improvements can be focused on various areas as health care is broad and diverse. Evaluations are often used to make future decisions.
2	Aims	Aims should be SMART (specific, measurable, achievable, relevant, and timely). Three specific types of aims that are used in quality improvement are process measures, outcome measures, and balancing measures.
3	Methods	Determine the methods and tools you will use for collecting data based on your aims. There are many different sources and methods to do this.
4	Data collection	The data collection process should be systematic and reliable to ensure the accuracy and validity of the evaluation findings that support believable and trustworthy results. Results should be collected ethically; remember issues related to privacy and confidentiality of patient data discussed in Chapter 10.
5	Analysis	The collected data should be analyzed in a way that addresses the evaluation objectives. This may involve descriptive or statistical analysis, thematic analysis, or other methods, depending on the nature of the data.
6	Dissemination	The final step is to communicate the evaluation results in a clear and comprehensive report to share with other people or organizations. The report should include an overview of the evaluation process, a presentation of the findings, and recommendations for future action based on the findings. As you will see in Chapter 12, dissemination can take many forms.

Formative Evaluation

Formative evaluations are primarily used during the development phase of health care projects, programs, policies, or interventions to refine and improve their design before full implementation or final summative evaluation. For example, let's say you are developing a smoking cessation program. Your team has gone through the EBP process, critically appraised the evidence, and found that there are many strategies that can be used in smoking cessation programs. How can you decide which one is best for your context and population?

Decision analysis focuses on enhancing decision-making processes by systematically assessing different options and their potential impacts before final actions are taken. You will use all your evidence and local data, such as patient demographics, along with organizational resources (time and money) to plan scenarios. Be sure to get all your stakeholders involved in scenario planning, which can allow them to foresee potential consequences, thus helping in making informed choices that mitigate risks and maximize benefits. Decision analysis is used in this example prior to beginning a project, but it is not a one-time activity. It can be used throughout the life of a project to revisit and refine decisions as more information becomes available. This iterative nature helps in adapting to changes and improving outcomes over time.

Another type of formative evaluation is process mapping and analysis. In our example of the smoking cessation program, a process map of the patient journey for those entering the smoking cessation program could be helpful to identify potential barriers and ensure all necessary resources and support systems are in place. See Chapter 9 for more on process mapping.

Process Evaluation

Process evaluations focus on the implementation process, checking if the intervention, program, or service is being delivered as intended, and identifying operational improvements. Examples of process evaluation are clinical audits.

The aim of a clinical audit for a smoking cessation program could be to evaluate the effectiveness and adherence to best practice guidelines of the smoking cessation program. Items that could be assessed using a review of a randomly selected number of patient records over a given time period might be these:

- Initial assessment: All patients enrolled in the smoking cessation program should undergo a comprehensive initial assessment, including smoking history, readiness to quit, and any relevant medical conditions.
- Intervention: Patients are offered evidence-based interventions such as behavioral therapy, pharmacotherapy, or a combination of both.
- Follow-up: Regular follow-up appointments are scheduled to monitor progress, provide support, and adjust treatment plans as needed.

For each of these criteria, you will determine if the criteria were met (yes/no). Calculate the percentage of patients meeting each criterion and compare the findings against the predefined standards. This type of audit can reveal areas of good practice and areas needing improvement. Regularly scheduled audits are a great way to monitor sustainability of a program, adherence to a new policy, or a practice change. Additional process evaluations are benchmarking and balanced scorecards, described in Chapter 9.

Summative Evaluation

Summative evaluations assess the outcomes and overall effectiveness of your program, policy, or practice change after it has been fully implemented to determine its impact and whether it should be continued or modified. An example of a summative evaluation for our smoking cessation program would be quit rate, measured as the percentage of all participants who are not smoking 6 months after the end of the program.

Another type of summative evaluation is patient-reported outcomes (PROMS). This type of evaluation would focus on the participants' experience and satisfaction with the smoking cessation program. Cost effectiveness analysis (CEA) and quality-adjusted life years (QALYs) might be a good choice for a longer term view of this program since the benefits of smoking cessation and the subsequent improvements in health may not be manifest until many years in the future (Mattock et al., 2023; see Chapter 7 for more information on CEA and QALY).

Importance of Ongoing Evaluation

Ongoing evaluation or regularly evaluating the outcomes of EBPQI initiatives is vital for several reasons. The safety, satisfaction, and health outcomes of patients are number one. Not only is it crucial to know if practice changes produce the intended results, but, ideally, the change(s) should do so without increased costs or workload. Evaluation of best practice, once changed, supports sustainability and continues to hold those involved accountable to the standard of care. It also fosters a culture of inquiry and continuous improvement. Often evaluation is important to determine whether regulatory standards or benchmarks are being met, as discussed in Chapters 2 and Chapter 9. Regular evaluation enables you to measure the impact of interventions and verify whether they are delivering the expected results.

Regular evaluation of practices will inform decision-making and strategic planning as new evidence or technologies become available. Best practice may need to change again! Sometimes initiatives can backslide, factors unrelated to the practice change become a priority, and the initiative can lose ground. Additional areas for improvement may be identified. It is important to know when this happens so that decisions can be made based on data. This is part of the continuous improvement process. The best practice is sustained practice.

Evaluation Measures

Evaluation measures or methods are the "how" of evaluation. See Table 11.2 for examples with descriptions. These should be familiar to you because many of the same methodologies are used in research. Each method has its strengths and limitations, and the choice of method depends on the specific evaluation objectives, available resources, and the nature of the EBP, QI, or EBPQI initiative being evaluated. Selecting appropriate and meaningful outcome measures can be a challenge. In addition, there may be issues related to the reliability and validity of measurement tools and difficulty in collecting accurate and complete data, so be sure to consider these factors when choosing your measures (Silver et al., 2016).

TABLE 11.2 Evaluation Measures/Methods and Descriptions

Evaluation Measures/ Methods	Description
Surveys/questionnaires	Used to gather data from patients, health care providers, or other stakeholders. They can assess knowledge, attitudes, behaviors, or satisfaction levels. These tools can be administered before and after implementation to evaluate changes over time.
Observation	Direct observation of health care practices can provide insights into adherence to EBP guidelines, practice or system changes, the nature of patient-provider interactions, or the processes involved in care delivery.
Patient record review	This involves systematically reviewing patient records to assess adherence to EBP guidelines, patient outcomes, and other quality indicators, as well as patient-oriented outcomes like BP reduction or laboratory results.
Audits	Clinical audits compare current practices against established standards or guidelines to identify gaps and areas for improvement. Audits can be particularly useful for evaluating adherence to EBP and its impact on the quality of care. Results of audits are often used as feedback to inform participants in the EBPQI about compliance with a practice change.
Feedback	Feedback from patients, health care providers, and other stakeholders can be collected through various methods, including interviews, focus groups, and feedback forms. Feedback can provide valuable insights into the perceived effectiveness and acceptability of EBPQI initiatives.
Clinical outcomes	This involves tracking specific outcomes related to the EBPQI initiative, such as rates of hospital-acquired infections, patient readmissions, or mortality rates. The selection of appropriate outcome measures is crucial for an accurate evaluation.
Statistical process control (SPC) charts	SPC charts are used to monitor and control processes in QI. They help identify variations in a process that may be due to specific causes and need intervention (see Chapter 9).
Benchmarking	This involves comparing an organization's performance or processes against industry standards or best practices. Benchmarking can help identify areas where an organization falls short and needs improvement (see Chapter 9).

You may find that your evidence includes EBP and QI endeavors that used pre-post analysis of data, for example baseline status of a benchmark and then a time-dependent assessment of the same benchmark after a practice change. Statistical analysis between the two time points may be performed and even a statistical significance reported. Beware that this design (pre-post) in EBPQI has significant limitations (Reynolds & Waldrop, 2024):

- **Lack of granularity**: Aggregated data can obscure important trends and fail to show month-to-month changes that more granular data can reveal. This can lead to missed opportunities for timely interventions.
- **Static nature**: Pre-post analysis treats QI as a one-time event rather than an iterative process. QI involves continuous monitoring and adjustments, which static analysis methods do not support.
- **Failure to capture iterative improvements**: Quality improvement is typically an ongoing process with multiple PDSA (plan-do-study-act) cycles. Pre-post analysis does not effectively capture the iterative nature of these cycles and their cumulative impact on improvement.
- **Misleading conclusions**: Without understanding the types of variation present in the data (common cause versus special cause), pre-post analysis can lead to incorrect conclusions about the effectiveness of interventions.

As described in Chapter 10, by focusing on dynamic data analysis methods like run charts and control charts, QI teams can gain a more accurate and actionable understanding of their processes and improvements.

Example: Low Vaccination Rates

Let's return to the examples in Chapter 3. You have implemented a practice change that includes nurses/nursing assistants and providers. To review, for the vaccination rate example, your aims were as follows:

Aim 1: Process measure—95% of children < 3 years old will be identified; the notification system will be used (blue sticky note on door)

Aim 2: Process measure—In 90% of vaccine eligible patients, documentation of a discussion will be present at 3 months post-practice change implementation.

Aim 3: Outcome measure—Vaccination rates for children < 3 will increase by 10% by 6 months after the implementation of the practice change(s).

Aim 4: Balancing measure—90% of providers report the practice change as feasible to implement.

How will you measure these?

Aim 1 is a critical step in the practice change. Nurses have a large quantity of things to document in patients' EMR when they prepare a patient before the provider sees them. You want this additional "flagging" of the patient to be seen as a simple thing to do that will take only 2 or 3 seconds, which is why you chose the low-tech option of a sticky note versus developing a best practice alert in the EMR or other electronic notification. Your team decides that they will start by doing a walkthrough once a day and check all roomed but not yet seen patient charts to determine if the sticky note is used as intended. Your clinic has five providers and 10 rooms. Most days you will have at least one chart to check. An audit sheet is developed to keep track on a weekly basis (Table 11.3).

TABLE 11.3 Example Process Audit Sheet

Patient	Date	Sticky Note Applied	
(Do not collect any PHI. Just use a number so you know how many records you have reviewed)	Or day of the week	Yes	No
3	Monday	1	2
2	Tuesday	1	1
2	Wednesday	1	1
1	Thursday	1	0
4	Friday	2	2
Total: 12		6	6
Percent		50%	50%

Aim 2 may be more difficult to monitor, but it is important. Consider the commonly used adage, "If it is not documented, it was not done." Also, if the practice change is not being done, it is very unlikely that the intended outcome will occur. So, immediately, you can start auditing patient records in the EMR and collecting data on whether providers documented their vaccination recommendation discussions. This is what we call a dichotomous variable. It was either done or not done, yes or no. You can use a simple chart or Excel spreadsheet to keep track of this information. Your practice sees an average of 50 patients a week ages 0–36 months. Do you need to review every single patient's record? Thankfully no. You can perform this audit using a sample of charts each time. You and your team will need to decide how many and how you will decide which ones to review. A couple of examples are to review all patients seen on one or two randomly selected weekdays or patients whose EMR number ends in the number 2 or 4. See Table 11.4 for an example of the first week of data collection (10 charts).

TABLE 11.4 Documentation Compliance Audit: Provider Vaccination Discussion

Patient (Do Not Collect Any PHI. Just Use a Number So You Know How Many Records You Have Reviewed)	Date (Week or Month, Depending on How Frequently You Decide to Audit the Process	Vaccination Conversation Documented (Yes/No)	
		Yes	No
1			X
2		X	
3			X
4		X	
5		X	
6		X	
7			X
8		X	
9		X	
10		X	
Total		7	3
Percent compliance		70%	30%

This data from your process aims (1 and 2) the first week can be visualized using a bar or pie chart (Figure 11.1). As you continue collecting this data, you can plot the weekly percent compliance on a run and then a control chart (see Figures 11.2 and 11.3.)

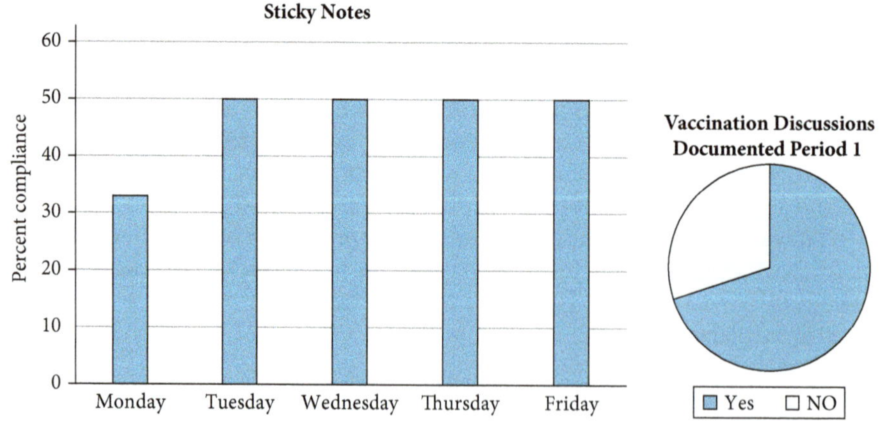

FIGURE 11.1 Week 1 process measures.

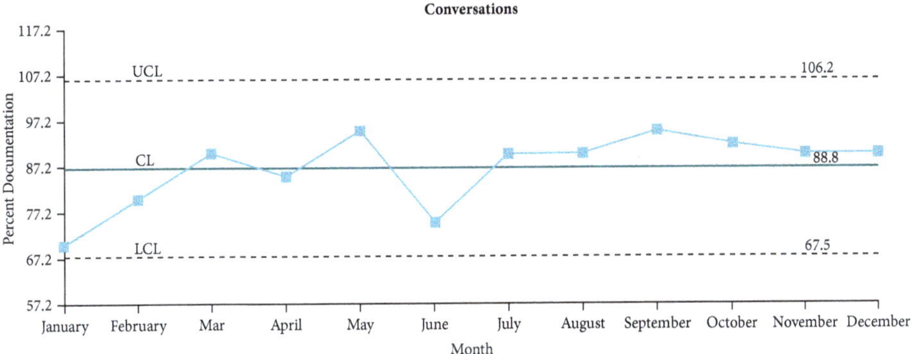

FIGURE 11.2 Percentages of conversations about vaccine hesitancy documented.

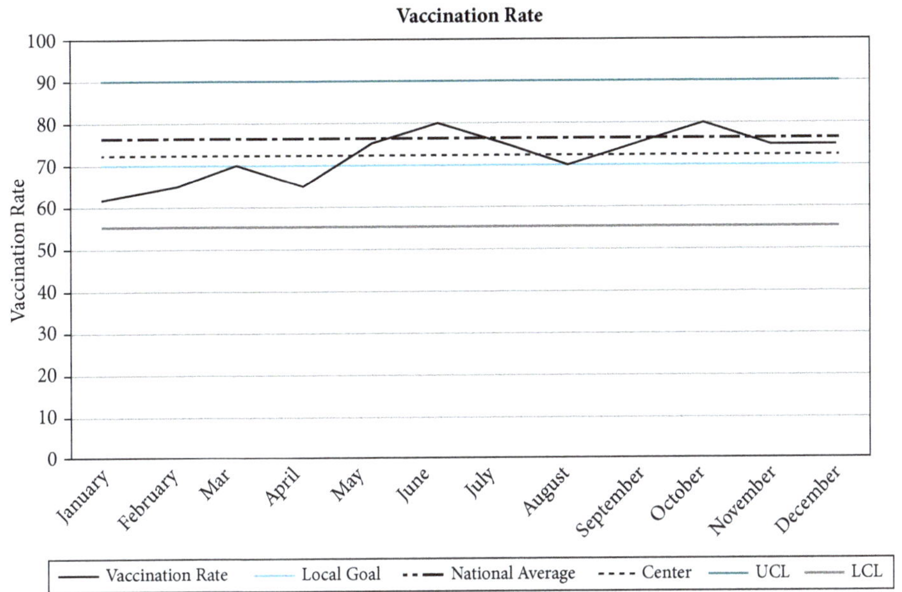

FIGURE 11.3 Vaccination rates.

Are you meeting your aims? What will you do about it? This is the great thing about EBPQI. You can continuously evaluate what is happening and make changes if needed. For example, the use of the sticky notes is not meeting your aim. As the persons responsible for this part of the practice change, you or a team member need to talk to the nurses (or nurse assistants) to find out what they think is keeping them from using the agreed-on system. You should also ask the providers charged with changing their practice what keeps them from documenting their vaccination conversations. You don't need to call anyone out; just ask a sampling of providers and see what information you receive. Maybe there is another problem that is unrelated to the vaccination discussion. Perhaps someone is out on vacation and the patient load has been higher than usual and this is something the providers chose to wait and discuss at a future visit. Maybe they have a suggestion about an easier way to document the conversation; for example, can you develop a smart phrase that can be used to improve consistency of documentation and save time (Anderson et al., 2020). Regardless of the reasons, it is the EBPQI team's job to work with those making the change to figure out how to keep improving and working toward the goal.

Since your organization already tracks vaccination rates, you automatically get a report each month. You may be able to ask your information technology and/or quality metric department to combine DPT, Polio, Measles, Mumps and Rubella (MMR), Haemophilus influenzae type B (Hib), and hepatitis B totals for all 3-year-olds (36 months of age), or you may have to calculate this yourself. Either way, the percentage of children who have completed the primary immunization series for these three vaccines is the outcome measure you have chosen. One thing to remember about all aims is that the people involved in the practice change want to know if what they are doing is making a difference, so the more frequently you can provide feedback, the better. You do have to balance this with the frequency of the occurrence of what you are monitoring and the time it takes to collect and analyze the data. Also, consider how many patients are included in the data frequency (the "n"); data with only a handful of patients reported on every week may not be helpful to your stakeholders because the compliance rate will appear to shift dramatically. If this is the case, consider stretching out the frequency of the reported data to every 2 weeks or monthly so there appears to be less dramatic fluctuation.

Aim 3 is your balancing measure. This measure can be very simple or more in-depth, depending on your resources and the willingness of your providers to take the time to share their feedback with your team on a regular basis. A simple example might be to directly ask providers in morning huddle once a week, "Was having a conversation about vaccine hesitancy feasible (yes/no), and do you have any suggestions for improving the process?" Or it could be a little more complex: an online survey asking for more information beyond yes/no, rationale for their choice, barriers, facilitators, and suggestions for improvement. There are more ways to collect evaluation information (Table 11.2). But remember, providers and other staff may tire of providing extensive feedback.

As you collect and analyze your data over the weeks and months of the project, you will develop a family of measures (Chapter 9). Be sure to share this information regularly with all those impacted by the initiative.

Figures 11.2 and 11.3 show what your family of measures looks like after 12 months. Did your team meet your aims? As you can see from the first chart in your family of measures, for the last 6 months of the evaluation period, providers have consistently documented their conversations with families about vaccine hesitancy above your aim of 90%. Everyone deserves recognition for this! The second chart demonstrates that vaccine series completion rate has also improved.

For the provider survey, you asked the feasibility question every month. The providers were not all sure it was feasible at first, but by the fifth month they were on board, and after 2 months at 100% they requested not be asked unless the compliance dipped below the aim level.

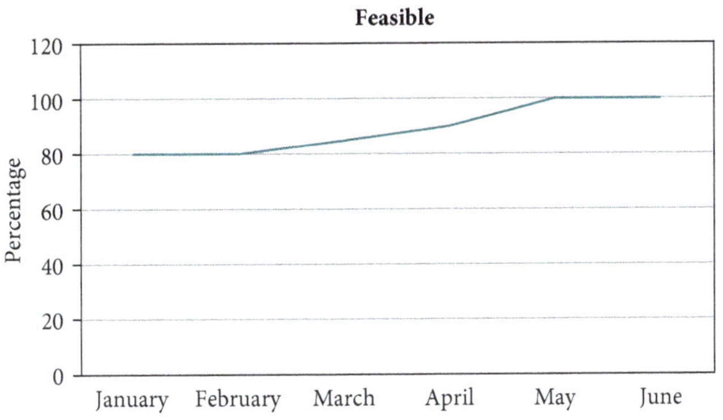

FIGURE 11.4 Provider survey/question.

Example: High Nurse Turnover Rates

The other example from Chapter 3 that you followed up with an implementation in Chapter 10 was the issue of high nurse turnover. In this example your aims were as follows:

> Aim 1: Process—50% of nurses will participate in one of the noneconomic benefits offered within 3 months of availability.
>
> Aim 2: Outcome—Nurse turnover will decrease at University Hospital by 5% by 6 months after the implementation of the practice change(s).
>
> Aim 3: Balancing—Workplace climate survey scores will remain stable (ideally, they should improve, but it will depend on the percentage of nurses who take advantage of the new benefits).

For aim 1, how can we measure the number of nurses who participate in the offered noneconomic benefits? There could be numerous ways to do this, but thankfully as a partner institution you have access to dashboards that track the number of nurses from your organization that sign up for the program and what aspects of the program they are participating in. This is one of the benefits to your organization: You don't have to budget for extra resources for developing a dashboard or other tracking system!

Aim 2 is easy. Your hospital's HR department already tracks this information monthly, so you can just request it. Your organization only conducts a climate survey semi-annually, so you won't get to track aim 3 data in the short-term. Overtime, though, you will be able to use this important information.

You can still produce a family of measures for this initiative even if you are receiving the data from another party or department. Aim 1 might include multiple run charts over time—one for overall participation and one for each of the five areas of focus: mental health, activity, rest, nutrition, quality of life, and safety. For aim 2 you could use a control chart to track turnover rate over time that includes your goal of 25%. As the program continues you will be able to add the employee climate survey results too.

Analysis: Evaluating the Impact of an EBPQI Initiative

In addition to interpreting your family of measures, other methods might help you and your stakeholders understand the impact of your EBPQI initiative. Additional evaluation strategies can be done using quantitative (numerical) and qualitative (stories) methods. These are the same methods you learned about in Chapters 5 and 6. Remember that any results that are numerical can be analyzed statistically. The choice of statistical analysis depends on whether the numbers represent categorical or continuous variables and assumptions about the distribution as well as the sample size. Table 11.5 provides the method and potential use for evaluation for quantitative methods, and Table 11.6 for qualitative methods.

TABLE 11.5 Quantitative Evaluation Methods

Method	How	Example
Surveys/ questionnaires	Closed questions (e.g., multiple choice) that can be scored numerically.	Patient satisfaction surveys Answers on a scale from 1 = disagree strongly to 4 = agree strongly.
Clinical outcome measures	Tracking specific numeric outcomes related to the practice change.	Percentage of patients with HgbA1C under 6.5%.
Benchmarking	Comparing numerical data with industry standards.	Vaccination rates.
Observation	Direct observation of activities or behaviors.	Suspect to the Hawthorne effect (see Chapter 5) but a very valid method for determining if an action is being performed or not.
Return on investment	Compares the cost of the practice improvement with its effects or the value in other ways that may be important to the organization.	Traditionally a monetary value is assigned. Alternatively, although not quantifiable monetarily, another metric could determine the value (e.g., patient satisfaction) or increased market share.

The data acquired through qualitative measures are analyzed differently than quantitative data, although sometimes descriptive (numerical) analysis can be done for some aspects of qualitative data (Sandolowski, 2000). For example, you might use descriptive statistics to describe the sample of nurses participating in your focus group. See Box 11.1. Most commonly, however, a thematic analysis (a type of qualitative analysis) is performed (see Chapter 6).

TABLE 11.6 Qualitative Evaluation Methods

Method	How	Example
Interviews	Interviews: Asking questions verbally can provide more in-depth insight into participants' experiences, perspectives, and reasons behind certain attitudes or behaviors.	Informal interviews may be used (e.g., in Chapter 7 during the pilot) or more formal interviews during which conversations are recorded and transcribed and analyzed using qualitative methods.
Focus groups	Interviews with a group of people can generate information about shared experiences, beliefs in a community, or norms of behavior.	A group of nurses discusses a practice change (again, this can be formal or informal).
Case studies	A detailed investigation of a single instance or event (a case) can provide an in-depth understanding of the complexity of an issue.	Full description of an adverse event. What happened before, during, and after from multiple perspectives? Information can be collected from multiple sources, people, and various documents.
Records review	Using text or documents to understand the context, processes or impacts of the practice change or quality improvement processes.	Evaluating notes or other documentation in the patient record.

BOX 11.1: EXAMPLE OF DESCRIPTIVE STATISTICS TO DESCRIBE A SAMPLE OF PARTICIPANTS

Ten nurse practitioners participated in two focus groups. Their ages ranged from 35–65 years old. Their years of experience fell into three groups. Four NPs had less than 2 years of experience, five had 2–10 years of experience, and one NP had over 10 years of experience. Seventy percent of the NPs were of White non-Hispanic ethnicity, and 30% were of other ethnicities. Five NPs expressed a positive attitude about the new practices to improve vaccination rates, and five were neither positive nor negative about the practice change, although all reported that it did not add any total time to their day.

The most suitable method will depend on the specific evaluation objectives, the nature of the practice change, and the resources available. Using a mix of quantitative and qualitative methods (a mixed-methods approach) can provide a more comprehensive understanding of the impact of evaluations, combining the "hard numbers" of quantitative data with the "rich stories" of qualitative data.

Challenges in Evaluating the Impact of EBPQI

Just as there are challenges in implementing a change in practice, there are challenges in evaluating whether the change is making a difference. Health care environments are complex and multifaceted, with various factors (e.g., patient characteristics, coexisting treatments, organizational culture) potentially influencing outcomes. Isolating the effects of a specific practice change can be challenging. Assessing the impact of EBPQI may often require substantial resources, including personnel for data collection and analysis, technology to support these processes, and training to ensure staff understand and can effectively contribute to evaluation efforts (Warren et al., 2016).

If the practice change is not applied consistently, it can be difficult to assess its true impact. Factors such as varying levels of staff training, resistance to change, or lack of support can lead to inconsistencies in adherence with the change. Clinicians also often operate under significant time pressures, which may limit their ability to participate fully in EBPQI evaluations. Some staff might resist evaluation efforts due to fear of criticism, increased workload, or skepticism about the value of the practice change or the evaluation process itself (Crawford et al., 2023).

Data collection and analysis for evaluation can be time-consuming as well as take a while to demonstrate an effect. It is possible that practice changes might not show immediate results; effects could become evident only over a longer period. Thus, assessment might require long-term follow-up, which could be logistically and financially challenging. Confidentiality and privacy must also be maintained when collecting and analyzing patient data (Chapter 10).

To overcome these challenges, it's essential to cultivate a supportive culture for EBPQI initiatives and evaluation, allocate sufficient resources, provide necessary training, and ensure transparent and effective communication about the evaluation process and findings (Barnsteiner et al., 2023).

When you reflect on the examples in this chapter, what do you think was the secret sauce that led to your project's success? Was it a unique aspect of implementation? Was it the way you collaborated with all the involved departments and leaders? Did you use a novel incentive strategy? Was there a critical point in the project where you had to pivot and do something different you were not expecting? Do you think other nurse leaders would benefit from learning about your efforts? They probably would! These are the insights you will use as you move on to summit the EBPQI mountain and disseminate your efforts. Chapter 12 will provide you with more information about all the ways you can make this happen.

Role of Electronic Health Records in EBP and QI

You have already seen in the vaccination rate example how electronic health records (EHRs) can be a valuable tool for evaluating EBPQI. EHRs provide a vast amount of provider and nurse documentation of patient data, including demographics, diagnoses, treatments, outcomes, and follow-ups. This data can be used to evaluate the impact of EBPQI initiatives, monitor trends over time, and identify areas for improvement. If you have determined there is not enough evidence yet to change practice, EHRs are also a rich source of data for research, which can contribute to the evidence base for future practice. Table 11.7 presents some examples of how data from EHRs can be used.

TABLE 11.7 Examples of Data for EBPQI

Type of Data	Example in EHR	Example Use
Quality metrics	EHRs may have built-in capabilities to track key quality metrics, such as readmission rates, medication errors, or adherence to preventive care guidelines.	These metrics can be used to evaluate the effectiveness of EBP and QI initiatives and to benchmark performance against external standards.
Audits	EHRs can be used to conduct audits to evaluate adherence to EBP guidelines.	For instance, you can check if appropriate tests were ordered or if evidence-based interventions were implemented consistently.
Clinical decision support	EHRs often include clinical decision support tools that guide providers and nurses in applying EBP.	These tools can also track compliance with these guidelines, offering insights for evaluation.
Patient outcomes	EHRs enable the tracking of patient outcomes, such as disease control measures (e.g., blood pressure or blood glucose levels) or complication rates.	These outcomes can be used to evaluate the impact of EBP or QI initiatives.
Population health management	EHRs can help identify patterns in large populations of patients, such as the prevalence of certain conditions or the effectiveness of interventions across different patient subgroups.	This information can be used to target and evaluate EBP and QI initiatives more effectively.

While EHRs can offer many advantages for EBP and QI evaluation, it's important to be aware of potential challenges, including data quality and integrity issues, privacy and confidentiality concerns, and the need for skills in extracting and analyzing EHR data. Moreover, EHRs capture data from routine clinical practice, which may not always align neatly with the data requirements for EBP or QI evaluations. Therefore, a combination of EHR data and other data sources or collection methods is often needed for comprehensive evaluations (Agency for Healthcare Research and Quality, 2018).

The Role of Feedback in EBP and QI

Feedback plays a critical role in EBPQI initiatives. It's a continuous process that provides information about performance and outcomes, helping identify areas for improvement and facilitating ongoing learning and development. Feedback is used to assess performance or adherence to a practice change. Feedback can motivate changes in behavior or practice, particularly when it highlights gaps between current and desired performance. By monitoring performance, areas that are working well and those that need improvement can be identified. Constructive feedback aids in learning and professional development, offering guidance on how to improve and sustain effective practices.

Regular feedback engages all stakeholders in continuous improvement, creating a sense of ownership and accountability. Ongoing feedback contributes to a culture of continuous improvement, and EBP and QI are seen as integral parts of everyday practice rather than one-off initiatives.

BOX 11.2: FEEDBACK EXAMPLE

Let's consider you are leading a hospital based EBPQI project to reduce patient readmission rates by improving discharge planning and postdischarge follow-up. To evaluate the effect of the improvements, the EBPQI team regularly collects data on (a) readmission rates, (b) adherence to the new discharge process, and (c) patient and staff experiences. They provide feedback to all involved staff every month.

This feedback might include data on changes in readmission rates, insights into the reasons for readmissions, and examples of successful discharges without readmission. It might also include qualitative patient feedback about their experiences with the discharge process and their ability to manage their conditions at home.

You and your EBPQI team then discuss this feedback with the staff, praising successes, identifying challenges, and brainstorming solutions for identified issues. For instance, if the feedback indicates that some patients are unclear about their medication regimens postdischarge, the team might decide to introduce a new step in the discharge process to ensure a thorough medication reconciliation and education. Through this process, the feedback not only informs the team about the progress of their QI initiative, but also drives ongoing learning and improvement, contributing to the goal of reducing readmissions.

AI is increasingly being utilized to evaluate and improve quality and safety in health care systems through various innovative applications. In particular, machine learning (ML) is being used to enhance diagnostic accuracy and reduce errors. For instance, ML algorithms can interpret medical images in fields like radiology and dermatology, often matching or surpassing human performance. This helps in early and accurate diagnosis, which is crucial for patient outcomes.

AI systems are being employed to improve patient safety by identifying and mitigating potential risks. AI can analyze vast amounts of data to detect patterns indicative of potential safety issues, such as medication errors or sentinel events (e.g., falls, wrong surgeries). These insights enable health care providers to take proactive measures to prevent such incidents. The use of AI in this context is supported by evidence suggesting that AI can enhance error detection and patient stratification, thereby improving overall patient safety (Choudhury & Asan, 2020).

The integration of AI in health care also requires robust governance to manage associated risks. Effective oversight is essential to ensure AI systems are safe, unbiased, and transparent. Recommendations include establishing strict AI governance frameworks at both institutional and federal levels to guide the ethical development and implementation of AI technologies in health care (Jeyaraman et al., 2023; World Health Organization 2021).

As AI technology continues to evolve, its role in health care will likely expand, offering even more opportunities to improve quality and safety across health care systems. Understanding the use of AI, its benefits and its potential biases and errors, is a new responsibility for nurses, especially those in advanced nursing roles.

Integrating and Sustaining the Practice Change

To make change stick, it needs to be hardwired into the system. Hardwiring may include permanent policy or protocol revisions. Revisions may need to be integrated into new employee orientation, annual training, competency evaluations, or required learning modules or skills fairs that provide ongoing mechanisms to support the practice change. Educational resources with clear guidance should remain available to all stakeholders. If you want to practice all the steps of an EBPQI initiative with yourself, see Appendix B and have some fun.

WRAPPING UP

In this chapter, you collected the data you needed to determine whether your team's initiatives met their aims. You used pilot data to adapt the practice change to fit your setting and continued to collect the data, and after time, you began to see that the practice change was being implemented more consistently and was making a difference in vaccination rates and, we anticipate, nurse turnover rates. Congratulations!

There is one more climb to reach the top of the EBPQI mountain summit. This climb involves disseminating your results! It is time to share the journey you have completed with others. This step determines the internal and external impact of your EBPQI work more than any other part of the process. In Chapter 12, you will be introduced to the importance of sharing information widely and learn about traditional and nontraditional methods to get your results into the hands of target audiences. But first, let's take a moment to consider intentional engagement in active (scheduled) rest so that you can sustain the longevity of momentum.

WELLNESS IN ACTION: BIRD WATCHING

My grandmother was an avid observer of nature but in particular birds. She passed this love of bird watching down to my father and he to me. Right now, as I write this, the day is just dawning, and because my windows are 85 years old, the bird songs are coming right into my home. Glorious! At one point in my bird-watching life, I started a bird list, a common practice among serious birders. But this list brought a sense of competition to my bird watching and stole some of the joy and awe that birding brought to my world, so I ditched it and brought my attention back to the beauty and wonder of a bird sighting, seeing the fleeting moments that a bird is visible to me as a gift.

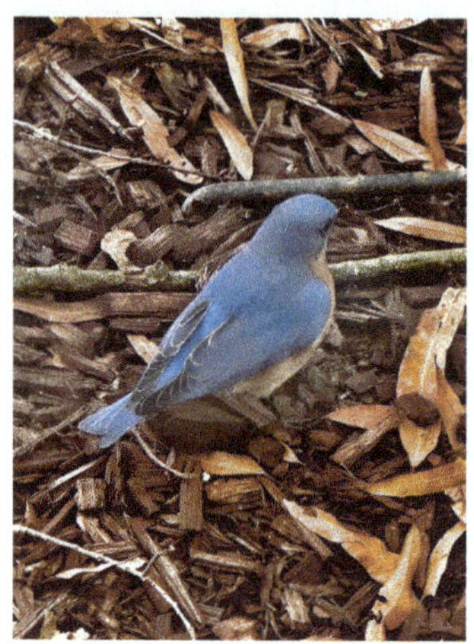
Image 11.1

If you can stop and listen or watch a bird for even 10 seconds you will start to feel a sense of calm and maybe even awe—depending on the bird. Bird watching can be a mindfulness activity that can reduce blood pressure and other benefits (Ratcliffe et al., 2013). People who watch more birds in their daily life experience less depression, stress, and anxiety (Huxley, 2016). Listening to birds also reduces stress and increases attention (Ratcliffe et al., 2013).

Bird feeders bring the birds to you. As long as you have a window, you can find a feeder that will allow you to share food with birds in exchange for observing them. My yard has multiple feeders with different types of food (of course I also feed the squirrels too). However, you can compound your benefits by going outside into nature and watching for birds.

REFLECTION QUESTIONS

1. What are the benefits of conducting a pilot of an EBPQI initiative?
2. Develop examples of family of measures charts for the example on nurse turnover.
3. Using the example in Box 11.2 on feedback for a hospital that implements an EBPQI project to reduce patient readmission rates by improving discharge planning and postdischarge follow-up, write one or more aims and develop strategies for collecting data to determine if the aims were met or not.
4. For either of the two examples, what are alternative ways to collect data to determine if you met the aims? Explain the who, what, when, how, and where for collecting the data.

REFERENCES

Agency for Healthcare Research and Quality (2018, November). *Optimizing electronic health records (EHRs) for quality improvement (QI).* https://www.ahrq.gov/evidencenow/tools/facilitation/qi-ehrs.html

Anderson, C., Tocchi, C. & Morrison, L., Rackley, C. (2020). A smart-phrase to improve documentation of supportive measures for idiopathic pulmonary fibrosis. *The Journal for Nurse Practitioners, 16*(2), 126–130. https://doi.org/10.1016/j.nurpra.2019.09.008

Barnsteiner, J., Beebe, S., Dicker, R., Halm, M., Hirsch, M., Taulbee, R., & Troy, D. (2023). Facilitating a culture of evidence-based practice and quality improvement excellence: Streamlining processes to improve care. *Journal for Nurses in Professional Development, 39*(4), 207–213. https://doi.org/10.1097/NND.0000000000000995

Choudhury, A., & Asan, O. (2020). Role of artificial intelligence in patient safety outcomes: Systematic literature review. *JMIR Medical Informatics, 8*(7), e18599. https://doi.org/10.2196/18599

Crawford, C. L., Rondinelli, J., Zuniga, S., Valdez, R. M., Tze-Polo, L., & Titler, M. G. (2023). Barriers and facilitators influencing EBP readiness: Building organizational and nurse capacity. *Worldviews on Evidence-Based Nursing, 20*(1), 27–36. https://doi.org/10.1111/wvn.12618

Huxley, J. S. (1916). Bird-watching and biological science: Some observations on the study of courtship in birds. *The Auk, 33*(2), 142–161, https://doi.org/10.2307/4072162

Jeyaraman, M., Balaji, S., Jeyaraman, N., & Yadav, S. (2023). Unraveling the ethical enigma: Artificial intelligence in healthcare. *Cureus, 15*(8).

Ratcliffe, E., Gatersleben, B. & Sowden, P. T. (2013). Bird sounds and their contributions to perceived attention restoration and stress. *Journal of Environmental Psychology, 36*, 221–228. https://doi.org/10.1016/j.jenvp.2013.08.004

Reynolds, S. S., & Waldrop, J. B. (2024). Optimizing quality improvement methods in practice: A case study approach. *Journal of Nursing Care Quality.* https://doi.org/10.1097/NCQ.0000000000000785

Sandelowski, M. (2000). Whatever happened to qualitative description? *Research in Nursing & Health, 23*(4), 334–340. https://doi.org/10.1002/1098-240x(200008)23:4<334::aid-nur9>3.0.co;2-g

Silver, S. A., McQuillan, R., Harel, Z., Weizman, A. V., Thomas, A., Nesrallah, G., Bell, C. M., Chan, C. T., & Chertow, G. M. (2016). How to sustain change and support continuous quality improvement. *Clinical Journal of the American Society of Nephrology, 11*(5), 916–924. https://doi.org/10.2215/CJN.11501015

Warren, J. I., McLaughlin, M., Bardsley, J., Eich, J., Esche, C. A., Kropkowski, L., & Risch, S. (2016). The strengths and challenges of implementing EBP in healthcare systems. *Worldviews on Evidence-Based Nursing, 13*(1), 15–24. https://doi.org/10.1111/wvn.12149

Wechsler, P. M. Liberman, A. L., Restifo, D., Abramson, E. L., Navi, B. B., Kamel, H. & Parikh, N. S. (2023). Cost-effectiveness of smoking cessation interventions in patients with ischemic stroke and transient ischemic attack. *Stroke, 54*, 229–1000. https://doi.org/10.1161/STROKEAHA.122.040356

World Health Organization. (2021, June). *Ethics and governance of artificial intelligence for health.* https://www.who.int/publications/i/item/9789240029200

CHAPTER 12

Dissemination Transcending the Discipline

Rosalie Mainous and Jayne Jennings Dunlap

KEY CONCEPTS

Dissemination

Authorship

Presentation

Publication

Media platforms and outlets

LEARNING OBJECTIVES

1. Review fundamental types of dissemination.
2. Describe various approaches to leading EBPQI dissemination.
3. Identify strategies for internal and external dissemination at the regional, national, and international levels.
4. Discuss innovative ways to expand the impact of EBPQI dissemination through advanced authorship and nontraditional outlets.

The goal of education is the advancement of knowledge and the dissemination of truth.

—John Fitzgerald Kennedy

Introduction

Welcome to the mountain pinnacle, the true culmination of the EBPQI process. In this chapter, we equip you with modern ways to disseminate your team's efforts so that they reach and significantly impact your target audience. All EBPQI process components are valuable, so if your team's initiative has proved successful, make sure it is shared! The optimal impact of EBPQI initiatives occurs when others learn of your accomplishment and transfer and adapt your improvement to their own organization or setting. As a role model and leader, you should fully embrace the goal of disseminating knowledge about improvement opportunities and successes, as well as challenges you have had and how to overcome them, so that others may benefit.

Any project or initiative that your team embarks upon should identify a sharing mechanism. In nursing school, you were taught "if it wasn't documented, it wasn't done," and the same is true of EBPQI: When there is no record of your work, it is as if your project was never conducted. Dissemination is critically important to the advancement of health care as it enables nurses and interdisciplinary partners across settings to promote practice changes that ensure optimal care. However, for you and your team, a rigorous, well-executed EBPQI initiative with system-level impact constitutes scholarship (i.e., high-level learning and academic achievement, which should include outcome output through dissemination) that can impact your future advancement as professionals. In this chapter, we explore ways to position your team to (a) have a demonstrated measurable impact and (b) to meet future expectations as their expertise expands with experience. We encourage you to take a forward-thinking stance as you delve into this chapter. Let's begin with a brief overview of dissemination basics.

Dissemination Types

Dissemination is the spreading of ideas (often widely) to individuals and/or groups; in the context of health care, dissemination involves the purposeful distribution of information or materials to a specific audience. The goal of disseminating EBPQI work is to increase evidence-based interventions and/or actions that result in sustained health improvements. With thoughtful and effective leadership, dissemination engagement can be a fun and exciting process. As a leader, you must consider which type(s) of dissemination will most effectively showcase your practice change to the right people. Passive dissemination involves one-way communication with targeted audiences; this is often a top-down approach to information sharing, generally taking the form of posted or published communications. Active dissemination, on the other hand, involves bidirectional interaction with target audiences, thus allowing you to impart key messages related to your work and entertain a back-and-forth exchange of ideas and questions in real time (LoBiondo-Wood et al., 2019).

Consider your dissemination options early and often. As you devise plans to share your team's initiative, try to incorporate elements of both passive and active dissemination. To reach internal audiences, for example, your team could present a luncheon webinar, display a poster within the unit, or routinely round to thank involved stakeholders and staff for their contributions to the new EBPQI success. Although important, such efforts must be combined with active dissemination to ensure a broad and sustained impact. To reach external audiences, your team could present a poster at a professional conference (e.g., sponsored by your state or national nursing association or a specialty organization) or interface with decision-makers from other health care systems to offer guidance on implementing new practices at their organizations.

Leading Your Team to the Right Audience

Before you decide how to disseminate your work, you must determine which group of people or professionals might be interested in using your improvement initiative or its various components in their settings. Whom to target is an important consideration, so take time to reflect on it. Audiences will differ depending on your topic or initiative focus, but you will want to target all audiences, both internal (e.g., local clinicians, clinical partners) and external (e.g., professional organizations, policymakers, community partners beyond your home organization), to whom your work might be relevant. Typically, EBPQI work on local and systems levels will be of interest to patients and clinical teams (including providers, nurses, and ancillary and leadership staff) as well as academic organizations, policymakers, and community partners. Your team might not realize that their successful EBPQI initiative may be broadly transferable to other departments or institutions. Furthermore, useful segments of your project (e.g., process, methodology, analysis of findings) can be disseminated for wider use.

Honesty in Reporting

Before we discuss various types of dissemination in greater detail, let's review actions to avoid. Plagiarism can take a variety of forms but basically entails claiming credit for someone else's work or ideas. Caution your team to avoid plagiarism under any circumstance, but also ensure that they understand when and how to credit others' work. Any material that is directly quoted (e.g., copied in the original author's exact words) must be enclosed in quotation marks to indicate that you are crediting not only someone's work, but their wording as well. Even if material is not quoted exactly, it is essential to provide a citation for all research, evidence, or information that is not your own, as well as for your own work if it has been published; each citation must have a corresponding reference, and each listed reference must have a corresponding citation. Failure to adhere to this rule constitutes plagiarism, and in the academic environment, plagiarism is regarded as (and treated as) academic dishonesty (i.e., intentional deception regarding the work of another; McClung & Gaberson, 2021).

Unfortunately, researchers and authors who lack knowledge of proper citation and reference guidelines often plagiarize inadvertently. For example, let's suppose that a member of your team copies and pastes information from a published study into a presentation but forgets to add a citation to the original source(s) along with a corresponding entry in the reference list. The lack of citation would imply to your audience that you were the source of the information that was copied and pasted. To avoid this pitfall, it is wise to have more than one team member cross-check citations and references. All team members should be aware that accurate citation is not only a courtesy to fellow evidence seekers (as it guides them to the material on which your work is based and related research), but also a form of currency (as the impact of one's work is often assessed to obtain professional advancement by counting the number of times it has been cited); for this reason, plagiarism can be regarded as a form of theft.

Consequences for plagiarism are varied and can be very serious: Your work could be discredited, and you could be penalized. Publishing your article in more than one journal (i.e., reusing text from your previously published work) constitutes self-plagiarism because the original journal or publication, not the individual author, generally owns the copyright to published work. Furthermore, it is considered unethical (as well as confusing to readers) for your team to publish parts of your project in multiple manuscripts to increase their number of published papers; this practice is sometimes referred to as "salami slicing" and is highly frowned upon. We recently came across an instance of salami slicing in published nursing literature, which reflected poorly on the authors and the discipline. If you want to be recognized as an empowered nurse leader whose teams conduct respected QI projects, it is critical that you understand and avoid all forms of plagiarism or unethical dissemination practices. Be vigilant and prevent even the perception of academic dishonesty.

Finally, your team must credit any and all funding sources (budgetary resources) at the time of dissemination. Funding sources include any monetary support received for the project or initiative. For example, grants (internal or external) or donations of in-kind support should be credited appropriately. Name your funding source(s) in a visible location and confirm that your team has fully complied with your institution's policy and the guidelines of the journal to which your team is submitting for publication. Acknowledging anyone whose efforts did not reach the level of authorship yet provided valuable reviews, feedback, or editing is a courteous strategy.

Ensuring Appropriate Authorship

Authorship involves creating new material, updating previously published material, or paraphrasing published material with an appropriate citation. Everyone listed as an author of the work should have substantially contributed to its completion. "Substantial" is the keyword here: for example, someone who contributes ideas and helps to write a work is an author; however, someone who reviews, edits, or critiques a finished work is not an author, not having contributed to its completion. Remember that personal and professional rewards, as well as a great responsibility for the work, accompanies authorship (Oermann & Hays, 2019). For this reason, the order of authorship is important and should be determined honestly and respectfully *from the start of the development of the scholarly work*. The first-listed (or primary) author is typically the initiative's leader and has contributed most substantially. Those who have contributed to the writing or presentation should be listed in order of contribution (work completed); for example, some expected contributions include conceptualization or writing/revising the content of drafts (works in progress). Make certain that the order of authorship truly reflects the standards of the International Committee of Medical Journal Editors. The ICMJE recommends that authorship be based on the following four criteria:

- Substantial contributions to the conception or design of the work; or the acquisition, analysis, or interpretation of data for the work; AND
- Drafting the work or reviewing it critically for important intellectual content; AND

- Final approval of the version to be published; AND
- Agreement to be accountable for all aspects of the work (ICMJE, 2024)

It is regrettable but true that some leaders in education or practice take advantage of their power differentials to request, or even demand, authorship without having made a corresponding contribution. This problem transcends nursing, but we can role-model integrity by holding one another accountable. If you ever witness such an occurrence, gather support and guideline evidence to present to your colleagues as a learning opportunity. For example, we once encountered a situation when a colleague of higher academic rank asked to be moved up in the authorship order, based not on their level of contribution but on their stated need for promotion; we politely cited the ICMJE guidelines and reminded this person that authorship is based on actual contribution to the work, and achievement of promotion is a separate responsibility. Given the information in the guideline, the individual agreed that the original authorship order accurately reflected each team member's contribution and role, and thus it remained unchanged. This transparent exchange empowered our team and helped to foster a healthy work environment.

Many journals now require that a credit statement disclosing each authors' contribution be included with the work at the time of submission. Be sure to carefully check the contributory itemization of all team members for accuracy. As a leader, it is your responsibility to ensure that all who meet the criteria for authorship are included and that the contributions of those who do not meet these criteria are acknowledged appropriately. Your team will look to you to role-model integrity and fairness by accurately crediting each person for their completed work.

Conflicts of interest occur when your personal interests have the potential to compromise your professional judgment. Any financial or competing interest that could cast doubt on your fairness or judgment constitutes a conflict of interest. For example, if you own a business that might be impacted by or receive a benefit from your EBPQI initiative, you must inform your audiences of this. Conflicts of interest or monetary relationships that are not disclosed for transparency may cause your disseminated work to be viewed skeptically when they are discovered. Disclosure enables your audience to respect the accuracy and value of your team's disseminated information and have confidence in your integrity as a scholar.

Dissemination Methods

Leaders must carefully consider your primary objectives of dissemination. This starts with exploring your dissemination method(s) with attention to your intended audience.

Traditional Methods

Let's focus on traditional dissemination methods first. These include but are not limited to oral presentations, poster presentations, and peer-reviewed publications.

Oral Presentations

You should impress upon your team that fellow professionals will want to know about their accomplishments and that presentations often provide high-level dialogue and ideas to improve messaging for future work. This has been our repeated experience throughout our nursing careers. A podium presentation is the gold standard in terms of impact for a presentation at a professional meeting. Teams should understand that the key to a successful presentation is a clearly articulated, accurate, and meaningful message delivered in an engaging way. Here is a piece of advice that we share with our doctoral students: It is okay to read, as long as the audience doesn't realize that you are reading! Your team should be encouraged to work from bullet points, but make eye contact with the audience. If space permits, they should walk around a bit. Mobile audio and video allow speakers to escape from behind the podium, which can feel liberating! We encourage practice partners to watch effective speakers and mimic their techniques, such as how they adjust their tone and voice inflections to increase engagement or accommodate special circumstances and situations. As an example, I (Jayne) attended one of Rosalie's virtual presentations. There were significant audio interruptions at one point, and without hesitation, Rosalie cheerfully quipped, "This should make for an interesting recording." The audience smiled and chuckled, and she continued to present without further issue.

Poster Presentations

Poster presentations can serve as a useful entry point to dissemination for team members who are in their early career. Inform your team that a key advantage of poster presentations is that they allow for one-on-one exchanges of information in a fairly private setting, which is a comfortable way for a nonseasoned speaker to gain the experience and confidence needed to present a timed oral presentation and open discussion before a large audience in a room tightly scheduled for successive activities. Ensure that your team follows the instructions for poster presentations and pays careful attention to details; if they do not adhere to the guidelines and required format for an abstract submission, it is unlikely that your poster will be selected for presentation. It is essential that your submission be appropriate for the audience, bold and easy to read, and concise, with a title that draws in readers (Errin & Bourne, 2007).

Include visual representations of your team's work as appropriate (e.g., evidence synthesis tables, run chart) to increase readability and understanding; perhaps sketch out your ideas digitally or on paper as a poster mock-up to organize preparation efforts. We have found that regardless of how a person or group may feel about a practice change, it is hard to argue with an evidence synthesis table (see Chapter 7)! Make sure that all components are clear and thoughtfully presented. A recent trend is to place a visible QR code on your poster for scanning; this allows viewers to make a copy of your abstract, poster, or material related to your initiative for future reference. The organization hosting the conference at which your team is presenting may require use of specific poster templates or have certain rules for presenting work publicly; encourage your team to check these closely and provide timely guidance to ensure that their presentation is clear and complete.

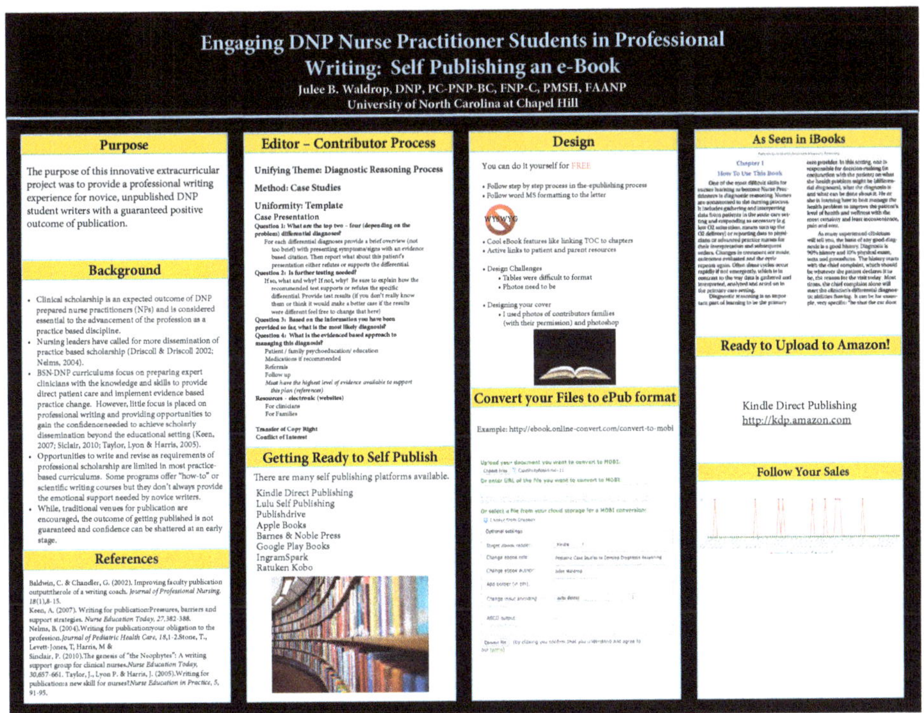

FIGURE 12.1 Example poster.

A DNP student was initially discouraged when I (Jayne) asked them to make several changes to their poster prior to a national audience presentation. However, 2 months later, they messaged me excitedly from the conference, attaching a stage photo of their acceptance of a poster award and cash prize. The award caused their EBPQI topic to be showcased to a larger audience than anticipated. The student also sent a photo of a handwritten note that an editor-in-chief had attached to the back of their poster; the note encouraged the student to submit the project presented on their poster to the association's high-impact, peer-reviewed journal for publication consideration. The student later reflected that the poster changes I had recommended, although challenging, had been necessary to ensure the rigor and accurate visibility of their team's EBPQI initiative and strengthen their future manuscript.

Developing and presenting a poster is a great first step toward writing a manuscript for publication. One of the coeditors of this book (Julee) presented the process for self-publishing at a conference first (Figure 12.1), then wrote an article on the same topic (Waldrop, 2018).

Writing a Manuscript for Peer-Reviewed Publication

As a leader, you should recognize that your service as an author and peer reviewer is important to the profession because it promotes high-quality, evidence-based dissemination. Readers depend on peer review to ensure the relevance, readability, and quality of articles (Morton, 2013). The most common type of peer review used by nursing journals is the double-blind peer review, in which the reviewers do not know (are "blind" to) the identity of the authors whose manuscript they are reviewing, and the authors are similarly "blind" to the identity of the peers who are reviewing their work (Waldrop & Likis, 2022). There is a trend in other disciplines to increase transparency in peer review by allowing the identity of authors and/or reviewers to be known. Reputable journals should have accessible and transparent author guidelines that inform potential authors of how their peer review process is conducted.

By sharing your team's EBPQI initiatives through publication, you contribute to the literature base so that others can potentially transfer/adapt your initiative to their local setting. Your team should consider using a structured guide that promotes EBP in an organized fashion as a tool to clarify and sharpen your message (Dean et al., 2021). As you choose journals to target, ask your team to consider where the leaders and decision-makers in your profession look for information. For example, the following are high-impact nursing journals that publish peer-reviewed articles on a variety of practice and education topics monthly, reaching a wide audience of nurses and nurse leaders: *Worldviews* (https://sigmapubs.onlinelibrary.wiley.com/toc/17416787/current) is a Sigma publication, and *Nursing Outlook* (https://www.nursingoutlook.org) is the official association journal for the American Academy of Nursing. You can also explore the International Academy of Nurse Editors Directory of Nursing Journals (https://airtable.com/shrjqveaKHtS9xku8/tblNXTxmTr18CC1If) for a current listing of vetted journals that have been authenticated by nurse editor leaders. Educate your team to use caution when selecting a target journal because predatory publications often use names similar to those of legitimate peer-reviewed journals. Sadly, many nurse leaders and teams have engaged in predatory publication unwittingly, thus compromising or invalidating their work and reducing their scholarly dissemination (Oermann et al., 2023).

Once you have targeted a journal, mentor your team on how to email a query to gauge the editor's interest in publishing an EBPQI manuscript on your specific topic. Your team should familiarize themselves with the journal's aims and read articles in its recent issues (in print or online) to identify exemplars. Alert your team to watch for special *calls* for manuscripts on specific topics of interest; these are usually located on the journal's homepage or circulated through leader electronic mailing lists. As with presentations, you must follow the journal's author guidelines closely to increase the chance of your work receiving a peer review rather than a desk rejection. A *desk rejection* occurs when an editor rejects the manuscript without sending it for peer review because the journal guidelines were not followed, the article was not deemed a good fit for that journal, or the journal recently published a paper on your submitted topic. It may take a few tries to find your work a good home, so encourage your team to persist and look for ways to strengthen the submission.

We strongly suggest that you ask a trusted colleague who is a seasoned writer, editor, and/or content expert to review your manuscript before you submit it for publication. Make this request a systematic part of your writing and dissemination process! We do this routinely and know many seasoned authors and editors who do the same because it can be difficult to see the strengths or weaknesses in your own work or judge it from another's point of view. Manuscripts are often accepted conditionally pending successful revisions (changes requested by peer reviewers and editors), so soliciting advice before submission may help you to anticipate reviewer concerns.

You may be invited to revise and resubmit your manuscript if the editor believes that your manuscript will be publishable when improved based on the reviewers' feedback. Make certain that your team follows their suggestions for revision closely and resubmits the revised manuscript within the allotted time frame. If more time is needed to complete a significant revision, proactively ensure that your team's corresponding author communicates with the editor to request an extension. Such communication is a basic courtesy as well as in your best professional interests: Editors and peer reviewers invest time in a manuscript that has publication potential; thus, they are colleagues working to strengthen your article and deserve your appreciation for and collaboration with their efforts. Accommodate all the suggestions that you can; if a reviewer's request seems unfeasible to you, politely explain why you cannot address it as suggested. Clearly itemize each of the changes requested by the reviewer(s) or editor along with your corresponding response. We strongly recommend organizing your itemized responses in a table format (see Table 12.1 for an abbreviated example). Your team can adapt our example or create a table by (a) copying/pasting each reviewer comment, (b) listing how the item was addressed (or the rationale and/or evidence succinctly detailing why your authorship team decided the particular request could not be accommodated), and (c) noting where the change is located (the page or line number in your revised manuscript) and/or pasting in a copy of the revised wording.

The publishing world is smaller than it seems, and you may be associating with the same colleagues in various capacities throughout your career: at conferences, on presentation panels, on committees, or as a reviewer or author. Remember that peer review is a voluntary professional service provided by your colleagues, and it is important to respect others' time and effort throughout the submission process. Coach your team to always be polite and professional in their dealings with editors and reviewers, even if they disagree with comments or a publication decision. If your team decides not to resubmit following a peer review, communicate your decision with the editor in a timely and collegial manner.

Predatory Journals

Predatory journals and publishers can be described as "entities that prioritize self-interest at the expense of scholarship and are characterized by false or misleading information, deviation from best editorial and publication practices, a lack of transparency, and/or the use of aggressive and indiscriminate solicitation practices" (Grudniewicz, et al., 2019, p. 211). There is a concerted effort internationally to find solutions to this growing problem. As reputable journals have moved into the open-access space, it has become harder to discern predatory journals from those that are under-resourced (Grundniewicz et al., 2019); however, a reputable journal will generally be a member of Open Access Scholarly Publishers' Association (OASPA). Check their website to see whether

TABLE 12.1 Sample Author Response Table

Reviewer Comment	Author Response	Revision Location
Reviewer 1		
This manuscript has importance for the academic community. It is generally written clearly. I have questions about two areas.	Thank you. We appreciate your support.	
On lines 67–70, why are italics used? Is this a quote? Please check the APA guidelines on italic font.	Per APA (7th ed.) style guidelines, italics should be used to highlight a key term rather than quotations (p. 158); as we feel the words in question are key terms, we have used italics.	Lines 70–73
When referencing Figure 2, has this been developed by the author, or is it from the developers of Figure 1?	Figure 1 and Figure 2 were developed by the first and second authors of this manuscript, which has a different focus than the original article currently in press at the *American Journal of Nursing*. We have clarified this in a citation below both figures.	Figures 1 and 2 citations
Overall, a well-written manuscript that should be of use to nursing faculty from the baccalaureate through doctoral levels.	Thank you!	
Reviewer 2		
The distinctions and interrelatedness of research, EBP, and QI are nuanced and thus can make it challenging for students across all nursing programs to learn and apply. I appreciate the authors' efforts to share tools for faculty that facilitate student understanding. The manuscript is well written and organized. The primary concern I have is the linear process between research—EBP—QI. It is not linear and unidirectional. And QI projects, while implemented within a local context, should include a critical review of the literature to ensure that changes to practice are based on evidence.	Thank you for your thoughtful comment. We believe our response has strengthened our manuscript. We have added content that clearly states that this process may be bidirectional. This was shown in Figure 1 through routes back to research at the EBP and QI levels, but we have added written content to clarify this as well. We agree that QI should include a critical review of literature; however, QI does not require it. You make an important point that supports why EBP and QI should not be uncoupled, as indicated in our unified framework (Figure 1).	Lines 84–85.

a journal is listed. Not all open-access journals are predatory, but all predatory journals are open access.

The consequences of publishing in a predatory journal can be terrible. In many universities and other settings, your work may be completely disregarded for promotion, tenure, or other advancement. Predatory journals usually seek manuscripts without rigorous review, and often without an editorial board; some might consider them "counterfeit journals" (Elmore & Weston, 2020). They lack transparency, misrepresent their publication practices, and often charge fees to publish. They are aggressive in seeking out publications, and their tactics often catch unsuspecting and junior scholars off guard. In a truly insidious form of parasitism, information from predatory journal publications can end up being cited and referenced in serious papers published by reputable journals, and thus their false content becomes interjected into the real scientific literature (Oermann et al., 2023).

An extremely valuable scoping review to determine the characteristics of empirical research on predatory publishing in health care literature was performed by Oermann et al. (2023). After screening, the authors reviewed 77 articles with empirical findings, of which most were in medicine and 11 in nursing. These studies highlighted that the articles in predatory journals were of lower quality, yet those in nursing were being cited frequently in legitimate journals. The authors concluded that the scourge of predatory publishing was so viral in the literature that it could be challenged only by rigorous institutional policies and other stringent measures. It is critical, therefore, that you make your team aware of this problem and caution them to avoid any publishing opportunity that appears suspect.

Nontraditional Forms of Dissemination

We recommend that formal dissemination methods, such as peer-reviewed publications, be augmented with nontraditional methods to reach the broadest audiences. Institutional repositories as a form of open access overseen by librarians have been used successfully to disseminate practice scholarship. You can use institutional, governmental, and discipline-specific repositories to maximize digital dissemination (Kesten & Hoover, 2022); one of the best is the Sigma Theta Tau International Honor Society of Nursing's Sigma Repository (www.sigmarepository.org/). Archiving lacks formal peer review but is still a method for dissemination and can make your work accessible to others.

Preprints (a word that is sometime used to mean the same thing as published ahead of print [hard copy of a journal] or assignment to an issue in an online journal) are an option to automatically post your work to a repository/online server such as SSRN (https://www.ssrn.com/index.cfm/en/nursingrn/). This is another nontraditional method of dissemination allowed by some journals upon submission for peer-review consideration. Authors may also choose to submit their preprint directly to a server, prior to or in lieu of publishing in a traditional journal. Be aware as a leader that research and other evidence posted initially on preprint servers has not undergone peer review (Waldrop, 2021). Authors must use caution as this makes your work publicly available via a search engine like Google prior to peer review. Originally used by other disciplines to disseminate research quickly, nursing as a practice profession has also begun to use preprints as a way to get EBPQI work disseminated more rapidly. For example, a DNP project focused article on the EBPQI framework used in this text, the mountain model (Wilson & McAlister, 2023), generated traffic and was cited by others prior to the work's peer review and ultimate acceptance and publication in 2024.

Blogs

Blogs are updated websites/pages that are informal but informational. In general, blogs associated with organizations or businesses may require you to sign up for access and often a fee. Personal blogs are more likely to be free. Pick your topic, then seek a blogging platform (web content home). Typically, a blog is not ideal for presenting a single piece of work; however, it can be suitable for presenting a series or examining a broad topic; long and short articles, updates, and breaking news are all acceptable. Although many bloggers try to develop their blog to support a revenue stream through advertising, such an endeavor is generally labor intensive and possibly costly, and it requires a lot of content. For some, however, it can be a dedicated way to build a professional presence (for an example see www.nursology.net).

Podcasts

Podcasts began as an alternative format to the written word and broadcast radio. They are a versatile means of presenting entertaining or educational information in a prerecorded audio format. Podcasts have increased in popularity over the past decade (Gotting, 2023), and there are many health-focused podcasts available to the public. They can be an excellent venue for dissemination, but securing an audience may be challenging. Because listeners must feel compelled to subscribe, you will likely need financial resources to develop and market your podcast. Generally, we approve of this means to reach a professional audience, and many nurses have used it successfully. If you search "nurse" on Apple or other podcast sites, you will find a variety of podcasts devoted to nursing topics.

Advanced Methods of Dissemination

Industry Partners

There can be both benefits and very specific pitfalls to working with industry as a nurse scholar. Nurses in advanced practice can serve as consultants to industry, take the lead on clinical application papers, and write in the professional literature about the usefulness of an industry's product. However, some nurses, while attempting to be helpful, have unwittingly relinquished their intellectual property. I (Rosalie) experienced this misfortune when I helped a company develop a biological sensor for preterm neonates. Never was I given credit for my testing or ultimate recommendations on their product development. Considering this experience, I recommend that you consider contract negotiations to protect your intellectual property when disseminating your work with industry. With reasonable precautions, working with industry can be a successful mechanism for dissemination. For example, I have great familiarity with industry specialties in biological measurement and have served on a consulting board for a biomedical company.

Elevator Speech

All professionals who wish to bring attention to their work should have at the ready an *elevator speech* (so titled because you should be able to give the entire speech on an elevator as you move from one floor to another). Elevator speeches can serve as a means of introduction, advocacy, or the dissemination of your work's key findings. Your speech should be crafted to a specific audience, so you may need several versions. Start by writing a draft with a clear opening, solid message, and effective closure. Practice speaking it within an approximately 3-minute time frame. Share your speech with a trusted colleague and ask for feedback on your delivery and messaging. You will need to describe who you are, what you do, and what you are asking of your audience. Elevator speeches have the potential to indelibly imprint your message on your target audience. Princeton University's Center for Career Development (n.d.) provides resources, including a useful template, for the development of an elevator speech. It also suggests that whether you are a student seeking a job or a capable professional looking to connect and network, an elevator speech is a quick and easy way to make a lasting impression.

Executive Summary

Another succinct way to communicate the key points of your EBPQI initiative is with an executive summary. You may have seen one attached to a business case, whitepaper, market analysis, or the findings from a task force or large collaborative. An executive summary is usually a document of no more than one or two pages that serves as a cover sheet for a comprehensive report. Like an abstract, the executive summary summarizes your more extensive report, so we suggest that you write it last. It usually has sections, including an introduction, the key points of the report with the findings, and conclusions; however, it must be able to stand on its own merit. Your executive summary should be formal and exact yet sufficiently interesting to engage an audience to read the full report.

Advanced Authorship Guest Editor/Editorial or Targeted Submissions

On occasion, a journal editor will put out a call for a special edition of a journal with a targeted focus. You will see these calls in advertisements in the journal or perhaps receive them by email. Although they usually have a short turnaround time for manuscript preparation, if you stay focused on the area of interest and produce a well-written paper, they offer a high likelihood of publication. If you are a seasoned writer, you might be offered the opportunity to serve as the guest editor of a particular journal issue. As such, you would solicit papers in a variety of ways to make a particular point in the literature (e.g., a treatise on a topic area, solicitation on diverging opinions, a review of the science). Finally, you may be asked to write an editorial on a topic in your specific area of expertise. One way to handle a call for an editorial is to put forward a call to action in your area of specialty and seek commentary on the issue.

Media

Social Media

Social media has introduced novel ways to enable rapid information sharing locally and globally. Some journals, and many professional nursing organizations, have social media channels. Nursing journals use social media to promote their content and increase engagement with their readers (Dunlap & Waldrop, 2021). Twitter (X) is the most used social media channel among nursing journals, followed by Facebook. Other types of social media used to promote nursing journal content include Pinterest, YouTube, and Instagram (Waldrop & Dunlap, 2021). If a journal posts about your article, share and comment on the post! Use hashtags to loop in others who may be involved in disseminating your work. Many nursing journals and PubMed Central have social media plugins that enable one-click sharing (Waldrop et al., 2022).

BOX 12.1: AMPLIFY YOUR VOICE AS A NURSE LEADER

- Follow nursing and health care peer-reviewed journals on your social media channels.
- Share relevant articles with your personal and professional networks.
- Include appropriate hashtags for related topics, audiences, and/or organizations that may be interested in your posted content. (Waldrop et al., 2022)

Speaking to the Media

Nurse leaders should consider sharing information with the media through lay outlets. Although this is one way to make the public aware of best practices or critical groundbreaking findings, speaking to the media can be challenging, even for the most experienced nurse or administrator. If you are approached by the media to showcase your work or provide commentary on a hot topic, proceed cautiously. You may need to obtain formal approval to speak with the media. First, we recommend that you ask your institution's communications and marketing department or association for their guidelines on media interviews. The communications department can usually help you produce a statement consistent with the institution's philosophy, which highlights your accomplishments or critique. Second, recognize that an interview with the press for a television or radio segment will likely be edited down to short sound bites that make the most impact; thus, it may not contain parts of your message. Third, ask whether the news agency will allow you to preview and edit the piece before it appears in print; if so, always take advantage of this opportunity to review the accuracy of the final piece and make any necessary changes. Fourth, listen carefully to what you are being asked and do not respond until the interviewer has finished asking their question. If you do not understand the question, or if you do not have a full and clear sense of what is being asked, request that the question be repeated or rephrased. It is possible that the interviewer has a hidden agenda or is seeking to support a view that their sponsor wants to represent. If you cannot provide an informed answer, do not hesitate to admit this; offer to get back to the interviewer as soon as possible or refer them to someone else.

Press Release

A press release is another method to translate the evidence or expand the reach of the results of your scholarship. There is no particular audience for a press release, so it must be crafted carefully. Public education campaigns often begin with a targeted press release on a particular topic; this can be a useful way to reach the broader population with important health information.

Changes to practice may necessitate policy changes, in which case your research findings must be brought to the attention of legislators, economists, public health officials, and the public. If your organization provides assistance, you may be able to use a template to inform the public of when and how to take advantage of the information that you are sharing. If you have access to someone in a public relations department, they can help you craft your message. You can also have PR Newswire or a similar company craft and release a press release for you (Nicholl, 2015). The headline must be accurate yet sensational enough to engage interest, and the press release should tell an engaging story about your work and its benefits to all who know about it (Nicholl, 2015). For a maximum impact, keep your message concise, clear, and compelling.

Op-Ed

According to Harvard Kennedy School's (n.d.) Communications Program, an op-ed is an opinion piece of about 800 words that is focused on a targeted audience and has a strong point of view; in addition to its description of this dissemination method, their website provides detailed instructions on how to write a successful op-ed. Op-eds generally are published in newspapers; thus, they can deliver your message to a wide audience and advocate for change based on your work (which you cite). An op-ed can both disseminate and mold the public's perception of your work, which can be particularly helpful if the subject matter is politically charged or has elicited widely different strong opinions. An op-ed allows you to have a voice in very relevant issues; however, to be credible, it must be steeped in current and reputable science and data.

Lay Literature

Practice-oriented projects are well suited for lay publications because the public is generally eager for evidence-based guidelines on health promotion and symptom management, screening guidelines, and anticipatory guidance for pediatric populations. Many lay publications have a large audience (readership) that is interested in the results of nursing practice scholarship. For example, *Reader's Digest*, *Family Circle*, *Women's Health*, *Men's Health*, and *Cosmopolitan* are among the most popular magazines in the country; each is a niche publication that may welcome a timely article steeped in evidence to support decision-making related to health practices. In addition, the publications in most clinics and health care provider's offices are purposeful in reaching the audience in their waiting room. It is important to remember that writing for the public is quite different than writing for the scientific community. For example, if your subject matter involves what to eat and drink to optimize a pregnancy, you should immerse yourself in the interests and concerns of your specific audience and choose a framework for dissemination that will be meaningful and accessible to them (Kaslow, 2015).

Advocacy

Professional Associations

There are many specialty organizations/associations within nursing, and each has a particular mission and population. For example, the American Association of Colleges of Nursing is the voice for baccalaureate and higher education within nursing; as such, it offers a wealth of resources to deans and their faculty on up-to-date issues of importance in higher education. Of note, it also offers many opportunities for dissemination! Additionally, there exist numerous organizations that address the needs and interests of nurses serving each population-specific specialty. For APRNs, there are specialty associations that have the best interests of the APRN at the forefront. Such associations offer a vast variety of methods of dissemination to specific audiences, including conference presentations, newsletters, journal articles, clinical guidelines, position statements, practice directives, webinars, and podcasts. Your objective is to choose the best means of ensuring that your message will be successful. For example, I (Jayne) and Julee, the coeditor of this textbook, engaged in a webinar to introduce the mountain model through Sigma Theta Tau, of which we are both members, to target global reach. Live attendees from 21 countries joined us in real time with high levels of audience engagement. The webinar was placed in the associations' repository, where it remains freely accessible. A post webinar viewer statistic link provided to us through this association revealed ongoing, widespread viewing by nurses at all levels.

Members of nursing associations are often asked to provide commentary or serve at the grassroots level for activism and advocacy within the political arena. They may be called upon by members of Congress, state legislatures, and other leadership factions in industry or service organizations to speak on issues of current importance as a means of dissemination. Some organizations offer individuals membership on various committees that serve the association and the profession. Dissemination in such cases can take the form of a special report, speech, or clinical bulletin or the development of discipline-specific directives on practice findings. At one point, this author (Rosalie) was a member of the American Academy of Pediatrics Committee on fetuses and newborns. As a member of that group, I was a coauthor of numerous population-specific clinical practice guidelines that define practice parameters and are currently used by neonatal intensive care units across the country.

State nursing associations, boards of nursing, chapters of Sigma Theta Tau, local and state chapters of the National Black Nurses Association, and the National Association of Hispanic Nurses produce newsletters and publications ranging from formal journals to brief communiques. Most health/hospital systems offer newsletters and various publications to the public on topics of interest and best health practices; some are peer reviewed, some require references, and some publish opinion pieces. Policy work can often be shared in these modalities; they are a great place to publish work that may be a bit controversial. All you need to do is query the editor with your idea to ensure a good fit, then follow the publication guidelines.

BOX 12.2: DISSEMINATION IN ACTION—DNP SCHOLARSHIP STANDARDS

You will recall that in Chapter 7, we noted that DNP-prepared nurses continue to fill faculty roles in increased numbers, often with practice time included in or added to their workload; therefore, thoughtful standards for DNP scholarship are needed to advance the nursing profession as a whole. Based on a PPCO question (see Table 7.10), we systematically explored scholarship standards for DNP-prepared faculty, which could be adapted and transferred across academic institutions to elevate faculty scholarship. Despite an extensive and iterative search, little research evidence investigating this problem was found. In the absence of available research evidence, other types of evidence were reviewed and synthesized (see Chapter 7). In addition, the diverse and collective expertise of the original authors was translated into recommendations using a new inclusive model of rigor for DNP-prepared faculty scholarship. This model can provide standards for the faculty member with a DNP degree or for the practicing nurse prepared with the DNP degree with one adaptation. Academic institutions are encouraged to use this work to expand the fundamental level of evolving scholarship, determine parameters, and provide clarity and support to DNP-prepared faculty and guidance for those in practice positions to facilitate their progress, as appropriate, within the local context (Dunlap et al., 2024). We hope this work informs and elevates the goals of the practice doctorate as originally envisioned (Mainous et al., 2023) so that DNP-prepared faculty are equipped and mobilized to target system-level health care improvements. Additionally, whether your setting is academic or practice focused, we encourage you to demonstrate the quantifiable impact of your team's work. Your disseminated works can be illustrated in a table. Tables 12.2 and 12.3 provide templates that you can personalize to meet your needs.

TABLE 12.2 Written Works (Disseminated)

Citation	Authorship	Citation Index	Journal Impact Factor or Book	Altmetrics	Mentorship	Other Evidence
Include full citation listing	Place in authorship order. For example, first, second, last, etc.	Number of traditional citations identified in a publication index such as Medline, Google Scholar, or Scopus	Include primary audience	Number(s) of complementary metrics, including social media shares and mentions, blogs, and mainstream media coverage	Structured or formal mentorship role on written work	List of works disseminated through nontraditional means, including policy or whitepapers that provide impact beyond academy in transforming health care

Source: Jayne Jennings Dunlap, et al., Selection from "Consistent Scholarship Standards among DNP-Prepared Faculty Needed: Actionable Insights," Journal of Professional Nursing, *vol. 51, p. 61. Copyright © by Jayne Jennings Dunlap, et al. (CC by 4.0) at https://www.sciencedirect.com/science/article/pii/S8755722324000206.*

TABLE 12.3 Presentations and Posters (Disseminated)

Presentation Title/Type	Organization	Reach	Attendance	Peer Evaluation	Special Recognition	Notes
Name of presentation; podium, poster, keynote, invited, peer reviewed; location	American Association of Colleges of Nursing, Sigma, National Organization of Nurse Practitioner Faculties etc.	Local, state, regional, national, or international	Number of attendees with specification of type of audience	Audience ranking, numeric scores	Any presentation awards or distinctions earned	Additional impact-related information

Source: Jayne Jennings Dunlap, et al., Selection from "Consistent Scholarship Standards among DNP-Prepared Faculty Needed: Actionable Insights," Journal of Professional Nursing, *vol. 51, p. 62. Copyright © by Jayne Jennings Dunlap, et al. (CC by 4.0) at https://www.sciencedirect.com/science/article/pii/S8755722324000206.*

Dissemination's Critical Element of Impact

Our dissemination described in Box 12.2 is the central piece of a new model that identifies the key components for maximum scholarly impact; it was originally intended for the environment of higher education but later adapted to fit higher education, practice, and policy (see Figure 12.2). One point of the star has been adapted to emphasize progression and depth of experience/expertise in the three arenas that are centrally depicted, thus highlighting the valuable ability to tri-focus. The rising star symbolizes the emergence and growing impact of DNP-prepared scholars in education, practice, and/or policy settings. The foundational criteria in the model should be incorporated into scholarship generated by DNP students (much can be leveraged from key assignments while matriculating), DNP-prepared academics, and clinicians in practice or who lead institutional EBPQI initiatives, or DNP-prepared professionals who are heavily involved in state or federal policy initiatives.

The work of the DNP-prepared nurse has the potential to achieve far-reaching impact and system-level change, with tremendous financial implications; therefore, when applying the model, first consider *quality* and *rigor*. The work of the nurse prepared with the practice doctorate should be of the highest quality, have integrity, and provide rigor within the scholarship paradigm. Although dissemination of work authored by DNP-prepared nurses is rapidly expanding (Cortez et al., 2021; Waldrop & Broome, 2024), there has been a drift from the essentials (AACN, 2021), which guides curriculum development and dissemination and serves as a framework for accreditation of Colleges of Nursing. We have seen many DNP projects that need greater quality and/or rigor; scholarship must have both in order to be respected and transferable. The importance of these criteria will be readily apparent when the outcomes are disseminated; without them, the work may be an exercise in futility.

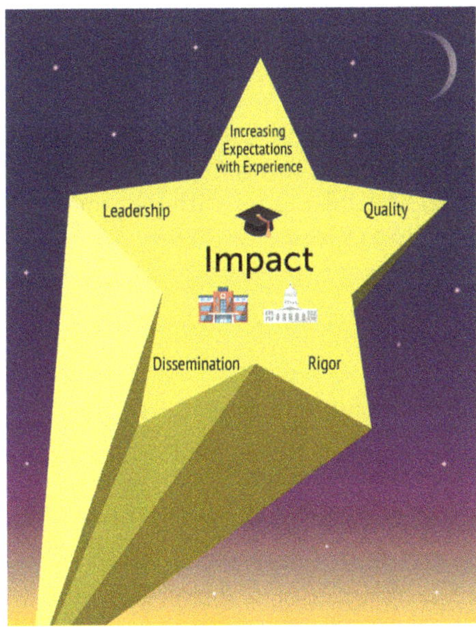

FIGURE 12.2 Foundational criteria for scholarship impact in academic, policy, practice, or policy settings.

Dissemination must (a) be reflective of the methods, thoughtful, and timely; (b) address a relevant issue or problem; (c) be defensible with regard to the process (rigor); and (d) reflect a high quality of effort. Work that is of poor quality or does not reflect doctoral-level preparation can be easily dismissed; however, such work may still appear in the literature. For this reason, doctoral education focuses on the careful scrutiny and evaluation of evidence. Serious scholars discard work that clearly lacks a discernable method or fails to address a problem or need.

Leadership is needed to increase the impact of scholarship. The DNP prepared nurse demonstrates leadership by ensuring that the work is optimally performed, prepared, presented, and promoted to an appropriate audience in order to serve an important purpose. The DNP prepared nurse leader maintains the expertise needed to align their work with current opportunities for dissemination. Too often, valuable evidence based on experiences and associated outcomes falls by the wayside. Although researchers may conduct projects to generate evidence, it is up to leaders in DNP education, policy, and practice to examine and report on that evidence in the literature, thus closing the evaluation loop. Finally, as one gains experience and expertise in a particular area, their work should become more refined, sophisticated, impactful, and successful at addressing health care and health system needs.

Strategies for High Visibility

When opportunity knocks, answer the door! We have each had numerous opportunities that did not seem worthwhile when first presented but eventually benefited us (overtly and covertly) as scholars. There are many ways to become recognized and stand out in a crowd. Consider the following suggestions:

- Volunteer: By volunteering, you uncover new areas of interest that can help you develop your knowledge and skill set. The more you are considered the expert in an arena, the more you will be asked for your opinion, and the more credible your message will become.
- Brand yourself: You can manage others' perceptions of you by striving to be engaged and authentic and always putting your best self forward. Many schools and programs offer advanced coursework on how to develop a self-brand. For example, the *Harvard Business Review* offers the following four steps to building a brand (Orduña, 2022): (1) define one's uniqueness as part of a personal brand; (2) align organizational goals with one's personal goals and those of the brand; (3) find colleagues with like interests to with whom to build a community; and (4) share or disseminate one's work, using the brand as a means to showcase what you know and can do.
- Seek and accept an invited speakership: Invited speakerships may not be paid and are not peer reviewed, but they allow you to expound on the outcomes of your latest project.
- Speak up in meetings: Meetings often offer opportunities to introduce or advance your agenda.
- Differentiate yourself and your message from all others: Know what makes you unique and leverage this knowledge in high-level discourse as appropriate and applicable.

By volunteering for every opportunity early in my career, I (Rosalie) was able to travel to McChord Air Force Base in Tacoma, Washington, to gain awareness of the rigors experienced by students who were participating in the Reserves Officers Training Corps (ROTC). During a program designed specifically for nursing faculty, I learned to rappel, was taught how to rescue trapped individuals by sawing off a car door, and was trained in marksmanship. This unique experience led to my deep interest and investment in supporting veterans; I saw needs in that population that compelled me to develop (at my next university) a psychiatric mental health nurse practitioner (PMHNP) program to assist veterans. The evidence I brought to the table to promote this solution was the high rate of student and veteran suicide, and this evidence proved critical to garnering support. The Veterans Administration hospital wholeheartedly agreed with my identified need, became a strong supporter of my solution, and funded faculty positions. The new PMHNP program (it was not a DNP program at that time) attracted the second largest number of students in the graduate program in my college! I share this example with you to show that many opportunities can leverage your work and significantly widen your influence.

Managing the Message

Be sure to network with other leaders at conferences; this is an effective way to identify future collaborators. Share your message/publication with colleagues who might be interested in your work; they may be willing to promote your work through their own outlets (Savor, 2021). Know how to control and manage your message (as opposed to letting your enthusiasm for the message manage you). It is important to choose language that presents your message clearly and carefully to avoid distortions, faulty interpretations, assumptions, or intentional misrepresentations; these semantic problems are called *doublespeak* (Walker et al., 2021) and can easily bias others against you or your message. Walker et al. (2021) offer the example of calling political protestors "activists" or "extremists"; such terminology, which is heavy with political connotations, would likely cause some listeners to reject the message without considering it. Your EBPQI work should influence the system to move toward positive change. If your work is misunderstood or leads to unintended conclusions due to poor messaging, your dissemination effort will have accomplished nothing positive.

WELLNESS IN ACTION: WRITING RETREATS

Writing retreats provide an opportunity to engage in focused writing projects outside of your normal setting or routine for a specific period. In addition to providing a creative (and often fun) mechanism for dissemination, a thoughtfully planned writing retreat can incorporate wellness elements such as physical activity, activities that foster creativity, and restorative experiences (Dunlap, 2024). In fact, the dissemination-in-action nurse team example presented in this chapter was written almost entirely during our writing retreat at a rented lake house. Between writing sessions, our authorship team explored the local city through shopping and dining experiences to create a rejuvenating mixture of productivity, rest, and creativity. Although we experienced some setbacks during our retreat (including sustained loss of power during a winter storm), we persisted and are excited to share the work we completed during that time through an open-access article in the *Journal of Professional Nursing* (Dunlap et al., 2024). Here are some practical recommendations for planning a writing retreat to engage with your team regarding disseminating your EBPQI work:

- Prepare for the retreat with set shared goals and clear guidance.
- Bring any needed supplies and an outline or draft of your paper (including the literature review).
- Divide and assign the writing assignments and provide opportunities for discussion and real-time peer review.
- Plan restorative breaks between writing sessions.
- Commemorate the completion of your retreat and eventual writing project in a meaningful way for your team.

WRAPPING UP

As a nurse leader, you can establish an essential role in your work setting by helping to guide EBPQI initiatives with new or seasoned nurses and other health care professionals. One mark of a great leader is commitment to team success rather than personal success. Guide your team by embracing modern modes of dissemination and role-modeling high standards and integrity. Be sure that your team(s) understand(s) that without successful dissemination, results have little or no impact.

Let your passion and excitement show! Others will become excited to work with you to bring the best possible care to deserving patients and populations. Given the rapidly evolving health care landscape, we have found that exploring potentially successful dissemination opportunities is personally and professionally rewarding. We sincerely enjoy guiding our teams, faculty, and students as they enter the scholarly realm toward the rewards of successful dissemination. As a leader, remain focused on sharing information throughout the EBPQI process, garner sustained support from your team and other important stakeholders, and always remember that effective dissemination ultimately benefits us all.

REFLECTION QUESTIONS

1. What barrier(s) and/or fear(s) could keep you from leading your team to disseminate their completed work to target audiences?
2. In addition to presentations and publications, what modern dissemination routes seem most realistic and potentially impactful for your team's current project?
3. How can you garner time and resources to most effectively help your team achieve EBPQI dissemination?
4. How can you negotiate/advocate for time to pursue scholarly outcomes in whatever environment you may be in?
5. As a nursing leader, when can you take steps toward amplifying the work of other teams?

REFERENCES

American Association of Colleges of Nursing. (2021). *AACN essentials*. https://www.aacnnursing.org/Essentials

Center for Career Development, Princeton University. (n.d.). *Developing your editing pitch*. https://careerdevelopment.princeton.edu/guides/networking/developing-your-elevator-pitch#Why-you-need-an-elevator-pitch

Cortez, S., Allen, S. , Balevre, P. , Rass, J., & Wechter, S. (2021). DNP-authored articles in peer-reviewed journals 2012-2018. *Nurse Educator, 46*(5), 290–294. https://doi.org/10.1097/NNE.0000000000000990

Dean, J., Gallagher-Ford, L., & Connor, L. (2021). Evidence-based practice: A new dissemination guide. *Worldviews on Evidence-Based Nursing, 18*(1), 4–7.

Dougherty, M. C., Freda, M. C., Kearney, M. H., Baggs, J. G., & Broome, M. (2011). Online survey of nursing journal peer reviewers: Indicators of quality in manuscripts. *Western Journal of Nursing Research, 33*(4), 506–521. https://doi.org/10.1177/0193945910385715

Dunlap, J. J. (2024). Writing retreats for nurses: Inspiration to share. *American Nurse*. Writing retreats for nurses: Inspiration to share

Dunlap, J. J., & Waldrop, J. (2022). An exploratory study of social media use and management by nursing journals. *Advances in Nursing Science, 45*(3), 218–226. https://doi.org/10.1097/ANS.0000000000000403

Dunlap, J. J., Waldrop, J., Mainous, R., Zellefrow, C., Beckett, C., Melnyk, B. M. (2024). Consistent scholarship standards among DNP-prepared faculty needed: Actionable insights. *Journal of Professional Nursing, 51*, 58-63. https://doi.org/10.1016/j.profnurs.2024.01.009

Elmore, S. A., & Weston, E, H. (2020.) Predatory journals: What they are and how to avoid them. *Toxicol Pathol, 48*(4), 607–610. https://doi.org/10.1177/0192623320920209

Erren, T. C., & Bourne, P. E. (2007). Ten simple rules for a good poster presentation. *PLoS Comput Biol, 3*(5), e102.

George, V., & Haag-Heitman, B. (2011). Nursing peer review: The manager's role. *Journal of Nursing Management, 19*(2), 254–259. https://doi.org/10.1111/j.1365-2834.2011.01225.x

Gotting, M. C. (2023). *U.S. podcasting industry—Statistics & facts*. Statista. https://www.statista.com/topics/3170/podcasting/ #topicHeader_wrapper

Grudniewicz, A., et al., (2019). Predatory journals: No definition, no defence. *Nature, 576*, 210.

Harvard Kennedy School. (n.d.). *How to write an op-ed or column*. https://projects.iq.harvard.edu/files/hks-communications-program/files/new_seglin_how_to_write_an_oped_1_25_17_7.pdf

Kaslow, N. J. (2015). Translating psychological science to the public. *American Psychologist, 70*(5), 361–371. https://doi.org/10.1037/a0039448

Kesten, K. S., & Hoover, S. N. (2022). Doctor of nursing practice dissemination through an open access repository. *Journal of Professional Nursing, 41*, 19–25.

LoBiondo-Wood, G., Haber., J., & Titler, M. G. (2019). *Evidence-based practice for nursing and healthcare quality improvement*. Elsevier.

Mainous, R. O., Dunlap, J. J., & Brewer, T. L. (2023). Realizing the DNP as envisioned: Moving toward consistent nomenclature, curricula, and outcomes. *Nursing Outlook, 71*(3), 101969. https://doi.org/10.1016/j.outlook.2023.101969

McClung, E. L., & Gaberson, K. B. (2021). Academic dishonesty among nursing students: A contemporary view. *Nurse Educ, 46*(2), 111–115. https://doi.org/10.1097/NNE.0000000000000863

Morton, P. G. (2013). Insights about the manuscript review process. *Nurse Author & Editor, 23*(3), 1–4. https://doi.org/10.1111/j.1750-4910.2013.tb00158.x

Nicoll, L. H. (2015). Writing a press release. *Nurse Author & Editor, 25*(1), 1–9. https://doi.org/10.1111/j.1750-4910.2015.tb00194.x

Oermann, M. H., & Hayes, J.C (2023). *Writing for publication in nursing* (5th ed.). Springer.

Oermann, M. H., Waldrop, J., Nicoll, L H., Peterson, G. M., Drabish, K. S., Carter-Templeton, H., Owens, J. K., Moorman, T., Webb, B., & Wrigley, J. (2023). Research on predatory publishing in health care: A scoping review. *Canadian Journal of Nursing Research, 55*(4), 415–424. https://doi.org/10.1177/08445621231172621

Orduña, N. (2022). How to build your personal brand at work. *Harvard Business Review.* Orduña, N. (2022). How to build your personal brand at work

Saver C. (2023). *Anatomy of writing for publication for nurses* (5th ed.). Sigma Theta Tau International.

Waldrop, J. (2018). Self-publishing: A novel incentive to write in graduate nursing education. *Nursing Education Perspectives, 39*(5), 315–316. https://doi.org/10.1097/01.NEP.0000000000000344

Waldrop, J. (2021) Preprints: New option for research studies at the journal for nurse practitioners. *The Journal for Nurse Practitioners, 17*(8), 901–902.

Waldrop, J., & Dunlap, J. J. (2021). Analysis of tweeting on journal usage and identification of nursing journals using social media. *CIN: Computers, Informatics, Nursing, 39*(6), 291–295. https://doi.org/10.1097/CIN.0000000000000774

Waldrop, J., & Dunlap J. J. (2024). A new question simplifies the search for evidence. *American Journal of Nursing, 124*(3), 34–37. https://doi.org/10.1097/01.NAJ.0001007676.91191.dd

Waldrop, J. B., Dunlap, J. J., & Kennedy, M. S. (2022). Social media and journals: Suggested best practices for nursing editors, authors, readers. *Nurse Author & Editor, 32*(1), 11–14. https://doi.org/10.1111/nae2.33

Waldrop, J., & Likis, F. (2022). Nurse editors' roles and practices. *Journal of Nursing Scholarship, 54*(4), 477–484. https://doi.org/10.1111/jnu.12745

Walker, A. C., Turpin, M. H., Meyers, E. A., Stolz, J. A., Fugelsang, J. A., & Koehler, D. J. (2011). Controlling the narrative: Euphemistic language affects judgements of actions while avoiding perceptions of dishonesty. *Cognition, 211.*

Wilson, J. E., & McAllister, E. (2023). *Implications for the mountain model for EBPQI in DNP education.* http://doi.org/10.2139/ssrn.4704982

IMAGE CREDITS

Fig. 12.1a: Copyright © 2012 Depositphotos/mikdam.

Fig. 12.1b: Copyright © 2019 Depositphotos/andreanissotti.

Fig. 12.1c: Screenshot generated with ebook.online-convert.com.

Fig. 12.1d: Screenshot generated with iBooks. Software Copyright © by Apple, Inc.

Fig. 12.1d.1: Julee Waldrop and Morgan Sabins, Selection from "Pediatric Case Studies to Develop Diagnostic Reasoning," *Pediatric Case Studies to Develop Diagnostic Reasoning.* Copyright © 2021 by Julee Waldrop.

Fig. 12.1e: Screenshot generated with Kindle Direct Publishing Order Report. Software Copyright © by Amazon.com, Inc.

Fig. 12.2: Adapted from Jayne Jennings Dunlap, at al., "Consistent Scholarship Standards among DNP-prepared Faculty Needed: Actionable Insights," *Journal of Professional Nursing,* vol. 21, p. 60. Copyright © by Jayne Jennings Dunlap, at al. (CC BY 4.0) at https://www.sciencedirect.com/science/article/pii/S8755722324000206?via%3Dihub#f0005.

CHAPTER 13

Leadership, Legacy, and Lifelong Learning in Advanced Nursing Practice

Jayne Jennings Dunlap and Paula Clutter

KEY CONCEPTS

Lifelong learning
Leadership
Self-awareness
Mentorship
Team building
Conflict management
Legacy

LEARNING OBJECTIVES

1. Connect EBPQI importance to leadership and management.
2. Define lifelong learning and legacy building.
3. Explore ways to promote project team building and conflict management.
4. Identify the importance of continual mentee and mentor participation.
5. Discuss future directions for EBPQI leadership that transcends the nursing discipline.

> Leaders become great, not because of their power but because of their ability to empower others.
>
> —John Maxwell

Introduction

EBPQI provides a framework for achieving and sustaining evidence-based health care improvements on organizational and system levels. When we realized that a textbook mapped to the AACN level 2 sub-competencies for ANP was urgently needed and could have a significant downstream impact on patients and populations in health care and related settings across the globe, we assembled a contributing author team comprised of representatives of every ANP role and specialty to present you with the first EBPQI fully merged model. We earnestly hope that you have learned how to scale the mountain of EBPQI initiatives and reach the summit to disseminate your work to your target audience, but your journey as an ANP leader does not end there.

Following the critical (and exciting) step of sharing your initiatives through dissemination, your commitment to EBPQI work and learning continues, and it will be career spanning. You will continue to grow both personally and professionally as you lead and oversee teams, set the tone and focus of important projects, and collaborate with others to improve health and health care. All of the information that follows is necessary for leaders to successfully implement and sustain EBPQI. We conclude our journey together with a call to lifelong learning, effective leadership and management, and meaningful professional legacy building. This chapter is devoted and dedicated to you!

Lifelong Learning

Let's begin by returning to the personal case study outlined in Chapter 1 (Box 1.2). Some information that we did not share is that the patient cherished her family (including her cats) and friends, was active in her church and community, and was employed as a store clerk. She suffered a needless and premature death during a hospital stay due to a system breakdown and below-standard care. The apology offered to the patient's family by the health care team's leader was sincere but could not bring back their loved one. I (Jayne) will always remember this patient's curiosity and friendliness, and I hope that sharing her story will serve as a warning and lesson. The patient's suffering and death severely impacted her family, the health care team and its leader, and the system. Monetarily, the final cost of this preventable health care outcome exceeded $600,000. Mistakes can be costly and powerful teachers, so we must try to learn from them. Preventable tragedies in health care inevitably propel professionals toward continual learning.

What does it mean to embrace lifelong learning as a leader? Intellectual curiosity enables nurses and teams to question the status quo and seek answers on a deeper level (Harper et al., 2019; Melnyk et al., 2017). We know that caring, curiosity, and critical thinking are essential to nursing roles; however, the relationships between these concepts, and the most effective strategies to cultivate curiosity, remain less understood and warrant further research (Nadelson et al., 2022). Nurses' curiosity and desire to understand on a deeper level have been linked to improved patient care (Scala et al, 2019). As leaders, we must consistently role-model a spirit of inquiry, which just happens to be the bedrock of EBPQI!

Table 13.1 presents some ideas (with examples) for promoting lifelong learning. We chose these suggestions to stimulate your desire to learn and illuminate a practical pathway on which to build into your professional goals, but there are many learning opportunities you can seek out as a nurse leader. For example, if neither of the certifications related to EBPQI in Table 13.1 suits your situation, find a certification that will specifically and directly benefit you and/or your institution and go for it! What is important is that you embrace learning and explore your interests, taking planned breaks when needed to renew your energy. Remember that organizations often provide leaders with full or partial reimbursement for continuing education with deliverables that align with their strategic plan, so if you ask for monetary assistance or support, be sure to articulate the benefits of your scholarly learning endeavors to the organization.

TABLE 13.1 Suggested Lifelong Learning Practices for Leaders

Suggested Learning Practice	Example(s)
Read regularly	Read books, scholarly works, and journal articles, and be sure to read for fun as well (for more information, review the wellness box in Chapter 1).
Enroll in continuing education opportunities that target your knowledge gaps	Take an implementation science course (e.g. https://epibiostat.ucsf.edu/online-certificate-implementation-science?utm_source=chatgpt.com) or course focused on leading QI (e.g., https://www.ihi.org/education/ihi-open-school/curriculum-and-ce-credits).
Apply for advanced leadership training or fellowships	Seek an additional structured leadership training academy or fellowship (e.g., https://www.sigmanursing.org/learn-grow/sigma-academies/; https://www.aonl.org/education/nursing-fellowships).
Pursue additional certification opportunities	Become certificated in health care quality (https://nahq.org/individuals/cphq-certification/).
Start ongoing leadership notes	Create an easily accessible (e.g., on a mobile device or Google Doc) list of lessons learned as a leader and add updates ASAP.
Write regular reflections	Keep a journal of reflections on problems, progress, and opportunities and update it as these come to mind. Connect the reflections to your values and allow them to inform your personal and professional decisions and commitments.
Serve as a mentor	Work with at least one individual mentee on a mutually beneficial project or goal toward which they aspire. Remember that learning often comes from teaching or guiding (this will be discussed in detail later in this chapter).

Creating a goal-oriented learning plan that is guided by your leadership values will help you determine items to place on your lifelong learning agenda. A learning plan serves as a practical guide to your learning agenda, helping you to translate your learning goals into specific actions over time. Identifying promising sources of information and ongoing learning opportunities can accelerate your progress toward your goals.

Leadership and Management

As we near the end of this journey together, we want to provide you with some advanced leadership and management strategies to support you as you prepare to lead EBPQI teams. Often, EBPQI initiatives are not effectively implemented or sustained due to team management issues signaling missed opportunities to improve care quality on a large scale. In a healthy work environment, leadership and management support all individuals' physical, mental, and social well-being, making them feel valued and respected. Effective EBPQI leaders cultivate a healthy work environment that promotes communication, collaborative teamwork, process improvement, and quality outcomes. They empower people and drive positive change through healthy team cultures. In your ANP role, you are an important leader in health care. Regardless of whether your leadership position is formal or informal, the art of inspiring and empowering others is an important aspect of your EBPQI leadership and management. Setting a positive tone will help you guide individuals and teams toward achievement of your organization's goals and initiatives. It is wise to take time to reflect on your experiences as a leader and identify your leadership and management strengths and values.

Leadership core values are fundamental to maintaining a healthy work environment and should align with the organization's purpose, mission, and vision. As a retired U.S. Air Force (USAF) Reserves Nurse Corps officer (Paula), I hold as my guiding principles the USAF core values of *integrity first*, *service before self*, and *excellence in all we do*. I believe we should do our best at all times, and leadership and management are vital in creating a culture of accountability and excellence.

Leadership integrity and an ethical compass in decision-making are foundational to creating healthy environments ripe for EBPQI initiatives. Honest, transparent, objective, and prompt communication about organizational initiatives, challenges, and successes is essential for building trust and creating an environment that values collaboration, productivity, and positivity. Lack of communication is detrimental to trust, transparency, productivity, and achieving organizational goals and initiatives because individuals tend to create their own narratives without timely and specific information. Role-modeling integrity includes communicating honestly about occurrences, providing facts, and avoiding blame.

Leaders must be responsible for their decisions and should ensure accountability from all individuals, especially those on their team. If you or your EBPQI team makes a mistake, immediately acknowledge and take responsibility for it; never try to conceal the error or shift the blame to others. Leaders who do not disclose errors risk lack of respect, loss of trust and credibility, employee disengagement, and retention problems. A recent literature review of 71 research studies that focused on the concept and correlates of leadership integrity at the individual, group, and organizational level found that perceived alignment of the leader's words and actions determines trust in the leader, which affects both individual and organizational outcomes (Nawaz et al., 2023). Most individuals do not want to work under a leader who lacks integrity or acts in a dishonest and unethical manner and will seek a work environment that better aligns with their personal values.

Effective leadership involves the ability to understand and manage your own emotions as well as those of others. Pause and think for a few moments about how you would describe your ability to recognize and understand your own emotions. What strategies do you use to control your emotions and manage stress? Effective leaders tend to have high emotional intelligence (EI; Goleman et al., 2002) and can create a healthy work environment with solid communication, teamwork, and conflict management. Important aspects of EI include (a) self-awareness, which refers to an individual's recognition of their own emotions and motivations; (b) self-regulation, or the ability to manage one's emotions and reactions by maintaining composure and controlling negative emotions in stressful situations; (c) empathy, which includes active listening and showing compassion; and (d) relationship management, or an understanding of interpersonal relationships (Goleman, 1995).

Effective EBPQI leaders possess strong soft skills (sometimes referred to as transferable skills); these are interpersonal competencies that promote communication and collaboration, and they are essential to inspire, motivate, and influence individuals and teams. EBPQI leaders must also possess hard skills—the technical competencies associated with education, knowledge, professional development, and work experience; however, inadequate soft skills can result in poor communication, low morale, and ineffective team synergy and cohesion, all of which adversely affect performance and productivity.

Building relationships and rapport to promote trust in the work setting is a key role of EBPQI leadership. Social connection fosters individual morale, satisfaction, engagement, and overall well-being (Meta & Gallup, 2023). Individuals who feel safe and connected are comfortable collaborating with others and sharing information and ideas; such interactions are important for stimulating creative EBPQI innovations and strategies on organizational initiatives. Psychological safety in the work setting is essential; individuals must be able to express their authentic self without fear of negative feedback. One of the cornerstones of the leadership role is creating an inclusive, supportive environment with appropriate resources and professional development opportunities to enhance EBPQI team skills.

Part of your professional journey is discovering your EBPQI leadership and management style and building on your leadership skills. I (Paula) have a background in EBPQI and lean toward being a situational leader—I adjust my leadership and management to meet the needs of the situation and individuals involved. Autocratic leadership provides direct instruction and guidance and is used in crisis management or to assist individuals who lack the knowledge and experience needed in a specific situation. I tend to be a democratic manager in that I value the input of team members. I have found that effective EBPQI leadership and management entails solid communication and interpersonal skills, active listening skills, and a commitment to creating an environment in which individuals feel that their voices are heard and valued.

The following websites provide resources that can assist you in enhancing your EBPQI leadership and management skills:

- The American Association of Nurse Practitioners (AANP) offers leadership and management publications and webinars as well as networking opportunities with other nurse practioners (www.aanp.org/).

- The American Nurses Association (ANA) provides leadership and management resources relevant to the nursing profession, including a section devoted to advocacy and continuing education resources for advanced nursing practice (www.nursingworld.org/).

Many non-nursing websites provide valuable leadership and management resources to expand your knowledge and skills to keep in mind as you lead EBPQI initiatives:

- Leadership Now (https://www.leadershipnow.com)
- TED Talks (www.ted.com)

EBPQI Team Building

There is no perfect setting, but leadership and management generally strive to hire and retain talented individuals who can be a "good fit" in a productive team. A cohesive team can work well during difficult and challenging times. Leadership role-modeling and adherence to core values provides a sense of assurance during times of uncertainty. Negativity breeds negativity; therefore, confident and affirmative leadership is vital for nurturing a positive daily mind-set among the team. The motivational speaker Jim Rohn offers a useful reminder: "Don't major in minor things" (Ndagba, 2023). Stay focused on what is significant and demands your attention as a leader. Unwise micromanaging or concentrating on insignificant details will drain both your own and your team's energy and joy. An effective leader role-models and creates an environment of hope and belief that positive outcomes are achievable and assists with problem solving issues if the timeline or goals veer off track. Remember to provide timely praise and honest appreciation (Reynolds, 2021) because a positive mind-set will help your team to persevere, demonstrate resilience and grit in challenging situations, work as a team to problem solve, and improve processes to maintain a culture of excellence. Repeated topics and themes in this chapter revolve around the importance of communication and collaboration in team building. Box 13.1 lists some practical team-building stepwise tips for forming and leading a high-performing team.

BOX 13.1: TEAM BUILDING TIPS

1. Form a team of individuals who have the skills needed to accomplish the task(s).
2. Provide professional development to enhance skills required for the task(s).
3. Understand and communicate the team purpose and goals for accomplishing the task(s).
4. Communicate and understand each team member's role and responsibility in achieving the goals and accomplishing the task(s).

5. Establish routine meetings to discuss progress, elicit feedback, and address questions or concerns related to tasks and timelines.
6. Communicate objectives and constructive feedback to ensure that the team accomplishes task(s).
7. Create an environment of respect and trust in which team members feel that their input is valued.
8. Promote quality improvement steps to include the use of evidence-based data in decision-making.
9. Maintain a positive mind-set and deal with challenges as they are presented.
10. Consult with leadership for guidance and keep your chain of command informed of issues and concerns.
11. Address concerns in a timely manner and work toward conflict resolution.
12. Acknowledge individual and team accomplishments and work efforts (positive verbal praise and recognition can have a powerful impact on motivation and productivity!).
13. Maintain individual and team accountability for contributions, quality of work, and timeline adherence.
14. Encourage creative problem solving to keep the team on track to accomplish tasks.
15. Find ways to have fun! These could include a potluck meal at work or a team meal outside the work setting (incorporating fun activities can enhance communication, collaboration, connection, commitment, and productivity).

Effective leaders ensure that initiatives remain on track by setting clear goals, a timeline, a plan of action, metrics, and respective individual roles. Individual, team, and leadership persistence as well as team building and engagement drive the achievement of EBPQI-focused organizational goals and initiatives.

Conflict Management

Diversity of thought is encouraged and valued in a healthy work environment that promotes EBPQI. Individual ideas, perspectives, and personality styles are enriching but can sometimes lead to conflict. Dealing with areas of conflict is a vital role of leadership. All team members contribute to success by accomplishing their respective tasks, so timely conflict management is essential to the achievement of organizational initiatives. Conflict issues rarely go away on their own but tend to escalate without proper intervention, so they must be addressed swiftly. Leaders often find themselves cast in the role of facilitator or mediator in conflict management issues. A useful "come to the table" intervention involves holding a group meeting to (a) ensure that everyone involved understands one another's individual perspective related to specific issues and (b) formulate a plan to move forward. Basic guidelines when dealing with a conflict issue are as follows:

- Assume positive intent (i.e., that individuals are performing at their best).
- Ensure active listening to all perspectives pertaining to the conflict issue. Consider each perspective equally and discard none until you have heard all.
- Depersonalize the conflict by focusing on the issue rather than on individuals.
- Manage emotions during communication and use objective data to address areas of concern. Emotional outbursts detract from resolving conflict.
- Avoid reading assumptions into emails. Misinterpretation of the tone of email messages can be prevented if individuals communicate issues in person or via a telephone call.
- Remember the goal: to work toward a resolution with the individuals involved and move forward in a positive manner with an agreed plan of action.

Routine communication with your supervisor/boss is an essential part of transparent communication and relationship building as it (a) keeps them informed of major issues that might warrant intervention at their level if not resolved, (b) allows you an opportunity to obtain their feedback and guidance, and (c) protects you by ensuring there can be no deniability of information about conflict issues that might require action to avoid negative outcomes in the organization.

An important part of the EBPQI leadership role is assuming responsibility to address unprofessional or inappropriate behavior in a timely manner so that issues can be resolved between the individuals involved without seeking external support. Effective leaders cultivate a healthy work environment by maintaining accountability for professional behavior and performance. Professional development can increase a leader's conflict resolution skills and comfort with addressing conflict.

Mentorship

Mentorship describes the powerful influence, direction, and guidance offered by an experienced person to a less experienced person over time to achieve an expected outcome. Mentors typically help their mentees obtain optimal growth, role development, and effectiveness (Hoover et al., 2020; Koon et al., 2020). In nursing practice, a mentor may be a trusted teacher or colleague who guides and facilitates EBP or some other endeavor (Melnyk & Fineout-Overholt, 2023). Mentors serve as role models; they embody leadership qualities that others wish to emulate, offer essential advice and candid feedback, and establish and maintain professional boundaries (Clark, 2015). Research has found that new graduate nurses are more likely to follow the practices of role models than recently learned, evidence-based patient care methods (Breckenridge-Sproat, 2015); this finding highlights the importance of trusted mentors who are willing to share their extensive EBPQI knowledge and skills.

BOX 13.2: EDITORS' MENTORSHIP IN ACTION

I (Jayne) began reading issues of the *Journal for Nurse Practitioners* as a nurse practitioner (NP) student, and I was compelled by the writing style of the journal editor, Julee Waldrop (coeditor of this textbook). I began searching for her work and was awestruck by her meaningful productivity and substantial contributions to the literature and the nursing discipline as a whole. At the annual American Association of Nurse Practitioners (AANP) conference the following year, I signed up to attend one of Julee's podium presentations, which focused on article authorship. My first manuscript had recently been published, and I wanted to learn more about this process that Julee had so clearly mastered. I immediately noticed that Julee was a skilled presenter: She easily engaged the audience with an authentic style that resonated with attendees. After the presentation, I gathered my courage and approached Julee to thank her for the presentation. She was kind and gracious, and I left longing to connect with her again, somehow, someday.

Two months later, I spotted Julee at another conference and approached her again. This time, I decided that I didn't have anything to lose, and I asked Julee if she would mentor me. She looked surprised, said that she would consider it, and asked me to email her my CV and some additional information. Later, I learned that Julee was considering whether and how mentoring me would benefit us both. Reciprocity is part of the mentor–mentee relationship that Julee instinctively knew to offer when approaching someone for mentorship; however, I had not yet learned this lesson. Julee emailed me back, and we arranged to meet on the last day of the conference. She greeted me with a warm but serious demeanor, agreed to mentor me, and invited me to be the social media director for the journal of which she was editor-in-chief; I would schedule social media posts for the journal on her behalf. I agreed and still remember what it felt like to shake Julee's extended hand. That firm handshake and all the interactions that followed would dramatically change the course of my professional career and positively impact my personal life.

Julee quickly initiated monthly mentorship meetings that were held virtually as we lived in different states. She led our first meeting by presenting a Google folder she had prepared outlining my future work at the journal, then asked what project I would like us to work on together. I didn't expect that we would be doing a project together immediately, but this set a productive tone that would permanently mark our mentor–mentee relationship. We have continued to work to deliver problem-informed, meaningful contributions that we believe are important for health and health care improvement. Although our work resides in shared folders and Google docs, and almost all of our meetings have been virtual, for the past couple of years, we have prioritized meeting in person at least once a year as a reward for our hard work.

The experiences and advice that Julee has gifted me have shaped me as a leader. I know that I can call on her if a leadership dilemma arises. She will challenge me, ask for rationales for my decisions, and care enough to tell me the truth in a kind and diplomatic way. These are qualities that I strive to emulate in my own role as a mentor.

While Julee and I were working on the prelicensure award-winning EBPQI nursing textbook that precedes this one, we met weekly rather than monthly and enjoyed our meetings immensely. You are holding this book in your hands right now because we knew it was needed but also because partnering on another book gave us a good reason to keep meeting every week instead of every month! I hope this book will help you as a leader because climbing a mountain is a perfect metaphor for my mentorship relationship with Julee: We continue to scale mountains, seeking ways to guide leaders of health care teams to new heights so that their EBPQI work can positively impact ever-larger populations in innovative and exciting ways.

Julee's impact and investment remind me of Dolly Parton's words: *If your actions create a legacy that inspires others to dream more, learn more, do more, and become more, then you are an excellent leader.* Knowing, learning from, and being inspired by Julee, who was brave enough to take me on as a mentee, has been a precious gift. I hope her generous investment is shared with you in some way through the contents of this textbook. I urge you to seek someone worthy of your emulation, work together with shared passion to accomplish more than you could separately, and enjoy the journey!

Mentorship should be a rewarding and mutually meaningful experience. As you consider the mentorship story outlined in Box 13.2, ask yourself which aspects of mentorship are most valuable to you. If your team members do not have access to internal EBPQI mentorship in your setting, consider the possibilities of obtaining an external mentor. External EBPQI mentorship in an academic setting has been associated with positive initial outcomes (Dunlap et al., 2023), and we believe this may hold true for practice and policy arenas as well. We challenge you to consider how you could best serve as a mentor in your ANP specialty or role, given your qualities and skills. Box 13.3 outlines some practical recommendations for service as a mentor.

BOX 13.3: PRACTICAL RECOMMENDATIONS FOR SERVICE AS A MENTOR

- Seek out mentees who are working on projects that could benefit from expertise you can share.
- Organize a plan for scheduled meetings and set SMART goals.
- Provide honest feedback for professional development purposes.
- Lead by example and be transparent about mistakes you have made and learned from.
- Connect your mentee(s) with stakeholders or notables in the field as appropriate and according to their specific needs.

Remember that if you can pilot the ship as a trusted leader, you will likely be asked to guide, oversee, and collaborate on many EBPQI projects and serve as a mentor to others. When approached with a new project and/or mentorship request, you should ascertain what the next steps will be and gather more information as appropriate. If you need time to think about your response, feel free to say that you are honored by the request but want time to consider it. Be sure to let the person or team know when you will follow up with your decision.

Living Your Legacy: Leading by Example

Because the focus of this textbook is EBPQI leadership, we want to end with some practical pearls from our nursing administration and practice leadership roles with evidence-based support. You are the architect of your professional career. Part of constructing your career can involve creating and implementing a self-stewardship plan. A self-stewardship plan allows you to identify areas for professional development and set goals to achieve your full potential.

Self-Stewardship and Self-Awareness

We have a responsibility to be mindfully aware and manage our emotions and personal resources in our leadership roles. One helpful means of doing this is by creating a self-stewardship plan to inform your decision-making effectiveness. Integrity involves knowing when and admitting that you need support. Survey the activities and responsibilities with which you have tasked yourself as a leader: Which ones are essential? Which ones can you let go? Which ones can you delegate? As your work progresses, regularly continue to assess your plan: What is working? What can you do less of? What can you amplify?

Every leader leaves a legacy and indelible imprint on the individuals they lead and on their organization. A leadership legacy identifies your values, beliefs, leadership style, and contributions. Your unique contributions are identified in your leadership legacy, so it is important to have clarity about who you are as a person and leader before leading others (Trepanier, 2023). Your hard and soft skills as a leader will define your legacy, so we encourage you to strive to have a positive, lasting influence on those you lead.

Take time to reflect on your professional journey. What do you want your leadership legacy to be?

BOX 13.4: PAULA'S LEGACY IN ACTION

I am sharing my reflections on my leadership legacy in the hope that they will inspire you to define your own EBPQI leadership approach and legacy. Throughout my 36 years in the nursing profession, I have let the USAF core values guide my leadership and management of others. Additional fundamental beliefs that hold significance for me and influence my leadership actions include the following:

- Embrace lifelong learning.
- Lead by example.
- Empower others.
- Create personal connections.
- Foster collaboration.
- Create a culture of accountability.
- Develop leadership in others.
- Maintain a work–life balance.

In my work as an EBPQI leader, I supported the principle of prioritizing service over self by placing the important needs of others, including those of the organization, ahead of my personal interests and desires. In my professional career, I have been asked to step up to serve in times of need and crisis, and I don't regret my past decisions to assist with these leadership opportunities. An effective leader seeks mutually beneficial outcomes and recognizes that, in most situations, doing so involves reaching a compromise on the best way to meet the organization's needs.

I have profound respect for Mother Teresa and her legacy. She was a servant leader and an exemplary role model of love, compassion, and selflessness in serving the sick and poor in India. Mother Teresa embodied love and valued every human being with her steadfast dedication to help others in need. Her impact was huge, and her example has inspired me and many others to be kind, charitable, and generous to those who are less fortunate.

Servant leadership focuses on serving others. Servant leaders believe in supporting team members for the collective good and success of the organization. The principles of servant leadership resonate deeply with me. Leading brings rewards as well as challenges and demands substantial effort and energy. Leadership opportunities may require time commitments and efforts that are physically and mentally fatiguing. As I reflect on past leadership and management roles, I realize that although declining opportunities to step up might have been easier or more comfortable, doing so would have meant missing out on invaluable growth experiences and disheartening my leadership chain of command. One strategy to handle the demands of leadership is to maintain a positive mind-set and surround yourself with optimistic individuals who provide support and inspiration and recharge your energy when it is depleted.

Effective leaders should empower and inspire others to reach their full potential. Offering opportunities for training, professional development, and mentorship is vital for fostering individual growth and advancement. Leaders should invest in human resources—which are the most valuable assets. They should allocate their time thoughtfully, not only addressing substandard performance or other problematic issues in a timely manner but also giving ample attention to recognizing and supporting high performance.

I encourage you to not let good opportunities slip by, even if they challenge you to step outside your comfort zone; consider them realistically, have courage, pursue ongoing development and learning, and embrace leadership and management professional growth opportunities with enthusiasm. For my willingness to step up and serve in leadership roles, I have earned recognition as an effective leader whose management skills and quality performance have led to advancement in administrative positions. Although leadership and management roles frequently come with challenging and complex responsibilities, the immense value and gratification of these opportunities cannot be emphasized enough; however, I want to be clear that it is okay to decline opportunities so that you do not overextend yourself because maintaining a healthy work life balance is crucial.

Self-care is essential to refuel your energy, and an effective leader should role-model self-care and create a work–life balance by setting boundaries that prioritize their physical and mental well-being. I am passionate about my work and enjoy what I do, but I make it a priority to place my family over work-related responsibilities. I am grateful for my supportive family, who recognize the significance of my work and understand its integral role in my professional fulfillment.

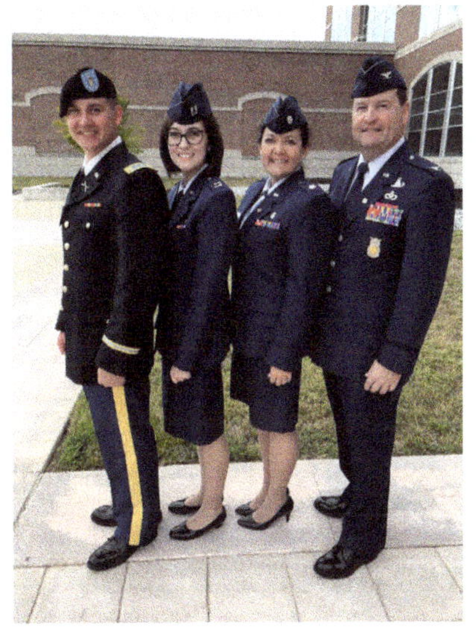
Image 13.1

The nursing profession greatly benefits from your APN leadership! Be a compassionate and effective leader, dedicated to fostering a culture of excellence and accountability and to empowering others to thrive and flourish. I firmly believe that your leadership will have a positive impact on others and your organization. Your potential for greatness is extraordinary, so be the best you can be!

WELLNESS IN ACTION: GRATITUDE

Pausing to reflect on the many people, things, and experiences for which we are grateful offers invaluable benefits, including reduction in depressive symptoms (Iodice et al., 2021). Even short-term gratitude interventions have been associated with sustained benefits over time (Bohlmeijer et al., 2021). Not only should we engage in grateful living, but as leaders, we should role-model demonstrations of gratitude to our teams. Gratitude is mutually beneficial for all participants in a giving exchange. Consider engaging in the following practices on a routine basis to strengthen your own well-being as well as that of your team:

- Ask others what they are most grateful for during a meal, meeting, or team-building activity as appropriate.
- Share your gratitude with others publicly and specifically. Individuals and teams typically desire and respond well to verbal praise.
- Send thank-you and congratulatory notes (handwritten and/or emailed) to your team to let them know that their achievements are noticed and appreciated.
- Learn what matters to your team members, and give them thoughtful tokens of appreciation in a timely manner.

WRAPPING UP

We hope this textbook has provided you with the fundamental information you need to lead EBPQI teams in current and future initiatives. EBP and QI allow nurses at all levels to make intentional and sound evidence-based decisions (Melnyk &

Fineout-Overholt, 2023; White et al., 2021) in practice, education, and policy. We must lead by example to achieve optimal care provision because we owe this to patients and populations across the globe. Adherence to EBP improves patient outcomes and returns on investment for health care systems (Conner et al., 2023); moreover, it is simply the right thing to do. As nurse leaders, we share a professional responsibility to improve the current state of health care through EBPQI.

Prioritizing lifelong learning in your personal and professional life will help you achieve your goals in the evolving field of health care. As leaders engaged in ANP, we welcome you to embrace a leadership role, be it formal or informal, and look forward to witnessing the far-reaching impact of your leadership on our profession. We hope that this textbook will fuel a persistent thirst for knowledge, a career-spanning investment in your leadership skills, a pursuit of excellence as you foster your own best practices, and a legacy of positive and productive leadership.

REFLECTION QUESTIONS

1. What are some practical ways you can cultivate a healthy EBPQI culture in your organization?
2. How can you role-model lifelong learning as an EBPQI leader?

REFERENCES

Breckenridge-Sproat, S., Throop, M. D., Raju, D., Murphy, D., Loan, L., & Patrician, P (2015). Building a unit-level mentored program to sustain a culture of inquiry for evidence-based practice. *Clinical Nurse Specialist, 29*(6), 329–337. https://doi.org/10.1097/NUR.0000000000000161

Bohlmeijer, E. T., Kraiss, J. T., Watkins, P. et al. (2021). Promoting gratitude as a resource for sustainable mental health: Results of a 3-armed randomized controlled trial up to 6 months follow-up. *J Happiness Stud, 22*, 1011–1032. https://doi.org/10.1007/s10902-020-00261-5

Clark, C. (2015). The power and potential of positive mentoring. *Nurse Educator, 40*(3), 109–110. https://doi.org/10.1097/NNE.0000000000000158

Connor, L., Dean, J., McNett, M., Tydings, D. M., Shrout, A., Gorsuch, P. F., ... & Gallagher-Ford, L. (2023). Evidence-based practice improves patient outcomes and healthcare system return on investment: Findings from a scoping review. *Worldviews on Evidence-Based Nursing, 20*(1), 6–15. https://doi.org/10.1111/wvn.12621

Goleman, D. (1995). *Emotional intelligence: Why it can matter more than IQ.* Bantam Books.

Goleman, D., Boyatzis, R., & McKee, A. (2002). *The new leaders: Transforming the art of leadership into the science of results.* Harvard Business Review Press.

Harper, M., Warren, J., Bradley, D., Bindon, S., & Maloney, P. (2019) Nursing professional development's spirit of inquiry focus areas. *Journal for Nurses in Professional Development, 35*(3), 118–124. https://doi.org/10.1097/NND.0000000000000515

Hoover, J., Koon, A. D., Rosser, E. N., & Rao, K. D. (2020). Mentoring the working nurse: a scoping review. *Human resources for health, 18*(1), 52. https://doi.org/10.1186/s12960-020-00491-x

Iodice, J. A., Malouff, J. M., & Schutte, N. S. (2021). The association between gratitude and and meta-analysis. *International Journal of Depression and Anxiety, 4*(24).

Koon, A. D., Hoover, J., Sonthalia, S., Rosser, E., Gore, A., & Rao, K. D. (2020). In-service nurse mentoring in 2020, the year of the nurse and the midwife: learning from Bihar, India. *Global health action, 13*(1), 1823101.

Melnyk, B. M., & Fineout-Overholt, E. (2023). *Evidence-based practice in nursing & healthcare: A guide to best practice* (5th ed.). LWW.

Melnyk, B. M., Gallagher-Ford, L., & Fineout-Overholt, E. (2017). *Implementing evidence-based practice competencies in healthcare: A practical guide for improving quality, safety, & outcomes.* Sigma Theta Tau.

Meta & Gallup. (2023). *State of social connections 2023 report.* https://www.circles.com/resources/social-connection-in-workplace-key-to-employee-engagement-and-wellbeing

Nadelson, S. G., & Nadelson, L. S. (2019). Connecting critical thinking, caring, and curiosity in nurse education: Exploring the beliefs and practices of nurse educators. *Journal of Nursing Education and Practice, 9*(8), 1–10. https://doi.org/10.5430/jnep.v9n8p1

Nawaz, A., Gilal, F., Channa, K., & Gilal, R. (2023). Going deep into a leader's' integrity: A systematic review and the way forward. *European Management Journal, 41*(6), 845–864. https://doi.org/10.1016/j.emj.2022.11.001

Ndagba, I. (2024). *Jim Rohn 100 greatest quotes*. Independently published.

Reynolds, S. S. (2021). How to win friends and influence people—as a nursing leader. *Nurse Leader, 19*(1), 87–89. https://doi.org/10.1016/j.mnl.2020.07.013

Scala, E., Patterson, B., Stavarski, D. H., & Mackay, P. (2019). Engagement in research: A clinical nurse profile and motivating factors. *Journal for Nurses in Professional Development, 35*(3), 137–143. https://doi.org/10.1097/NND.0000000000000538

Trepanier, S. (2023). Leadership legacy. *Journal of Continuing Education, 54*(4), 152. https://doi.org/10.3928/00220124-20230310-03

White, K. M., Dudley-Brown, S., & Terhaar, M. F. (2021). *Translation of evidence into nursing and healthcare* (3rd ed.). Springer.

Appendix A: Competency Index

American Association of Colleges of Nursing: New (2021) Essentials: Core Competencies for Advanced Nursing Education

Essential EBP-related Competencies and Level 2 Sub-Competencies for the Professional Nurse Addressed by Chapter

The American Association of Colleges of Nursing's (AACN, 2021) core competencies for professional nursing education provide 10 domains of competence that constitute the expectations of the practicing nurse with integration of the concept of EBP throughout all domains and quality and safety with its own designated domain:

- Domain 1: Knowledge for Nursing Practice
- Domain 2: Person-Centered Care
- Domain 3: Population Health
- Domain 4: Scholarship for the Nursing Discipline
- Domain 5: Quality and Safety
- Domain 6: Interprofessional Partnerships
- Domain 7: Systems-Based Practice
- Domain 8: Informatics and Healthcare Technologies
- Domain 9: Professionalism
- Domain 10: Personal, Professional and Leadership Development

This textbook will provide you with the knowledge and tools to demonstrate several AACN competencies and level 2 sub-competencies beyond entry-level practice related to EBP and QI expected of the advanced-level nurse. While you learned much about EBPQI leadership throughout this book, remember that you set the tone for interdisciplinary team project participation that transcends the nursing discipline.

Domain	Competency	Sub-Competency
1	1.1 Demonstrate an understanding of the discipline of nursing's distinct perspective and where shared perspectives exist in other disciplines.	1.1g Integrate an understanding of nursing history in advancing nursing's influence in healthcare.
1	1.2 Apply theory and research-based knowledge from nursing, the arts, humanities and other sciences.	1.2i Demonstrate socially responsible leadership. 1.2e Translate theories from nursing and other disciplines into practice.
1	1.3 Demonstrate clinical judgment founded on a board knowledge base.	1.3d Integrate foundational and advanced specialty knowledge into clinical reasoning.
4	4.1 Advance the scholarship of nursing.	D 4.1h Apply and critically evaluate advanced knowledge in a defined area of nursing practice. 4. 4.1i Engage in scholarship to advance health. 4.1 4.1j Discern appropriate applications of quality improvement, research and evaluation methodologies. r444.1k Collaborate to advance one's scholarship 44 4.1m Advocate with the interprofessional team and with other stakeholders for the contributions of nursing scholarship.
4	4.2 Integrate best evidence into nursing practice.	4.2h Address opportunities for innovation and changes in practice.
9	9.1 Demonstrate an ethical complement of one's practice reflective of nursing's mission to society.	9.1i Model ethical behaviors in practice and leadership roles.
9	9.2 Employ participatory approach to nursing care.	9.2h Foster opportunities for intentional presence in practice. 9.2i Identify innovative and evidence-based practices that promote person-centered care. 9.2k Model professional expectations for therapeutic relationships. 9.2l Facilitate communication that promotes a participatory approach.
9	9.5 Demonstrate the professional identify of nursing.	9.5f Articulate nursing's unique professional identity to other interprofessional team members and the public 9.5h Identify opportunities to lead with moral courage to influence team decision-making.
10	10.1 Demonstrate a commitment to personal health and wellbeing.	10.1c Contribute to an environment that promotes self-care, personal health, and well-being.

Domain	Competency	Sub-Competency
1	1.2 Apply theory and research-based knowledge from nursing, the arts, humanities and other sciences.	1.2g Apply a systematic and defendable approach to nursing practice decisions. 1.2h Employ ethical decision making to assess, intervene, and evaluate nursing care. 1.2i Demonstrate socially responsible leadership.
1	Demonstrate clinical judgment founded on a broad knowledge base.	1.3d Integrate foundational and advanced speciality knowledge into clinical reasoning. 1.3e Synthesize current and emerging evidence to influence practice 1.3f Analyze decision models from nursing and other knowledge domains to improve clinical judgment.
2	2.2 Communicate effectively with individuals.	2.2e Apply individualized information, such as genetic/genomic, pharmacogenetic, and environmental exposure information in the delivery of personalized healthcare. 2.2j Facilitate difficult conversations with disclosure of sensitive information.
2	2.5 Develop a plan of care.	2.5h Lead and collaborate with an interprofessional team to develop a comprehensive plan of care. 2.5i Prioritize risk mitigation strategies to prevent or reduce adverse outcomes. 2.5j Develop evidence-based interventions to improve quality and safety.
3	3.1 Manage population health.	3.1k Analyze primary and secondary population health data for multiple populations against relevant benchmarks. 3.1l Use established or evolving methods to determine population-focused priorities for care.
4	4.1 Advance the scholarship of nursing.	D 4.1k Collaborate to advance one's scholarship. 4. 4.1a Demonstrate an understanding of the different approaches to scholarly practice. 4.1 4.1e Participate in scholarly inquiry as a team member. 4.1
4	4.2 Integrate best evidence into nursing practice.	4.2g Use diverse sources of evidence to inform practice 4.2j Articulate inconsistencies between practice policies and best evidence.

(*Continued*)

CHAPTER 2: *(Continued)*

Domain	Competency	Sub-Competency
4	4.3 Promote ethical conduct of scholarly activities.	4.3h Implement processes that support ethical conduct in practice and scholarship.
5	5.1 Apply quality improvement principles in care delivery.	5.1i Establish and incorporate data driven benchmarks to monitor system performance. 5.1j Use national safety resources to lead team-based change initiatives.
5	5.2 Contribute to a culture of patient safety.	5.2g Evaluate the alignment of system data and comparative patient safety benchmarks. 5.2h Lead analysis of actual errors, near misses and potential situations that would impact safety. 5.2i Design evidence-based interventions to mitigate risk.
5	5.3 Contribute to a culture of provider and work environment safety.	5.3e Advocate for structures, policies, and processes that promote a culture of safety and prevent workplace risks and injury. 5.3f Foster a just culture reflecting civility and respect. 5.3g Create a safe and transparent culture for reporting incidents. 5.3h Role model and lead well-being and resiliency for self and team.
6	6.3 Use knowledge of nursing and other healthcare professions to address healthcare needs.	6.3d Direct interprofessional activities and initiatives.
6	6.4 Work with other professions to maintain a climate of mutual learning, respect and shared values.	6.4e Practice self-assessment to mitigate conscious and implicit biases toward other team members. 6.4f Foster an environment that supports the constructive sharing of multiple perspectives and enhances interprofessional learning. 6.4g Integrate diversity, equity, and inclusion into team practices.
7	7.1 Apply knowledge of systems to work effectively across the continuum of care.	7.1f Participate in system-wide initiatives that improve healthcare delivery and/or outcomes. 7.1g Analyze system-wide processes to optimize outcomes.
9	9.1 Demonstrate an ethical comportment of one's practice reflective of nursing's mission to society.	9.1i Model ethical behaviors in practice and leadership roles.

Domain	Competency	Sub-Competency
9	9.3 Demonstrate accountability to the individual, society and profession.	9.3i Advocate for nursing's professional responsibility for ensuring optimal care outcomes. 9.3j Demonstrate leadership skills when participating in professional activities and/or organizations. 9.3k Address actual or potential hazards and/or errors. 9.3l Foster a practice environment that promotes accountability for care outcomes. 9.3m Advocate for policies/practices that promote social justice and health equity.
9	9.4 Comply with relevant laws, policies and regulations.	9.4d Advocate for policies that enable nurses to practice to the full extent of their education. 9.4e Assess the interaction between regulatory agency requirements and quality, fiscal, and value-based indicators. 9.4h Participate in the implementation of policies and regulations to improve the professional practice environment and healthcare outcomes.

CHAPTER 3: Comprehensive Clinical Questions and Specific Aims

Domain	Competency	Sub-Competency
1	1.2 Apply theory and research-based knowledge from nursing, the arts, humanities, and other sciences.	1.2g Apply a systematic and defendable approach to nursing practice decisions.
2	2.5 Develop a plan of care.	2.5h Lead and collaborate with an interprofessional team to develop a comprehensive plan of care. 2.5j Develop evidence-based interventions to improve outcomes and safety.
3	3.1 Manage population health.	3.1l Use established or evolving methods to determine population-focused priorities for care.
4	4.1 Advance the Scholarship of Nursing.	4.1h Apply and critically evaluate advanced knowledge in a defined area of nursing practice. 4.1i Engage in scholarship to advance health. 4.1k Collaborate to advance one's scholarship. 4.1m Advocate within the interprofessional team and with other stakeholders for the contributions to nursing scholarship.

(Continued)

CHAPTER 3: *(Continued)*

Domain	Competency	Sub-Competency
4	4.2 Integrate best evidence into nursing practice.	4. 4.2a Use diverse sources of evidence to inform practice.
6	6.1 Communicate in a manner that facilitates a partnership approach to quality care delivery.	5t 6.1j Communicate nursing's unique disciplinary knowledge to strengthen interprofessional partnerships. 6. 6.1k Provide expert consultation for other members of the healthcare team in one's area of practice.
7	7.1 Apply knowledge of systems to work effectively across the continuum of care.	Gf 7.1e Participate in organizational strategic planning.
10	10.2 Demonstrate a spirit of inquiry that fosters flexibility and professional maturity.	2d 10.2g Demonstrate cognitive flexibility in managing change within the complex environment. 10.2i Foster activities that support a culture of lifelong learning.

CHAPTER 4: Leading Literature Searches

Domain	Competency	Sub-Competency
1	1.2 Apply theory and research-based knowledge from nursing, the arts, humanities, and other sciences.	1.2g Apply a systematic and defendable approach to nursing practice decisions.
1	1.3 Demonstrate clinical judgment founded on a broad knowledge base.	1.3e Synthesize current and emerging evidence to influence practice.
2	2.6 Demonstrate accountability for care delivery.	2.6i Apply current and emerging evidence to the development of care guidelines/tools.
3	3.4 Advance equitable population health policy.	3.4f Identify opportunities to influence the policy process. 3.4h Engage in strategies to influence policy change.
4	4.1 Advance the Scholarship of Nursing.	4.1i Engage in scholarship to advance health.
4	4.2 Integrate best evidence into nursing practice.	4. 4.2f Use diverse sources of evidence to inform practice. E 4. Address opportunities for innovation and changes in practice.
10	10.2 Demonstrate a spirit of inquiry that fosters flexibility and professional maturity.	2d 10.2i Foster activities that support a culture of lifelong learning.
10	10.3 Develop capacity for leadership.	10.3 Influence intentional change guided by leadership principles and theories.

CHAPTER 5: Leading Critical Appraisal of Quantitative Evidence

Domain	Competency	Sub-Competency
1	1.2 Apply theory and research-based knowledge from nursing, the arts, humanities, and other sciences.	1.2f Synthesize knowledge from nursing and other disciplines to inform education, practice, and research. 1.2i Demonstrate socially responsible leadership.
1	1.3 Demonstrate clinical judgment founded on a broad knowledge base.	1.3d Synthesize current and emerging evidence to influence practice.
4	4.1 Advance the scholarship of nursing.	D 4.1i Engage in scholarship to advance health. 4.1 4.1k Collaborate to advance one's scholarship. 4.1 4.1m Advocate within the interprofessional team and with other stakeholders for the contributions of nursing scholarship.
4	4.2 Integrate best evidence into nursing practice.	4.2g Lead the translation of evidence into practice.
7	7.3 Optimize system effectiveness through application of innovation and evidence-based practice.	7.3e Apply innovative and evidence-based strategies focusing on system preparedness and capabilities.

CHAPTER 6: Leading Critical Appraisal of Qualitative Evidence

Domain	Competency	Sub-Competency
1	1.2 Apply theory and research-based knowledge from nursing, the arts, humanities, and other sciences.	1.2f Synthesize knowledge from nursing and other disciplines to inform education, practice, and research. 1.2i Demonstrate socially responsible leadership.
1	1.3 Demonstrate clinical judgment founded on a broad knowledge base	1.3d Synthesize current and emerging evidence to influence practice.
4	4.1 Advance the scholarship of nursing	D 4.1i Engage in scholarship to advance health. 4.1 4.1k Collaborate to advance one's scholarship. 4.1 4.1m Advocate within the interprofessional team and with other stakeholders for the contributions of nursing scholarship.
4	4.2 Integrate best evidence into nursing practice	4.2b Evaluate appropriateness and strength of the evidence. 4.2c Use best evidence in practice.
7	7.3 Optimize system effectiveness through application of innovation and evidence-based practice.	7.3e Apply innovative and evidence-based strategies focusing on system preparedness and capabilities.

CHAPTER 7: Leading Appraisal of Other Evidence to Inform Best Practice

Domain	Competency	Sub-Competency
1	1.2 Apply theory and research-based knowledge from nursing, the arts, humanities, and other sciences.	1.2f Synthesize knowledge from nursing and other disciplines to inform education, practice, and research. 1.2i Demonstrate socially responsible leadership.
1	1.3 Demonstrate clinical judgment founded on a broad knowledge base.	1.3d Synthesize current and emerging evidence to influence practice.
4	4.1 Advance the scholarship of nursing.	4. 1.b 4.1c A 4.1i Engage in scholarship to advance health. 4.1 4.1k Collaborate to advance one's scholarship. 4.1 4.1m Advocate within the interprofessional team and with other stakeholders for the contributions of nursing scholarship.
4	4.2 Integrate best evidence into nursing practice	4.2g Lead the translation of evidence into practice. 4.2f Use diverse sources of evidence to inform practice.
7	7.3 Optimize system effectiveness through application of innovation and evidence-based practice.	7.3a 7 7.3e Apply innovative and evidence-based strategies cu focusing on system preparedness and capabilities.

CHAPTER 8: Patient Preferences and Values

Domain	Competency	Sub-Competency
1	1.2 Apply theory and research-based knowledge from nursing the arts, humanities and other sciences.	1.2i Demonstrate socially responsible leadership.
2	2.1 Engage with the individual in establishing a caring relationship.	2.1d Promote caring relationships to effect positive outcomes. 2.1e Foster caring relationships.
2	2.2 Communicate effectively with individuals.	2.2g Demonstrate advanced communication skills and techniques using a variety of modalities with diverse audiences. 2.2h Design evidence-based, person-centered engagement materials.
2	2.5 Develop a plan of care.	2.5h Lead and collaborate with an interprofessional team to develop a comprehensive plan of care.

Domain	Competency	Sub-Competency
3	3.2 Engage in effective partnerships.	3.2e Challenge biases and barriers that impact population health outcomes. 3.2g Lead partnerships to improve population health outcomes.
4	4.2 Integrate best evidence into nursing practice.	4.2f Use diverse sources of evidence to inform practice.
9	9.2 Employ participatory approach to nursing care.	9.2h Foster opportunities for intentional presence in practice. 9.2i Identify innovative and evidence-based practices that promote person-centered care. 9.2j Advocate for practices that advance diversity, equity, and inclusion. 9.2k Model professional expectations for therapeutic relationships. 9.2l Facilitate communication that promotes a participatory approach.

CHAPTER 9: Advanced Quality Improvement Competencies

Domain	Competency	Sub-Competency
5	5.1a Apply quality improvement principles in care delivery	5.1i Establish and incorporate data driven benchmarks to monitor system performance. 5.1j Use national safety resources to lead team-based change initiatives. 5.1m Lead the development of a business plan for quality improvement initiatives. 5.1n Advocate for change related to financial policies that impact the relationship between economics and quality care delivery.
6	Perform effectively in different team roles, using principles and values of team dynamics.	6.2g Integrate evidence-based strategies and processes to improve team effectiveness and outcomes. 6.2h Evaluate the impact of team dynamics and performance on desired outcomes.
7	7.1 Apply knowledge of systems to work effectively across the continuum of care.	7.1d Participate in system-wide initiatives that improve care delivery and or outcomes. 7.1g Analyze system-wide processes to optimize outcomes.
7	7.3 Optimize system effectiveness through application of innovation and evidence-based practice.	7.3e Apply innovative and evidence-based strategies focusing on system preparedness and capabilities. 7.3f Design system improvement strategies based on performance data and metrics. 7.3g Manage change to sustain system effectiveness.

Domain	Competency	Sub-Competency
1	1.3 Demonstrate clinical judgment founded on a broad knowledge base.	1.3a Integrate foundational and advanced specialty knowledge into clinical reasoning. 1.3f Analyze decision models from nursing and other knowledge domains to improve clinical judgment. 1.3b Integrate nursing knowledge (theories, multiple ways of knowing, evidence) and knowledge from other disciplines and inquiry to inform clinical judgment. 1.3c Incorporate knowledge from nursing and other disciplines to support clinical judgment.
2	2.6 Demonstrate accountability for care delivery.	2.6e Model best care practices to the team. 2.6f Monitor aggregate metrics to assure accountability for care outcomes. 2.6g Promote delivery of care that supports practice at the full scope of education. 2.6 Ensure accountability throughout transitions of care across the healthcare continuum.
4	4.2 Integrate best evidence into nursing practice.	4.2g Lead the translation of evidence into practice.
4	4.3 Promote the ethical conduct of scholarly activities.	4.3e Identify and mitigate potential risks and areas of ethical concern in the conduct of scholarly activities. 4.3f Apply IRB guidelines throughout the scholarship process. 4.3g Ensure the protection of participants in the conduct of scholarship. 4.3h Implement processes that support ethical conduct in practice and scholarship.
5	5.1 Apply quality improvement principles in care delivery.	5.1k Integrate outcome metrics to inform change and policy recommendations. 5.1l Collaborate in analyzing organizational process improvement initiatives.
6	6.2 Perform effectively in different team roles, using principles and values of team dynamics.	6.2g Integrate evidence-based strategies and processes to improve team effectiveness and outcomes. 6.2j Foster positive team dynamics to strengthen desired outcomes.

CHAPTER 11: Advanced Evaluation of Outcomes

Domain	Competency	Sub-Competency
2	2.6 Demonstrate accountability for plan of care.	2.6h Contribute to the development of policies and processes that promote transparency and accountability. 2.6l Apply current and emerging evidence to the development of care guidelines/ tools.
2	2.7 Evaluate outcomes of care.	2.7d Analyze data to identify gaps and inequities in care and monitor trends in outcomes. 2.7e Monitor epidemiological and system-level aggregate data to determine healthcare outcomes and trends. 2.7f Synthesize outcome data to inform evidence-based practice, guidelines and policies.
3	3.4 Advance equitable population health policy.	3.4f Identify opportunities to influence the policy process. 3.4g Design comprehensive advocacy strategies to support the policy process. 3.4i Contribute to policy development at the system, local, regional, or national levels. 3.4j Assess the impact of policy changes. 2.4k Evaluate the ability of policy to address disparities and inequities within segments of the population.
4	4.2 Integrate best evidence into nursing practice.	4.2i Collaborate in the development of new/revised policy or regulation in the light of new evidence. 4.2k Evaluate outcomes and impact of new practices based on evidence.
5	5.1 Apply quality improvement principles in care delivery.	5.1k Integrate outcome metrics to inform change and policy recommendations. 5.1l Collaborate in analyzing organizational process improvement initiatives.
6	6.2 Perform effectively in different team roles, using principles and values of team dynamics.	6.2f Evaluate the impact of team dynamics and performance on desired outcomes.
7	7.3 Optimize system effectiveness through application of innovation and evidence-based practice.	7.3f Design system improvement strategies based on performance data and metrics. 7.3g Manage change to sustain system effectiveness.

CHAPTER 12: Dissemination that Transcends the Discipline

Domain	Competency	Sub-Competency
2	2.2 Communicate effectively with individuals.	2.2g Demonstrate advanced communication skills and techniques using a variety of modalities with diverse audiences. 2.2h Design evidence-based, person-centered engagement materials.
3	3.4 Advance equitable population health policy.	3.4d Contribute to policy development at the system, local, regional, or national levels.
3	3.5 Demonstrate advocacy strategies.	3.5h Engage in relationship-building activities with stakeholders at any level of influence, including system, local, state, national, and/or global.
4	4.1 Advance the scholarship of nursing.	4.1l Disseminate one's scholarship to diverse audiences using a variety of approaches and modalities.
4	4.3 Promote the ethical conduct of scholarly activities.	4.3i Apply ethical principles to the dissemination of nursing scholarship.
5	5.1 Apply quality improvement principles to in care delivery.	5.1o Advance quality improvement practices through dissemination of outcomes.

CHAPTER 13: Lifelong Learning, Leadership and Mentorship for Advanced Nursing Practice

Domain	Competency	Sub-Competency
6	6.1 Communicate in a manner that facilitates a partnership approach to quality care delivery.	6.1l Demonstrate the capacity to resolve interprofessional conflict.
6	6.2 Perform effectively in different team roles, using principals and values of team dynamics.	6.2g Integrate evidence-based strategies and processes to improve team effectiveness and outcomes. 6.2i Reflect on how one's role and expertise influences team performance. 6.2j Foster positive team dynamics to strengthen desired outcomes.
6	6.4 Work with other professions to maintain a climate of mutual learning, respect, and shared values.	6.4e Practice self-assessment to mitigate conscious and implicit biases toward other team members. 6.4f Foster an environment that supports the constructive sharing of multiple perspectives and enhances interprofessional learning. 6.4g Integrate diversity, equity and inclusion into team practices. 6.4h Manage disagreements, conflicts and challenging conversations among team members. 6.4i Promote an environment that advances interprofessional learning.

Domain	Competency	Sub-Competency
9	9.5 Demonstrate the professional identity of nursing.	9.5g Identify opportunities to lead with moral courage to influence team decision-making. 9.5i Engage in professional organizations that reflect nursing's values and identity.
10	10.1 Demonstrate a commitment to personal health and wellbeing.	10.1 Contribute to an environment that promotes self-care, personal health, and well-being
10	10.2 Demonstrate a spirit of inquiry that fosters flexibility and professional maturity.	10.2g Mentor others in the development of their professional growth and accountability. 10.2i Foster activities that support a culture of lifelong learning. 10.2j Expand leadership skills through professional service.
10	10.3 Develop capacity for leadership.	10.3j Provide leadership to advance the nursing profession. 10.3k Demonstrate leadership skills in times of uncertainty and crisis. 10.3q Advocate for the nursing profession in a manner that is consistent, positive, relevant, accurate, and distinctive.

Source: Adapted from "The Essentials: Competencies for Professional Nursing Education," by American Association of Colleges of Nursing, 2021, https://www.aacnnursing.org/Portals/42/AcademicNursing/pdf/Essentials-2021.pdf

Appendix B: Evidence-Based Personal Improvement Plan

Looking beyond engagement with the evidence-based wellness activities included at the end of each chapter, we encourage you to lead by example through addressing challenging wellness areas of your personal life through the creation of a customizable, evidence-based personal improvement plan (EBPIP) of your own. As nurse leaders and people, we can personalize evidence-based recommendations anecdotally and then track our progress toward health and wellness improvements (Reynolds & Waldrop, 2024). An EBPIP uses many but not all of the steps of EBP:

1. Identify the problem.
2. Search for evidence.
3. Develop a plan.
4. Implement.
5. Evaluate.

To help you identify the problem and search for evidence, we adapted the PPCO question. Rather than stand for population, the second P in PPCO stands for "person" when used for EBPIP. That person is a unique individual, and the emerging nurse leader is you!

Here, we offer two of our personal EBPIP examples in the hope that sharing them will help you on your wellness journey. Check it out and see what you think!

Julee

1. Person: Me (Julee)
2. Problem: Low protein intake. I had hired a coach to help me train for my first 50-mile run, and based on my diet history, she recommended an increase in my daily protein intake to support my muscles adaptation to training.
3. Search for evidence: The International Society of Sports Medicine recommends 1.6–2.5 grams per kilogram body weight per day. Minimum per day for me was 90 grams, more on long run days.
4. Plan:

    a. Trial various protein supplements.
    b. Include foods high in protein in my diet daily.
    c. Keep a daily record of my protein intake: goal 90 gms or more a day.

5. Implementation:

    a. I downloaded an app: In the app I was able to document my daily protein intake, look up the amount of protein in food sources, and set a timer to remind me to document each day.
    b. I recorded my protein intake as I tried various ways to increase my intake in the app and in my Google document that I shared with my running coach. Some things I tried were protein powder in my coffee (no way!), protein powder in my cereal (not too bad, and this was something I did most days), high-protein yogurt or a serving of almonds for snacks, and one serving of fish or chicken daily.

6. Evaluate: After 30 days I evaluated the effectiveness of my plan using the calendar in the Protein Pal app. Just for fun I made a run chart for you with the goal line (just like in QI).

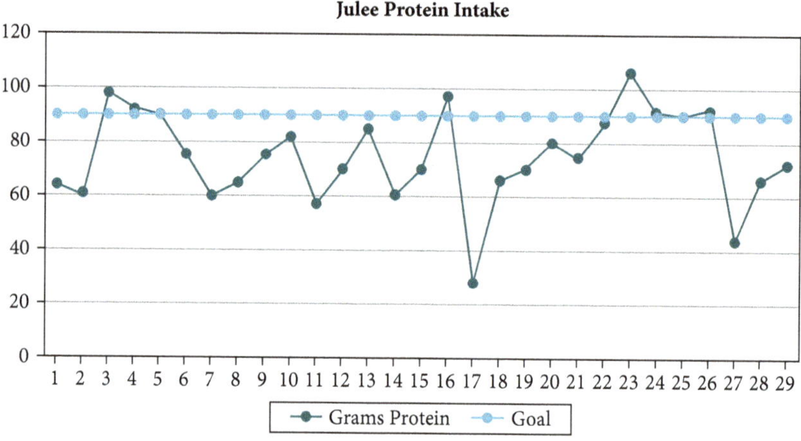

FIGURE B.1 Julee: Protein intake.

What do you think? I met my goal a few days, and they were on the weekends when I had long runs, so that was a positive, but overall there is still room for improvement.

Jayne: Regular Physical Activity

1. Person: Me (Jayne)
2. Problem: Inconsistent physical activity. With the publication of the prelicensure-focused EBPQI textbook while taking over interim oversight of a DNP program, my daily free time shrunk. At the same time, our children's activities ramped up as I began increasingly driving them to

the basketball courts, auditoriums, or the swim center. As I sat watching them practice weekly and month after month regularly, I realized that I had become relatively sedentary. As my movement and exercise decreased, I noticed muscle wasting, and very mild back and neck pain. When I would try to run or swim once or twice per week (at most), I was breathless and uncomfortable. For the first time in my life, physical activity didn't feel good anymore. I decided to take my advice and search the literature for practical ways to get back on track that might work in my unique life phase, when my children remain the priority commitment.

3. Search the evidence: What interventions were used to mitigate this issue?

    a. Exercise routine/consistency (Warburton et al., 2006; Ruegsegger & Booth, 2018)
    b. Physical activity variability (World Health Organization, 2022)

4. Plan:

    a. Consistent exercise routine
    b. Adaptable physical activity based on location

5. Implementation:

    a. Plan an hour of daily movement while ensuring I can still take my kids to their practices. This required that I pack tennis shoes, and after I checked my daughter into the swim center, I did laps walking or jogging around the building and parking lot. When my son had basketball practice, I watched him from the windows while riding the exercise bike and/or elliptical and simultaneously reading a book for fun. On those days, I did some lightweight exercises and a core workout. Once or twice per week, when my parents could help transport a kid, or on the weekends, my husband and I exercised together.

6. Evaluate:

    a. A couple of weeks into this new routine, I experienced dramatic improvements, increased energy, and noticeably more physical endurance within a few months. I also think more clearly with improved focus. Although my husband pushes me physically when we exercise together, and I don't always like it at the moment, we genuinely enjoy the time together and feel good afterward. These improvements have been sustained for almost a year since this writing.

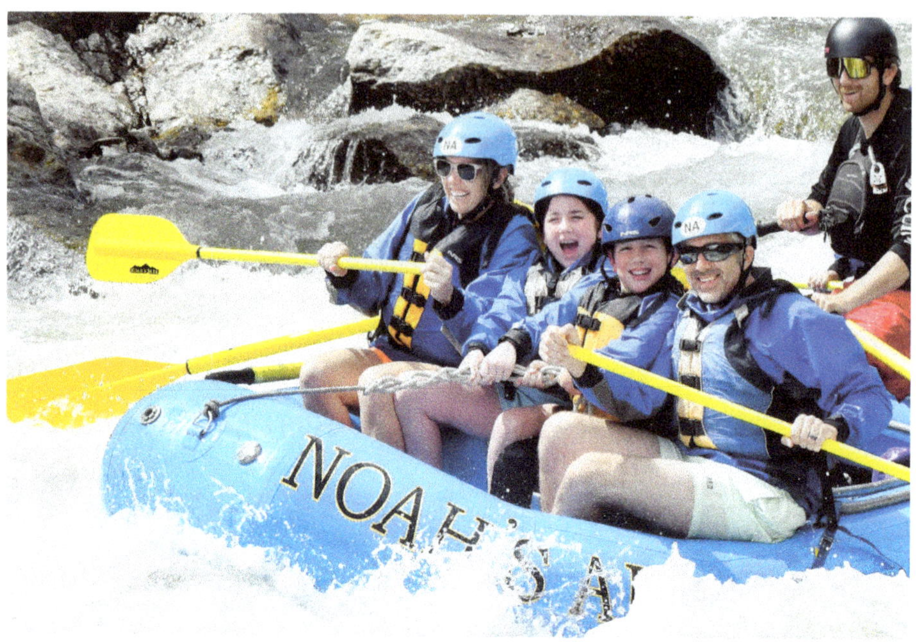

FIGURE B.2 Physical activity with family.

REFERENCES

Reynolds, S., & Waldrop, J. (2024). Optimizing quality improvement methods in practice: A case study approach. *Journal of Nursing Care Quality.* Advance online publication. https://doi.org/10.1097/NCQ.0000000000000785

Ruegsegger, G. N., & Booth, F. W. (2018). Health benefits of exercise. *Cold Spring Harbor Perspectives in Medicine, 8*(7), a029694. https://doi.org/10.1101/cshperspect.a029694

Tiller, N. B., Roberts, J. D., Beasley, L., Chapman, S., Pinto, J. M., Smith, L., Wiffin, M., Russell, M., Sparks, S. A., Duckworth, L., O'Hara, J., Sutton, L., Antonio, J., Willoughby, D. S., Tarpey, M. D., Smith-Ryan, A. E., Ormsbee, M. J., Astorino, T. A., Kreider, R. B., McGinnis, G. R., ... & Bannock, L. (2019). International Society of Sports Nutrition position stand: Nutritional considerations for single-stage ultra-marathon training and racing. *Journal of the International Society of Sports Nutrition, 16*(1), 50. https://doi.org/10.1186/s12970-019-0312-9

Warburton, D. E., Nicol, C. W., & Bredin, S. S. (2006). Health benefits of physical activity: The evidence. *Canadian Medical Association Journal, 174*(6), 801–809. https://doi.org/10.1503/cmaj.051351

World Health Organization. (2022). *Physical activity.* https://www.who.int/news-room/fact-sheets/detail/physical-activity

IMAGE CREDITS

Appendix C: Critical Appraisal Tools

As you learned throughout Chapters 5–7, critically appraising the evidence is a systematic process. Remember that critical appraisal involves use of a checklist tool to assess the quality and strength of evidence. We use checklists because they help us do things in a systematic way and remind us to be diligent to all of the critical aspects of a process. The information included in this appendix will provide you with a stepwise approach to guide you through five different types of critical appraisals through freely available tools you can access on your own through the QR codes provided. Because we believe examples are needed to really put all the pieces together, we are incorporating five corresponding examples to facilitate your quest for competency as an EBPQI team leader. Let's begin with a critical appraisal of a systematic review and meta-analysis. Remember the evidence pyramid? The systematic review and meta-analysis are at the top, but that doesn't necessarily mean it will be appraised as the highest quality!

How to Use the Critical Appraisal Skills Programme (CASP) Checklist for Systematic Reviews and Meta-Analysis

Step 1. Download a copy of the fillable document from the CASP website.

https://casp-uk.net/casp-tools-checklists/systematic-reviews-meta-analysis-rcts/

Step 2. Have a copy of this article as the reference example we will use.

Feng, Y., Lin, Y., Ningning, Z., Jiang, X. & Zhang, L. (2021). Effects of animal-assisted therapy on hospitalized children and teenagers: A systematic review and meta-analysis. *Journal of Pediatric Nursing*, *60*, 11–23. https://doi.org/10.1016/j.pedn.2021.01.020

Step 3. Read the article and answer the questions.

The CASP checklist includes 10 (sometimes multicomponent) questions to help you make sense of an SRMA. There are instructions within the checklist that this example will help you interpret.

The three big questions that you want to answer when critically appraising any piece of evidence are generally the same, and the questions in sections A, B, and C of the CASP checklist for SRMA help you answer them. Most of the questions (except 7, which asks about precision) are answered with a yes, can't tell, or no, but the real appraisal information that will help you remember why you answered the way you did should be placed in the comments box. Also, do not make any assumptions about what the researchers did or did not do. If it is not reported, it is a no or can't tell. After reading the article, see if you agree with what we put in the boxes.

Section A

Is the basic study design valid for a systematic review?

> Validity is appraised based on the study designs and has to do with how the study was conducted.

Section B

Is the systematic review methodologically sound?

> Results are the actual outcomes of the study based on the data collected in this study.

Section C

Are the results of the systematic review trustworthy?

Section D

Are the results of the systematic review relevant locally?

> Only you can determine if the results are applied to the patients you care for in your setting.

Section E

Will the implementation of the results represent greater value for your service users or population?

Section A.

Question 1 answer:
Yes
Comments:

> The researchers provide evidence in the introduction that the effectiveness of AAI has not been quantitatively analyzed, especially in a broad group of hospitalized patients.
>
> A PICOT question was not included. However, one can deduce (not assume) the question from the purpose statement.

Purpose: "To quantitatively analyze experimental studies on AAT and synthesize its effects on medical outcomes, including pain, anxiety, depression, stress, BP, and HR in hospitalized children and teenagers, including those with cancer."

P: Hospitalized children and adolescents

I: AAT

C: Usual care (no AAT)

O: Pain, anxiety, depression, stress, BP, and HR

Question 2 answer:
Yes
Comments:

RCT or quasi-RCT

Section B

Question 3 answer:
Yes
Comments:

All relevant databases were searched, and Open Gray Literature and Google Scholar were used for primary studies.

Inclusion criteria: Evaluation of pain, anxiety, depression, stress, BP or HR ages 3–18; admitted to a treatment ward

Exclusion criteria: Animals used were not real; cognitive impairments

The authors used the *Cochrane Handbook* for SR of interventions and PRISMA. Two authors reviewed and extracted data, with disagreements arbitrated by a third author.

Question 4 answer:
Yes
Comments:

Used the Cochrane Risk of Bias Tool (Table 4)

Question 5 answer:
Yes

Comments:

Reported in the Results selection

Data is presented in Tables 1, 2, and 3.

Section C

Question 6 answer:
Yes
Comments:

Different outcomes had different numbers of studies included in the analysis.

Heterogeneity was calculated using the I(2) statistic: Table 5

Pooled effect sizes were calculated with standard mean difference (SMD) and confidence intervals at 95%. Forest plots in Figures 1–8.

Question 7 answer:
Yes
Comments:

Limitations were reported.

Only biomedical outcomes were evaluated.

AAT was not the only intervention (including medical therapies), so it was difficult to interpret the specific effects.

Effects based on only two studies should be considered preliminary.

Studies with bias were reported: random-sequence generation, lack of control for confounding factors. Medium risk of bias overall.

No librarian involved.

Section D

Question 8 answer:
Only you can determine if the results can be applied to your local population, setting, or context.

Section E

Question 9 answer:
Only you can determine if the results represent greater value for your population.
Question 10 answer:
Only you and your team can determine if the findings would be of enough value to change your practice.

What is your conclusion about the SRMA? Can it be used to support decision-making?

Appraisal Summary

Positive	Negative
Quality is high. Methodological rigor. Accurate reporting of results. No harms reported.	Included studies had moderate risk of bias. Total number of studies was small. The small number of studies in the pooled SMD calculations.

The quality of this SRMA is high. There was methodological rigor and accurate reporting of results. The primary studies included were rated as having moderate risk of bias, which you might expect given the obvious nature of ATT as an intervention. The number of total studies and the small number of studies in the pooled SMD calculations limits the confidence in the results for all outcomes except maybe BP and pain.

How to Use the CASP Checklist for Randomised Controlled Trials

Step 1. Download a copy of the fillable document from the CASP website.

https://casp-uk.net/casp-tools-checklists/

Step 2. Have a copy of this article as the reference example we will use.

Khalili, S., Shirinkam, F., Ghadimi, R. & Karimi, H. (2021). The effect of group walking program on social physique anxiety and the risk of eating disorders in aged women: A randomized clinical trial study. *Applied Nursing Research*, *64*, 151555.

Step 3. Read the article and answer the questions.

This CASP checklist includes 11 (sometimes multicomponent) questions to help you appraise a RCT. There are instructions within the checklist that this example will help you interpret.

The three big questions that you want to answer when critically appraising any piece of evidence are generally the same, and the questions in sections A, B, C, and D of the CASP checklist for RCT help you answer them. Most of the questions are answered with a yes, can't tell or no, but the real appraisal information that will help you remember why you answered the way you did should be placed somewhere in the answer box. After reading the article see if you agree with what we put in the boxes.

Section A

Is the study valid?

> Validity is appraised based on the study design and has to do with how the study was developed.

Section B

Was the study method sound?

> Was the study method appropriate for the research question and conducted rigorously?

Section C

What are the results?

> Results are the actual outcomes of the study based on the data collected in this study.

Section D

Will the results help locally?

> Only you can determine if the results be applied to the patients you care for in your setting.

Let's go!

Section A

Question 1 answer:
Yes
Comments:

> The hypothesis was stated: A group walking program would positively affect the risk of EDs and SPA, ED subscale, and BMI in aged women.
>
> The research question is focused, but a PICO was not used. It can be helpful to determine if the research question or hypothesis is focused by applying the PICO.
>
> P: Aged women
>
> I: Walking program
>
> C: No walking program
>
> O: ED, SPA, and BMI

Question 2 answer:
Yes
Comments:

Cluster sampling occurred first, then random allocation but participants were matched in terms of age and BMI.

Computer-generated random sequence upon admission to either unit 1 or 2 by personnel who were not aware of the allocation nor took part in the study.

Question 3 answer:
Yes
Comments:

All participants were accounted for in the CONSORT diagram in Figure 1.

Section B

Question 4 answer:
No
Comments:

The participants were not blind to the intervention. This can be difficult with an obvious intervention and when it is difficult to prevent participants from socializing in the community.

There is no mention of blinding of the researchers or those who analyzed the data.

Question 5 answer:
Yes
Comments:

Yes, in Table 1 baseline characteristics between the groups are presented, and there are no significant differences between the groups

Question 6 answer:
Yes
Comments:

The components of the intervention were clearly described, and follow-up intervals were the same for each group.

Section C

Question 7 answer:
Yes
Comments:

A power analysis was done and determined to be 60 (30 per group). Data was analyzed on 62 participants. Results were reported for each outcome at each follow-up, and there was no missing or incomplete data used. There were no significant differences in drop out between groups.

One potential source of bias was not being able to blind the intervention and thus of having contamination between the different groups.

The outcomes analyzed were clear, and the measures were valid and reliable. (See section on measures.)

Multiple statistical analyses were used. ANCOVA and MANCOVA were used to compare the outcome measures.

Question 8 answer:
Yes
Comments:

P values of < .05 were considered statistically significant (Table 3).

Question 9 –answer:
Yes
Comments:

No effect size for the intervention was reported. The intervention produced statistically significant results in the primary outcomes of reducing SPA and ED.

No harms or unintended consequences were reported.

No cost analysis was conducted.

Section D

Question 10 answer:
Only you can determine this based on the patients you care for.
Question 11 answer:
Only you and your team can determine if the findings would be of enough value to change your practice.

Appraisal Summary

This is a low-cost intervention that improved SPA and ED in aged women in Iran. It may or may not be feasible in your practice setting or health care delivery system

How to Use the NHLBI Quality Assessment Tool for Observational Cohort and Cross-Sectional Studies

Step 1. Download a copy of the fillable document from the JBI website.

https://www.nhlbi.nih.gov/health-topics/study-quality-assessment-tools

Step 2. Have a copy of this article as the reference example we will use.

White, L., Waldrop, J., & Waldrop, C. (2016). Human papillomavirus and vaccination of males: Knowledge and attitudes of registered nurses. *Pediatric Nursing*, *42*(1), 21–35.

Step 3. Read the article and answer the questions with either yes, no, CD = cannot determine, NR = not reported, or NA = not applicable).

Question 1 answer:
Yes
Comments:

> "The purpose of this research study is to identify knowledge and attitudes of registered nurses and potential barriers to achieving adequate HPV vaccination rates in males."

Question 2 answer:
Yes

Faculty

Current graduate students

Alumni

STTI members

BSN, RN, > 18 years old

Question 3 answer:
No
The survey response rate was 7.5%

Question 4 answer:
Yes
See answer to question 2.

Question 5 answer:
No
A power analysis or determination of sample size was not reported.

Question 6 answer:
NA
not a cohort study

Question 7 answer:
NA
not a cohort study

Question 8 answer:
NA
not a cohort study
Question 9 answer:
Yes Independent variables were clearly defined (demographic variables), valid, reliable, and requested from each participant.

Question 10 answer:
NA
not a cohort study

Question 11 answer:
Yes
Outcome measures (dependent variables) of knowledge statements were adapted from a previous study (Daley et al., 2010) and attitude statements from another study (Weiss et al., 2010) and current literature. The measures have face and expert validity. Cronbach's alpha was 0.54–0.74.

Question 12 answer:
NA
not a cohort study

Question 13 answer:
NA
not a cohort study

Question 14 answer:
NA
not a cohort study
Quality rating: Good, fair or poor

Assess the risk of bias in the study due to flaws in study design or implementation. Only six questions apply to a cross-sectional study, and five of six were answered yes. Number 5 is related to the sample size required to generalize the results. In addition, the sample was likely mostly from a similar geographic area, and therefore the results must be viewed with caution.

A second concern is that the measures used for the outcome variables have not been rigorously validated or tested for reliability with psychometric measures and so it cannot be certain how well they measure what they are proposed to measure.

We rate the quality of this study as fair.

Generally, a good study is one with the lowest risk of bias and valid results, whereas a fair study may have some susceptibility to bias but not enough that the results are invalid. The fair rating category may be broad and have studies with varying strengths and weaknesses. A poor study is one that has significant bias resulting in untrustworthy results.

How to Use the CASP Checklist for Qualitative Research

Step 1. Download a copy of the fillable document from the CASP website.

https://casp-uk.net/casp-tools-checklists/

Step 2. Have a copy of this article as the reference example we will use.

Vandrevala, T., Montague, A., Boulton, R., Coxon, K., & Jones, C. E. (2024). Exploring the implementation of an educational film within antenatal care to reduce the risk of cytomegalovirus infection in pregnancy: A qualitative study. *BMC Pregnancy andCchildbirth*, *24*(1), 524. https://doi.org/10.1186/s12884-024-06715-5

Step 3. Read the article and answer the questions.

This CASP checklist includes 10 (sometimes multicomponent) questions to help you appraise a qualitative research study. The checklist includes instructions that this example will help you interpret.

The three big questions that you want to answer when critically appraising any piece of evidence are generally the same, and the questions in sections A, B, and C of the CASP checklist for a qualitative study will help you answer them. All but the last question are answered with a yes, can't tell, or no, but the real appraisal information that will help you remember why you answered the way you did should be placed in the comments box. After reading the article, see if you agree with what we put in the boxes.

Section A

Are the results valid?

> Validity is appraised based on the study design and how the study was developed. In qualitative research, if the design is not appropriate to address the purpose of the study, it may not be worth continuing your appraisal.

Section B

What are the results?

Results are the actual outcomes of the study based on the data collected in this study.

Section C

Will the results help locally?

Only you can determine if the results be applied to the patients you care for in your setting.

Let's go!

Section A

Question 1 answer:
Yes
Comments:

The aim of this study was to explore the transition and adjustment of African immigrant women, particularly Ethiopian immigrant women (EIW), as they navigate the U.S. health care system and their ability to access and utilize health care services.

Question 2 answer:
Yes
Comments:

This was a qualitative design using a semi-structured interview guide and using a phenomenological approach to explore the women's experiences, perceptions and challenges. The authors note that it is the appropriate approach because there is no adequate information on the health care experiences of EIW and the need for an in-depth examination of the complexity of the issues in EIW's lived experience.

Question 3 answer:
Yes
Comments:

Yes, to explore perceptions of EIW.

Section B

Question 4 answer:
Yes
Comments:

> This population was described as "hard to reach," so a mix of purposive and snowball sampling was used.

Question 5 answer:
Yes
Comments:

> Data was collected through a one-time, in-depth interview that lasted 45–90 minutes. The semi-structured interview guide that was pilot tested. All interviews were audio recorded and transcribed verbatim with identifiable information removed from the transcripts. Saturation of the data was reached, and no further interviews were conducted.

Question 6 answer:
No
Comments:

> The researchers did not examine the potential bias their role or life experience might have on the conduct of the study or the interpretation of the results.

Question 7 answer:
Yes
Comments:

> Yes, this study was approved by the ethics committee (IRB), and informed consent occurred. Interviews were conducted in a private space, and data was anonymized.

Question 8 answer:
Yes
Comments:

> An inductive thematic analysis process was used with a five-step approach:
>
> 1. Data was transcribed and cleaned.
>
> 2. Deidentified transcripts were read repeatedly, and memos were kept.
>
> 3. Potential themes and patterns were built, and a codebook was used to code each transcript in NVivo12 software.

4. Interpretations were assessed and developed.

5. Structural and textural description of what the EIW experienced in accessing health care was provided.

Question 9 answer:
Yes
Comments:

Findings were developed into clear themes with subthemes, which were clearly supported by example quotes. Discussion presented the results in the context of prior studies and identified areas for application and future research.

Section C

Question 10 answer:
Only you can determine this based on the patients you care for.

Note: This tool does not have a scoring system or a validated benchmark of what constitutes a poor-, moderate-, or high-quality report. In this case there was only one no answer related to researcher bias, and the answer to question 10 is up to you. However, in general, this study describes findings that need further validation but that may contribute to practice now. For example, how might you consider approaching/communicating with EIW in your practice or organization based on this study? Would you need more evidence to change your practice? Depending on how similar your population and setting are, you may or may not decide to include this study as evidence that supports a proposed EBPQI initiative.

How to Use the EBPQI Critical Appraisal Tool

Step 1. Download a copy of the fillable document from the article to learn how to use it and then a blank copy of the tool, which is linked as supplemental digital content within the article.

https://pubmed.ncbi.nlm.nih.gov/39072449/

Step 2. Have a copy of this article as the reference example we will use.

Luzum, N., Beckius, A., Heinrich, T., & Stoner, K. (9900). Implementation of an evidence-based treatment protocol and order set for alcohol withdrawal syndrome. *Journal for Healthcare Quality*. https://doi.org/10.1097/JHQ.0000000000000452

Step 3. Read the article and identify if the EBPQI initiative met the criteria.

In this critical appraisal tool, there are 20 criteria. The criteria are evaluated by determining if the item is *present* (2 points), *partially present* (1 point), or *not present* (0 points). Including comments or notes can be helpful when returning to use the appraisal in your evaluation of the body of the evidence. In the end the local context and potential transferability is considered. This tool has a scoring rubric, which can aid in providing a quality judgment of low, moderate, or high.

Criteria 1
Partially met (1)
Comments:

> The problem in general is clearly identified, but no information is provided on the incidence or prevalence of the problem in the local context.

Criteria 2
Met (2)
Comments:

> A nice synthesis of the evidence to support the practice change is presented.

Criteria 3
Not met (0)
Comments:

No PPCO or PICOT question or literature search was performed to identify the best solutions to the problem.

Criteria 4
Not met (0)
Comments:

Since there was no evidence synthesized because there was no search, there was also no critical appraisal and synthesis.

Criteria 5
Partially met (1)
Comments:

Best evidence was not supported by a search, but a multidisciplinary team was involved in updating the order sets for treatment of acute alcohol withdrawal.

Criteria 6
Not met (0)
Comments:

Patient preferences or values were not considered in this initiative.

Criteria 7
Partially met (1)
Comments:

Baseline data was collected retrospectively but not presented prior to order set change as evidence of the local problem.

Criteria 8
Not met (0)
Comments:

There were no SMART aims for this EBP initiative. The only purpose stated was "to monitor clinical outcomes and prescribing habits after initiation of a new order set."

Criteria 9
Not met (0)
Comments:

A pre-post retrospective method was used, which is not a QI methodology.

Criteria 10
Met (2)
Comments:

"study"* took place at a large 766 bed academic hospital in the Midwestern region of the United States in an urban/suburban setting.

*study is associated with research, not an EBPQI initiative.

Criteria 11
Met (2)
Comments:

A multidisciplinary team was engaged, including hospital medicine, psychiatry, trauma surgery, pharmacy, social work, and nursing.

Criteria 12
Not met (0)
Comments:

No tests of change were conducted due to retrospective analysis and pre-post design.

Criteria 13
Met (2)
Comments:

Outcomes were measurable: Prescribed medications, ICU transfer, LOS, readmissions at 72 hours and 30 days, all-cause mortality.

Criteria 14
Partially met (1)
Comments:

In quality improvement data should be collected at regular intervals and run charts or statistical process control charts should be used to determine improvement. In this study data was only collected before and after and only as pre-/postcomparisons and statistical analyses with significance level of 0.05 was used. This can result in clinically significant improvements being missed.

Criteria 15
Met (2)
Comments:

Results were provided for all outcomes selected.

Criteria 16
Partially met (1)
Comments:

A table was used to report statistical analysis/significance, but a bar chart was used to visualize the difference in orders for medications.

Criteria 17
Met (2)
Comments:

Results were discussed and compared to prior evidence.

Criteria 18
Met (2)
Comments:

Limitations were inappropriate for an EBPQI study but given the pre-post design could be considered.

Criteria 19
Met (2)
Comments:

Sustainability of the practice change (order set) will include continued educational efforts, data surveillance, and updates.

Criteria 20
Met (2)

Conclusions are based on the results.

Total Score: 23 points.
Rating: High quality: 27–40
Moderate quality: 14–26
Low quality </= 13

This EBP initiative is rated as **moderate quality**. The primary reasons it was rated down were because of the methods.

Suzy Lockwood, PhD, MSN, RN, FAAN

Texas Christian University, Harris College of Nursing & Health Sciences, Associate Dean for Nursing & Nurse Anesthesia, Professor

Early in my practice as a nurse I recognized that I had lots of questions and wanted to better understand the "why" behind the day-to-day clinical decisions I made as a nurse. This period of questioning and wondering aligned with my transition from a bedside, clinically based nurse to that of a director for a seven-member physician group. These same physicians served as the clinical faculty for a large OB-GYN residency program and were actively engaged in research themselves. The medical director encouraged me to be active in the various research activities that were being conducted. With his support and encouragement, I was able to merge so many of my passions (oncology, policy, administration) into a program of research that examined participation in cancer screening and impact of health policy. At this same time, I began serving as an adjunct faculty for the nursing program where I am now associate dean. Upon completing my PhD, I was approached by the dean of that program about a full-time position. The same individual who encouraged and supported me towards pursuit of a PhD gently nudged me to make the move. Over time and with a few incredible mentors, I have learned that teaching and preparing the next generation of nurses is my "calling." The opportunity to not only continue to explore the "why" but also work alongside nurse scientists in an academic setting is a gift. Daily I am able to impact directly and indirectly the delivery of care and best practice by supporting colleagues who are passionate about nursing and EBP and knowledge generation.

Rosalie Mainous, PhD, APRN, FNAP, FAANP, FAAN

University of Kentucky, Dean and Warwick Professor

My career progression is due to my motto: When opportunity knocks, answer the door. I completed an associate's degree nursing program in a regional university after someone approached me at freshman registration and asked me if I wanted one of the two remaining program openings. I said yes and embarked on a 45-year career that started in the operating room, went to the surgical ICU, and eventually went to the NICU. I went back and got a BSN, MSN, then a PhD. Following the award of the MSN, I worked two jobs—one in the hospital and one in academia. As I was finishing my PhD, I let go of the practice but decided I wanted to become a neonatal nurse practitioner—so, 2 weeks after I defended my dissertation, I embarked on three semesters of a postgraduate NNP program, ultimately becoming certified. I had a clinical practice in a 95-bed NICU and was appointed the director of the NNP program. I was thrilled with the direction my career had taken. Then the dean left for another job, the associate dean moved up, and I became an associate dean. When was asked if I wanted the opportunity, I didn't waiver. Several years later I decided I wanted a deanship and moved to Ohio to take one. Now in my third deanship and with a productive stint at the American Association of Colleges of Nursing in Washington, DC, as the director of academic nursing development, I find that I have found my niche.

About the Editors

Jayne Jennings Dunlap, DNP, APRN, FNP-C, CNE, EBP-C

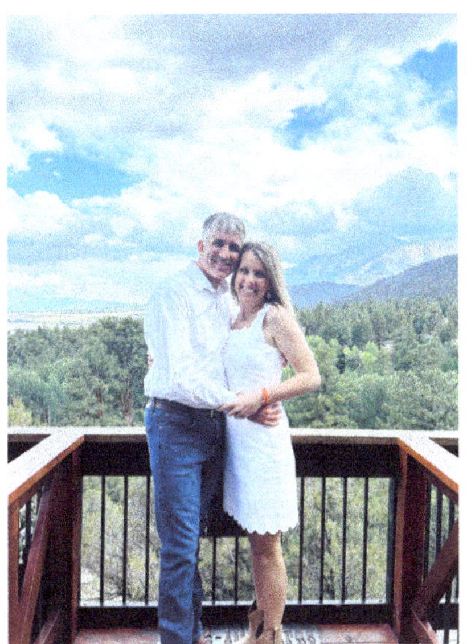

Image 0.1

Texas Woman's University, DNP Program Director, Associate Clinical Professor

Baylor Scott and White Heath, Family Nurse Practitioner

The Journal for Nurse Practitioners, Associate Editor

I worked as a new nurse in the neonatal intensive care unit and immensely enjoyed this position. What a privilege to care for the tiniest patients in the healthcare system while supporting their families. When my own family began to grow, I realized that continued night and weekend shift work would be an increasing challenge. I also became frustrated with some limitations impacting patient care improvements in my bedside and charge nurse roles.

I enrolled in a Family Nurse Practitioner (NP) program to learn to provide sustained care for families on a schedule more conducive to my life stage. Upon graduation, I had a few job opportunities. After completing interviews, instead of the position with the best clinic hours, I decided on the primary care NP role with the strongest collaborating physician who was a gifted teacher and NP champion. This remains one of the wisest career decisions I ever made. I still remember how exciting it was to knock on the door to see my first patient as an NP.

After a few years of clinical practice, I pursued my Doctor of Nursing Practice (DNP) degree to engage in healthcare improvement targeting a practice gap across clinics affecting a vulnerable group. My collaborating physician ultimately inspired me to become an educator with the privilege of helping shape future nurse leaders who will go on to touch countless lives. I continue to practice and precept students as an NP and still get excited when I (or we) knock on patient room doors.

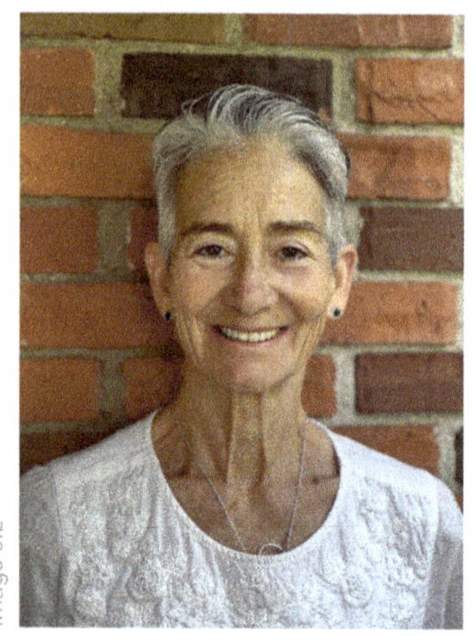
Image 0.2

Julee Briscoe Waldrop, DNP, PNP, FNP, CNE, EBP-C, NC-BC, FAANP, FAAN

Professor Emeritus, The University of North Carolina at Chapel Hill School of Nursing

Consulting Associate, Duke University School of Nursing

The Journal for Nurse Practitioners, Emerging Scholars Editor

While working as a nurse in a family-centered care unit (at that time, it described labor and delivery, newborn nursery, and postpartum unit), I was exposed to both the Clinical Nurse Specialist (CNS) and the NP role. The CNS in the hospital where I worked was my idol; she was an expert in everything. Her role was to support nurses to provide the best care possible for patients, and she did this well, but it was a big job. I was also working in a rural area with no advanced education opportunities at the time. I was exposed to the NP role, particularly women's health NPs.

I continued working as a nurse, then a nurse manager, and then a nurse educator. Because of my husband's career and my children, I did not have the option to apply to a graduate program and move somewhere, so when the University of Illinois at Chicago College of Nursing was awarded funding from the federal government to bring their FNP program to the rural parts of the state, I was excited to apply. Our small cohort of four people attended class in person, using photocopied outlines for notetaking as we listened to lectures over the phone! It was a prototype of the now common delivery of distance-based education. As we sometimes find when we begin a new educational endeavor, we don't know what we don't know, and what I didn't know was that I would fall in love with and become passionate about pediatric primary care!

About the Contributors

Kathy A. Baker, PhD, APRN, ACNS-BC, FCNS, FAAN

Texas Christian University, Harris College of Nursing & Health Sciences, Professor
Editor-in-Chief, *Gastroenterology Nursing*

Two years into my practice, I was not completely satisfied as a bedside critical care nurse. Though I loved caring for my patients and their families and the fast pace of the critical care setting, I was dissatisfied with the "routine" of a registered nurse and yearning for additional opportunities to learn and grow. As a novice nurse, I had experienced learning alongside a clinical nurse specialist (CNS) who impressed me with her knowledge, skills, expertise, and confidence. She was everything I wanted to be as a nurse. As I explored the CNS role further alongside other advanced practice roles, I realized the broader focus of the CNS on patients, nurses/nursing, and the organization suited my interests and personality. I relished the opportunity to consult on complex patients for direct patient care issues, and I loved teaching and mentoring other nurses and serving on organizational committees that gave me an opportunity to directly impact the health care system and patient outcomes. The CNS is a change expert, and that got me excited! Another key CNS responsibility is supporting evidence-based practice (EBP). As someone who loves reading nursing research and expanding my clinical expertise through immersion in nursing literature, I knew this was the advanced practice role that would maximize my passions and allow me to continue to grow. Eventually, I pursued my Doctor of Philosophy (PhD) degree and am privileged to now teach advanced practice nursing students in both Doctor of Nursing Practice (DNP) and PhD programs.

Tracy L. Brewer, DNP, RNC-OB, CLC, EBP-C

University of Tennessee, Knoxville, DNP Program Chair, Clinical Professor

I started my nursing career as a labor and delivery nurse and have always respected the opportunity to help women through one of their life's most challenging yet rewarding experiences. My ultimate dream was to become a certified nurse midwife (CNM), and I was thrilled to be accepted to attend a prestigious university to begin midwifery studies. Unfortunately, I suffered a severe knee injury while providing patient care and had to undergo four surgeries, ultimately leading to complex regional pain syndrome, resulting in my withdrawing my admission. However, I refused to abandon my graduate school ambitions. Instead, I reflected on my enjoyment of teaching others as a preceptor. I received a master's degree in nursing education and a DNP in educational leadership. These two degrees led to a fulfilling 2-decade academic career sharing my passion and experiences in maternal, newborn, and pediatric nursing. As a novice educator, I received exceptional mentorship and encouragement from nursing and academic leaders. I now serve as a director of a DNP program at a large land grant university. With my extensive knowledge and involvement in EBP and quality improvement, I assist doctoral students and novice faculty by teaching, advising, and mentoring them to impact patient care. My story intends to share that you will face challenges through graduate studies. I hope you find strength in my perseverance to overcome and succeed in your graduate studies despite any obstacles you may face. I am grateful for the guidance and support I received and am committed to paying it forward to others like you.

Garry J. Brydges, PhD, DNP, MBA, MHA, APRN, CRNA, ACNP-BC, FAANA, FAAN

UT MD Anderson Cancer Center, Director, Quality & Safety in Anesthesiology, Critical Care, & Pain Medicine

Embarking on the journey of advanced nursing practice (ANP) has been a profoundly enriching and transformative experience for me. Inspired by the remarkable career based on multifaceted expertise from clinical anesthesia to groundbreaking work in predictive analytics using machine learning, I have found my passion for elevating health care through advanced leadership and innovation. My commitment to education, leadership, and global health care initiatives has motivated me to pursue excellence in my professional journey. In my roles as vice president of the National Council on Certification and Recertification for Nurse Anesthetists, president of the American Association of Nurse Anesthetists, and significant contributions to nurse anesthesia globally, I am inspired to engage actively in shaping the future of health care policy and practice.

My focus on cost-effective care, quality improvement, and the application of innovative strategies, such as time-driven activity-based costing, resonates with my belief in the importance of data-driven decision-making in health care leadership. I am committed to making meaningful contributions as I navigate the challenges and opportunities within ANP. I continue to be passionate about ANP, leadership, and pursuing knowledge that transcends traditional boundaries. I am eager to apply the principles and insights gained from my career path, contributing to health care advancement and patients' well-being.

Ninotchka Brydges, PhD, DNP, MBA, APRN, ACNP-BC, FNAP, FAAN

UT Medical Branch Division of Pulmonary Critical Care Medicine, League City and Clear Lake Campuses, Department of Internal Medicine, Lead Advanced Practice Provider

UTMB School of Nursing Graduate Program, Assistant Clinical Faculty
Philippine Nurses Association of America, Accredited Provider Program Director

My pursuit of ANP is rooted in a genuine passion for delivering comprehensive health care that extends beyond conventional boundaries. Working in the intensive care unit (ICU) for over 2 decades, I've witnessed firsthand the evolving landscape of health care and the increasing complexity of patient needs across health care settings. My critical care experience has fueled a desire to contribute more substantively to patient outcomes and prompted me to seek advanced education and give back through teaching. As a nurse practitioner, I have spent years navigating the dynamic environment of critical care settings, where each moment demands swift, precise decision-making and a nuanced understanding of complex health conditions. I am drawn to taking a leadership role in patient management and EBPQI. The dynamic nature of adult acute care demands a practitioner who is not only adept in clinical skills but also capable of leading EBPQI initiatives that enhance and sustain the overall quality of care provided. ANP leadership aligns with my commitment to lifelong learning, which is not just a personal goal but an ethical responsibility.

Heather Carter-Templeton, PhD, RN, NI-BC, FAAN

West Virginia University, School of Nursing, Adult Health Department, Director of Evaluation, & Associate Professor

Deputy Editor, *CIN: Computers, Informatics, Nursing*

Throughout my formative years I was always interested in science and technology. Thankfully and gratefully, I landed in nursing school in college. Once licensed, I found myself seeking to work in more high-tech environments such as critical care areas. At the same time, electronic health records were coming online in many places and the need for quality data management was being identified in the field. My work led me to administrative positions and even a research position in which I could see the necessity for wide-scale information technology that supported decisions driven by data to support patient care. I quickly realized informatics, a relatively new specialty area at the time, was a good fit for my interests. I attended a graduate school that offered informatics courses that were not available in all nursing programs. I later found myself in a position to teach nursing students in the clinical setting, which led to a full-time faculty position. I enjoyed the role in addition to the reading, writing, and learning that accompanied it. I wanted to be certain I could continue to grow and contribute to academia; therefore, I chose to enter a doctoral program. As a PhD student I had the opportunity to study information literacy and was immersed in this work through my doctoral studies and my role on a funded grant. I have remained in academia, where I have been able to pursue my interests related to research, writing, and teaching in a discipline that has been so good to me.

Paula Clutter, PhD, MSN, RN, CNL, CNE, EBP-C, CENP, CMSRN

Texas Woman's University, Interim Dean for Nursing; Professor

I have always valued lifelong learning, and I am grateful for my parents who instilled the core values to be kind, respect others, work hard, and always to do your best. I entered active duty in the U.S. Air Force (USAF) Nurse Corps upon graduation of my Bachelor of Science in Nursing degree. I was fortunate to obtain an Air Force Institute of Technology assignment to pursue a master's degree in adult health nursing from the University of Florida. My husband was working on his PhD in aerospace engineering at the University of Florida, and we were able to enjoy the graduate student journey together and participate in the joint nursing and engineering graduation ceremony. Go Gators! During my military career, my advanced nursing knowledge was used in a variety of clinical, educational, and administrative roles. I served 13 years in active duty and then separated from the USAF to complete my PhD in nursing science. I had an 8-year service gap before I entered the USAF Reserves Nurse Corps to continue my military service. I retired from the USAF Reserves in 2016, ending with one of my favorite career opportunities: serving as the chief nurse of a medical squadron. I continue to learn things in my current academic role and cherish the joy of learning. I have encountered some challenging times in my nursing career and appreciate growth that comes through difficult periods. I truly treasure the personal and professional rewards, which have been immeasurable.

Bradi B. Granger, PhD, RN, FAHA, FAAN

Duke University School of Nursing, Professor

Director, Duke Heart Nursing Research Program

Faculty, Duke Margolis Center for Health Policy

The reason I became a nurse was to be able to work with patients and peers (nurses) on scientific evidence to promote health and support new developments in health behaviors through nursing science. I began my nursing career on a cardiothoracic step-down unit in Charleston, West Virginia, in 1986, after graduating from University of Tennessee. The following year I transferred to Duke to attend graduate school and work as a critical care nurse, earning a master's degree from Duke in 1991 and a PhD from University of North Carolina at Chapel Hill in 2004. Currently, I serve as a clinical nurse specialist and director of the Heart Center Nursing Research Program at Duke and am core faculty at the Duke Margolis Center for Health Policy.

Throughout my career, I have retained the same objective and goal: work with patients and peers to advance nursing science. This passion has led me to grow the Heart Center Nursing Research Program at Duke and to serve and lead 23 staff nurse research studies and the "International Study Buddies" program, a program developed to mentor international nurses in developing research programs abroad. My career focus has been in helping nurses think differently about their practice using a unit-based, team-centered model. My own research focuses on improving patients' health behaviors to reduce mortality and hospital readmissions and to implement strategies for safe care transitions across settings of care, from hospital to home and community-based settings. I feel fortunate to work with the patients and nurses who make each day worthwhile!

Melissa Hessock DNP, APRN, FNP-C, EBP(CH)

The University of Tennessee, Knoxville, Post-Master's DNP Concentration Coordinator, Clinical Assistant Professor

Women's Health Clinic, Student Health Center, University of Tennessee, Knoxville, Nurse Practitioner

In the first half of my nursing career, frequent moves allowed me to work in different specialties and settings. However, I always gravitated to the care of women and families. After several years of practice in labor and delivery, NICU, and various perinatal settings, I had the opportunity to seek additional training and become a lactation consultant. While I genuinely enjoyed working with families to meet their individual feeding goals, I thrived on the autonomy and challenge of the "detective work" of assessing, diagnosing, and developing plans of care. I decided to pursue a role that would allow this same autonomy and challenge but with a broader population. After considering my options, I elected to pursue an MSN and become a family nurse practitioner (NP).

Early in my practice as an NP, I noticed that women's concerns, particularly as relates to sexual and reproductive health, were often unaddressed, minimized, or perceived as taboo, even in the medical setting. Education and care were too often driven by opinion, bias, and "the way we have always done it" instead of EBP. Frustrated by the barriers to impacting change, I pursued a DNP degree to develop the knowledge and skills to promote best practices, influence change, and improve outcomes for women. As graduation approached, it occurred to me that I could more widely impact change by sharing this knowledge and skill with aspiring RNs and APRNs. Thus began the current chapter of my nursing career. It is a true privilege and honor to continue to practice as an NP and, as a nurse educator, share my passion for normalizing sexual/reproductive health care and EBP improvement.

Staci S. Reynolds, PhD, RN, ACNS-BC, CCRN, CNRN, SCRN, CPHQ, FAAN

Duke University School of Nursing, Associate Clinical Professor

Journal of Nursing Care Quality, Editor-in-Chief

During high school, I enjoyed biology classes—so much so that I took extra science classes to learn more. Upon graduation, I knew that I wanted to continue in a field where I could further study biology. Nursing was a very practical option, as it included not only additional science classes, but would also allow me to make a significant, caring impact on patients and families. After serving as a staff nurse in the neuroscience ICU, I furthered my education and became a CNS. My mentors encouraged me to become an advanced practice RN so that I could have a broader impact on nursing care quality. Over the last decade, I have served as a neuroscience CNS and an infection prevention CNS. In both practice areas, I was able to enact change through leading quality improvement projects, developing policies and procedures, and assisting with education and staff professional development. I went on to obtain my PhD in nursing clinical science to continue my ability to effect change. One mentor encouraged me, saying, "As an ICU nurse, you can make a difference in one to two patients each shift. As a CNS, you can affect change at the unit or hospital level. With a PhD, you can influence quality at an international level." Now as a faculty member and researcher, I am able to influence the quality of nursing care in multiple ways, including mentoring the future leaders of health care.

Elizabeth Miller Walters, DNP, CPNP, RN

American Nurses Association, Assistant Director of Operations, Advanced Practice Initiatives and Certification Outreach

After several years of working as an infection preventionist, I found myself longing for the direct patient care I had once been so passionate about. The transition back to graduate school was a pivotal moment in my career, driven by a deep desire to reconnect with the core of nursing—caring for patients. My passion for adolescent medicine became a guiding force, as I recognized the profound impact of this work on young lives during such a critical period of development.

Adolescent medicine is not just a specialty; it is a calling that allows me to make a meaningful difference in the lives of young people. This field requires a unique blend of compassion, understanding, and expertise, all of which I am eager to contribute. Being part of an interdisciplinary team is equally important to me, as it fosters a collaborative approach to patient care. Working alongside professionals from various disciplines enhances our ability to provide holistic care, ensuring that each patient receives the comprehensive support they need.

Returning to school and pursuing APN has reignited my commitment to patient care and allowed me to serve in a role that aligns with my values and aspirations. The journey has been challenging, yet immensely rewarding, and I am honored to be a part of a profession that continuously strives to improve the lives of others.

Jennifer Woo, PhD, CNM, WHNP, FACNM

University of Texas Arlington, Assistant Professor

Parkland Memorial Hospital, Certified Nurse Midwife

Faith has always been an important part of my journey, and in my BSN program at the University of Pennsylvania, I happen to get a work-study job in the midwifery program as one of their administrative assistants. I was introduced to the world of midwifery, and one faculty stood out to me, Sister Teresita Hinnegan. She was a Catholic nun who had dedicated her life to serving mothers and babies in Africa for much of her adult life and now was teaching in the midwifery program. Her passion for social justice and empowering women through midwifery practice lit a fire in me, and I changed from being interested in pediatric oncology to midwifery. I loved the continuity of care with mothers and families that certified nurse midwives (CNMs) had, along with the impact you could make on communities. I had the privilege of being one of the first CNMs at a federally qualified health center in the westside of Chicago. I implemented a group prenatal care program known as Centering Pregnanc,y and that is when I saw the power of community and the potential for positive health change come to life. My experiences as a new graduate CNM working in a predominantly Medicaid/uninsured patient population inspired me to get my PhD and to try and make a difference in the maternal health disparities in Black women. That is what fuels my research agenda to this day, and as APRNs and nurse leaders we should all be striving to be leaders in achieving health equity.

Index

D

E

R

S

www.ingramcontent.com/pod-product-compliance
Ingram Content Group UK Ltd.
Pitfield, Milton Keynes, MK11 3LW, UK
UKHW050139280726
14058UKWH00006B/730